FRONTIERS OF DIABETES RESEARCH:

CURRENT TRENDS IN NON-INSULIN-DEPENDENT DIABETES MELLITUS

Frontiers of diabetes research:

Current trends in non-insulin-dependent diabetes mellitus

Proceedings of the Symposium on NIDDM:
Research and Clinical Frontiers in Diabetes,
New York, 4–7 May 1989

Editors:

K.G.M.M. Alberti
School of Clinical Medical Sciences, University of Newcastle upon Tyne, UK;
Director of WHO Collaborating Centre for Research in Laboratory Techniques
in Diabetes

R.S. Mazze
Department of Family Practice and Community Health, The School of Medicine,
University of Minnesota; Head, WHO Collaborating Centre in Behavioral
Medicine and Computer Science in Diabetes, International Diabetes Center,
Minneapolis, MN, USA

 1989

EXCERPTA MEDICA, AMSTERDAM – NEW YORK – OXFORD

International Congress Series No. 859
ISBN 0-444-81127-3

Published by:
Elsevier Science Publishers B.V.
(Biomedical Division)
P.O. Box 211
1000 AE Amsterdam
The Netherlands

Sole distributors for the USA and Canada:
Elsevier Science Publishing Company, Inc.
655 Avenue of the Americas
New York, NY 10010
USA

This book is printed on acid-free paper

Printed in The Netherlands

Foreword

This volume represents the proceedings of 'Research and Clinical Frontiers in Diabetes', a meeting held in May 1989 in honour of two of the great figures in international diabetes: Professors Harold Rifkin and Harry Keen. Both have made significant contributions in wide areas of clinical diabetes research and practice. Both are Directors of WHO Collaborating Centres in Diabetes, both have served in their respective national diabetes associations, as well as in the higher echelons of the International Diabetes Federation. Their contributions have encompassed many fields, but have, perhaps, had their greatest impact on non-insulin-dependent diabetes mellitus (NIDDM). The selected theme for the meeting was therefore frontiers of research in NIDDM. The programme covered the molecular to the epidemiological, included basic concepts as well as clinical applications, and was contributed to by researchers from throughout the world. The contents of this volume will serve, we trust, as a state-of-the-art synopsis of cutting-edge research and clinical practice in NIDDM. We owe a particular debt of gratitude to the Diagnostics Division, Miles, Inc., for a generous educational grant which made this meeting possible.

K.G.M.M. Alberti
R.S. Mazze

Introductory address

To the Distinguished Members of the 1989 Symposium on Research and Clinical Frontiers in Diabetes convened in New York City

On behalf of the International Diabetes Federation, I would like to convey to the members here assembled my best wishes for a stimulating and inspiring meeting, and for an increase in our knowledge about diabetes.

The International Diabetes Federation would also like to congratulate the two Guests of Honour, Professor Harold Rifkin and Professor Harry Keen. It is quite appropriate to honour these two physicians during the year celebrating the 100th anniversary of Minkowski. The perceptive mind of the latter was able to make essential advances in the fundamental approach to the disease called diabetes. Clinical as well as epidemiological advances have been achieved by the two Guests of Honour. Progress in diabetes care does depend upon this interaction of research and clinical acumen. This symposium on Research and Clinical Frontiers in Diabetes is achieving just this goal. The prospects are also bright for the next meeting of the Federation, which will be in Washington in 1991, under the invigorating and enlightened leadership of Professor Harold Rifkin.

The sponsors and organizers should also be congratulated for their courage in arranging this meeting, made possible by a remarkable educational grant.

With best and most respectful regards.

Joseph J. Hoet
President, International Diabetes Federation

Contents

Foreword
K.G.M.M. Alberti and R.S. Mazze   v

Introductory address
J. Hoet   vii

Epidemiology

Chapter 1
Diabetes epidemiology, a frontiersman's tool
H. Keen   3

Chapter 2
Genetics of NIDDM: pilgrim's progress
S.W. Serjeantson and P. Zimmet   21

Chapter 3
The prevalence and incidence of non-insulin-dependent diabetes mellitus
G.K. Dowse and P.Z. Zimmet   37

Chapter 4
Hyperandrogenicity and insulin resistance as predictors for non-insulin-dependent
diabetes mellitus in women
P. Björntorp   61

Chapter 5
Epidemiology of complications of NIDDM
E. Eschwège, A. Lacroux, L. Papoz, A. Fontbonne and D. Castagliola   71

Chapter 6
Risk factors for vascular complications of NIDDM
P.H. Bennett, R.G. Nelson, D.J. Pettitt and W.C. Knowler   89

Chapter 7
Primary prevention of non-insulin-dependent diabetes mellitus: a dream or
reality?
J. Tuomilehto   101

Screening for non-insulin dependent diabetes mellitus

Chapter 8
Screening for undiagnosed non-insulin-dependent diabetes
M.I. Harris   119

Chapter 9
To screen or not to screen for NIDDM
D.M. Nathan   133

Chapter 10
Glycated hemoglobin: is it a useful screening test for diabetes mellitus?
D.E. Goldstein, R.R. Little, J.D. England, H.-M. Wiedmeyer and E. McKenzie   141

Biochemical aspects of NIDDM

Chapter 11
Regulation of glucose transport in diabetes
B.B. Kahn and S.W. Cushman   155

Chapter 12
Insulin resistance, abnormal free fatty acid metabolism, and fasting
hyperglycemia in patients with non-insulin-dependent diabetes mellitus
G.M. Reaven   167

Complications of NIDDM

Chapter 13
Non-insulin-dependent diabetes and hypertension
E. Barrett-Connor   177

Chapter 14
Antiplatelet drugs and the prevention of progression of macrovascular disease in
diabetes mellitus
J.A. Colwell   193

Treatment of NIDDM

Chapter 15
What should be controlled in non-insulin-dependent diabetes: the use of insulin
and the European consensus
P.J. Watkins   207

Chapter 16
Model care 1989: some thoughts from the United Kingdom
P.D. Home   215

Chapter 17
Model care of NIDDM: an American perspective
R. Bergenstal, D. Etzwiler, P. Hollander, M. Spencer, E. Strock and R. Mazze   223

Chapter 18
Diet USA
A.I. Vinik   233

Chapter 19
Diet and NIDDM: a view from the Old World
R. Tattersall   263

Chapter 20
Exercise and non-insulin-dependent diabetes mellitus
E.S. Horton and J.T. Devlin   271

Chapter 21
Acarbose and related compounds for the treatment of diabetes mellitus
W. Creutzfeldt   285

Chapter 22
The role of inhibitors of lipolysis and lipid oxidation in the treatment of
non-insulin-dependent diabetes
G.R. Fulcher and K.G.M.M. Alberti   297

Chapter 23
The clinical significance of insulin resistance in NIDDM: studies with continuous
subcutaneous insulin infusion
E. Cerasi, B. Glaser, G. Del Rio, S. Sasson and L. Della Casa   309

Conclusions

Chapter 24
Four decades of clinical research and care: reflections of a clinical diabetologist
H. Rifkin   323

Author index   331

Epidemiology

© 1989 Elsevier Science Publishers B.V. (Biomedical Division)
Frontiers of diabetes research: current trends in non-insulin-dependent diabetes mellitus
K.G.M.M. Alberti and R. Mazze, editors

CHAPTER 1

Diabetes epidemiology, a frontiersman's tool

H. KEEN

Unit for Metabolic Medicine, UMDS, Guys Hospital, London SE1 9RT, U.K.

Introduction

Diabetes epidemiology, the study of the disease in its population or community setting, has proved to be a powerful and productive method in diabetes research. It has opened new perspectives, created new methodologies, generated many new questions and provided some new answers relevant to the understanding of diabetes. Diabetes epidemiology grew, as did much other clinical epidemiology, out of shrewd, impressionistic, incomplete but nonetheless vital observations such as Elliot P. Joslin's comments on the rarity of diabetes among the Pima Indian tribe of Native Americans whom he visited while he convalesced from tuberculosis in Arizona early this century [1]. The present-day application of standardized methods to defined populations to answer specific questions usually starts from astute observations, often made in the clinic or at the bedside.

The disciplines of epidemiology have been extended in a number of directions important to diabetes. They include the methods and purposes of the clinical trial. In the rapidly advancing field of molecular biology and molecular genetics, the laboratory techniques of the basic scientist are being fashioned and adapted to the purposes of epidemiology. We shall certainly see more multidisciplinary epidemiological collaborations including the techniques of molecular biology and genetics. Health Service research has also greatly benefited from its conjunction with epidemiology in such areas as bias-free sampling, case-control studies, the use of power calculations and the application of statistical analytical methods evolved for the interpretation of population-based data. My presentation reflects some aspects of this still evolving multidisciplinary interplay.

The doctrine of 'continuous variation'

My own involvement in clinical science and particularly its clinical epidemiological dimension sprang from my association as a student and as a research fellow with Professor Sir George Pickering. His preoccupation was with blood pressure [2], not blood glucose. Well on in his distinguished career, largely concerned with the search for 'the cause' of hypertension, he came upon epidemiology and measured blood pressure in several thousand people under fairly standardized conditions [3]. His findings led him to the conclusion that the quality, hypertension, was an arbitrary category, imposed upon a continuously varying quantity, blood pressure [4]. On average, pressures rose with age and differed between the sexes, but in no age or sex category was he able to find in the frequency distribution of pressures a natural break which separated hypertensive subjects from the rest (Fig. 1A).

My chance to ask in a population setting the same questions of diabetes (as a quality) and glucose tolerance/intolerance (as a quantity) came with the Bedford Survey in 1962 [5]. When the glycaemic responses to an oral glucose load measured on a stratified random sample of about 500 Bedford citizens were analysed by age and sex the continuous distributions of the responses resembled those for arterial pressure. Mean values rose with age, frequency distributions appeared to be continuous in each; in none was there a natural division demarcating a normal from an abnormal group either at the then recommended diagnostic cut-off level or, for that matter, at any other. The US National Health Survey of post-load blood glucose responses measured in a much larger sample of the North American population [6] gave a similar pattern, namely an apparently single, positively skewed, but continuous distribution (Fig. 1B).

These conclusions are presented in a diagrammatic way in Fig. 2. Although these and other cross-sectional studies suggest a 'loss' of glucose tolerance with increasing age, there is relatively little evidence on the lifetime movement of individuals across the spectrum of glucose tolerance/intolerance. We do not know whether individuals ultimately destined to finish with 'diabetes' run higher in the blood glucose range throughout their prior life. Being identified on one occasion with impaired glucose tolerance (IGT) gives some predictive information but, although the chance of progression to unequivocal diabetes is greater the higher the glycaemic response [7, 8], there are many exceptions and much unaccountable reversion of glucose intolerance to normality.

Pimas, Nauruans and South Asians

This generalization about the possible nature of NIDDM in a population as an arbi-

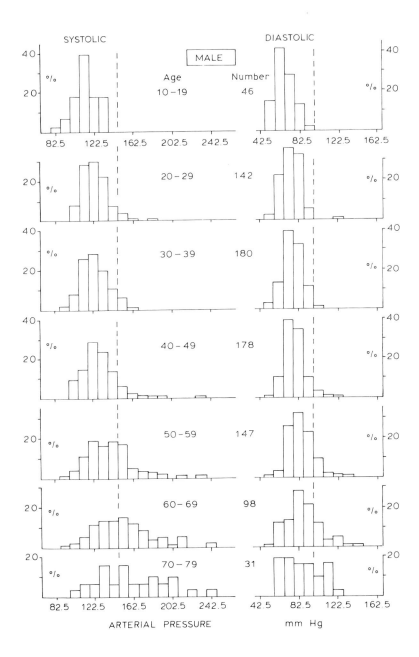

Fig. 1A. Frequency distribution histograms of arterial pressure (systolic and diastolic) by decade of age in ambulant 'CV-neutral' male outpatients. There is a clear trend to increasing values and upward skewing in successive age groups. There is no clear division of distributions into 'normal' and 'hypertensive' subgroups at levels commonly accepted as defining hypertension (vertical dashed lines) or at any other.

6

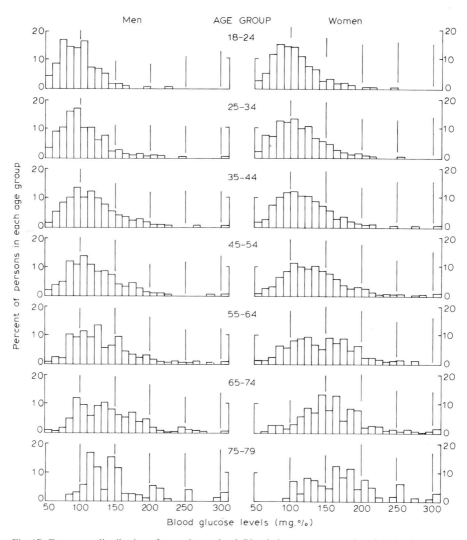

Fig. 1B. Frequency distribution of post-glucose load. Blood glucose concentrations in US adults (1960–62) by age-group and sex. As with arterial pressure (Fig. 1A) concentrations rise and skew increasingly positively in successive age groups, with no 'natural' divisions into normal and diabetic subsets at conventionally accepted or other diagnostic cut-off values.

trarily defined extreme segment of a continuously varying spectrum of glucose tolerance/intolerance should not be extrapolated outside the population groups on which it is founded. Among the Pima Indian people living near Phoenix, Arizona, where, decades before, Dr. Joslin regained his health, Peter Bennett and his colleagues reported a different blood glucose spectrum [9]. Not only had diabetes prevalence now

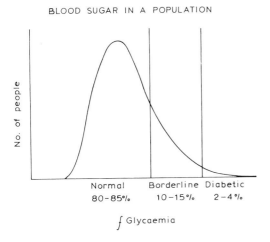

BLOOD SUGAR IN A POPULATION

No. of people

Normal   Borderline Diabetic
80–85%   10–15%   2–4%

∫ Glycaemia

Fig. 2. Diagrammatic representation of frequency distribution of blood sugar (glucose) or of glucose tolerance responses (glycaemia) in large mixed Westernized population samples. The distribution is positively
skewed. The vertical lines depict the diagnostic limits imposed on the distribution following the Bedford
survey (1962). The 'borderline' segment is the forerunner of today's category of 'impaired glucose tolerance' (IGT).

come to be very high, but when the population was systematically submitted to oral
glucose tolerance testing in successive age groups, the blood glucose responses separated out into two clear subdistributions, with a progressive proportionate rise with
age in the size of the upper population. Clear bimodality of glucose tolerance emerges
with age though with a degree of overlap between the two subpopulations. Many
thousands of miles away in the South Pacific, Zimmet and colleagues have made very
similar observations [10] in the isolated Micronesian population of the island of
Nauru. Their very high diabetes prevalence and bimodal glycaemic distribution
closely resemble the Pima pattern.

These two well-studied populations share some common features. First, they are
inbred, geographically or culturally isolated communities with a relatively restricted
gene pool. The possession of a gene or a cluster of genes which might be rendered
detrimental by altered conditions is thus less likely to be 'diluted out' by genetic admixture [11]. Second, both populations have, for different socio-economic reasons,
a very high prevalence of massive obesity of relatively recent origin. Here, perhaps,
are the altered environmental conditions (overnutrition/obesity) interacting with relatively homogeneous genetic constitutions. These considerations led to an explanatory hypothesis that, in these two genetically restricted populations, the general im-
position of obesity unmasks a diabetes-susceptible subset, probably genetically
determined; at a particular age (or after a particular duration of exposure to obesity)

8

susceptible individuals transfer from the lower (normal) to the higher (diabetic) blood glucose population. Evidence of bimodality has also been advanced in Mexican Americans, another relatively high diabetes prevalence population [12]. While the argument about the quantitative versus the qualitative nature of the (non-insulin-dependent) diabetic state has some of the philosophical reverberations of the Pickering-Platt debate [13], it is nonetheless of fundamental importance in determining investigative and perhaps therapeutic strategies.

The increased liability of expatriate South Asian Indian people to NIDDM by comparison with other local ethnic groups has been abundantly documented but it is difficult to explain their predisposition for diabetes on the same basis as for the Pima and Nauruan peoples. They are neither so genetically restricted nor so outstandingly obese. Using the crude but epidemiologically robust tool of the door-to-door enquiry, Dr. Hugh Mather and I [14], assisted by a splendid group of multiethnic volunteers, enquired into the prevalence of known diabetes in the very large population of Asian Indian immigrants settled in the West London suburb of Southall. In this setting, also, we found diagnosed NIDDM considerably more prevalent among the approximately 30,000 Asian Indian inhabitants of Southall than among the roughly similar number of Southall Europids. We were impressed by the early age at diagnosis of NIDDM among these Indian people, and by the substantial excess of men over women with diabetes. We were, however, surprised when our colleague, Narendra Verma Singh, using ascertainment techniques identical to ours, conducted a house-to-house enquiry in Darya Ganj [15], a middle-class suburb of New Delhi. He found a pattern of known diabetes prevalence extraordinarily similar to that of the Southall Indians and differing from reports elsewhere in the Indian subcontinent (Fig. 3). This brings me to my first set of questions:

(a) Is NIDDM in Europids the 'same disease' as in Pimas, Nauruans, Mexican Americans or S. Asians?
(b) Can NIDDM susceptibility be dependent on a single gene of major effect in all families of all populations?
(c) If it is, is it the same gene for all?

Glucose intolerance and arterial disease risk

One of the questions which arose from the findings of the Bedford Survey took the following form: In the absence of any natural diagnostic division in the distribution of GTT responses, is it possible to establish an 'operational' diagnostic definition of diabetes mellitus by identifying a degree of glycaemic abnormality associated with increased risk of the vascular complications of the disease? More simply stated, is there a degree of glucose intolerance at which it starts to do people harm? In order to explore this notion, after characterizing the Bedford population by their OGTT responses, we divided the observed range of glucose tolerance/intolerance into three rather than two categories (Fig. 2). 'Diabetes mellitus' was defined as the degree of glucose intolerance (summarized in the blood glucose concentration 2 hours after an oral glucose load) at which all observers agreed that the diabetic state was present. We identified similarly a lower level below which all observers agreed that diabetes was absent. The zone of the diagnostic uncertainty between the two, which we originally called 'borderline diabetes', has come to be known as the category of 'impaired glucose tolerance' (IGT) [16]. At baseline in Bedford, with increasing degrees of glucose intolerance there appeared to be a gradient of arterial disease prevalence based

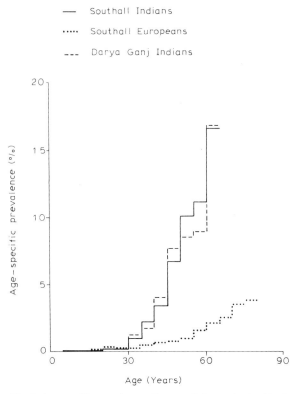

Fig. 3. Age-specific prevalence of known diabetes obtained by house-to-house enquiry in a geographically defined population in a suburb of London, England. There were approximately similar-sized groups (approx. 30,000) of European and South Asian Indian inhabitants. Rates are strikingly higher in Southall Indians than Europeans, and closely resemble rates estimated by identical ascertainment methods among Indian residents of Darya Ganj, a suburb of New Delhi, India.

10

upon positive WHO questionnaire history of angina pectoris, myocardial infarction and intermittent claudication and Minnesota-coded ECG findings [17]. A mortality analysis after 10 years of follow-up also suggested that total mortality and the proportion of it attributed to coronary heart disease (CHD) also rose with increasing glucose intolerance categories [18].

Another large population group of about 24,000 male civil servants aged 40 years and over, studied in the mid-1970s [19], were characterized at baseline, inter alia, by their capillary blood glucose concentration measured 2 h after an oral load of 50 g glucose, then the standard challenge dose in the UK. Cardiovascular mortality over subsequent years was ascertained by automatic reporting from the central death registry. When coronary heart disease mortality was related to the baseline 2 h blood glucose concentration, there appeared to be a sudden doubling of rates which occurred in individuals above the upper 95th percentile of the baseline 2 h blood glucose distribution [20]. In addition, this group also showed higher mean values of arterial pressure with increasing degrees of glucose intolerance (Fig. 4). Reaven et al. [21]

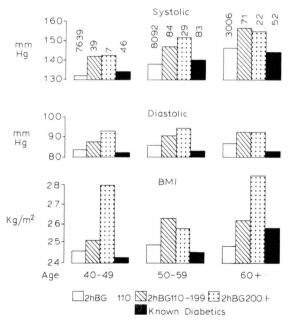

Fig. 4. Mean arterial pressures (systolic and diastolic) and body mass index (BMI) by age group in approximately 19,000 male civil servants aged 40 years or more participating in the Whitehall survey. Mean values tend to show a progressive rise with age and, within age groups, from normal two-hour blood glucose (measured 2 h after 50 g oral glucose load), through borderline or impaired glucose tolerance (110–199 mg/dl) to diabetic glucose intolerance (> 200 mg/dl). Mean pressures in the known diabetic subjects, however, do not exceed those of the normoglycaemic subjects.

have shown that increasing degrees of glucose intolerance are associated with rising levels of insulinaemia (Fig. 5), attributable to increasing degrees of insulin resistance [22]. Epidemiological findings in this field have therefore prompted the questions, currently of great interest, of the possible role of insulin resistance, the accompanying raised plasma insulin concentrations and the associated metabolic disturbances in the genesis of the raised blood pressure [23] and increased cardiovascular risk of glucose intolerance and NIDDM [24].

Insulin resistance, NIDDM and arterial disease risk

Some new epidemiological insights into the important contemporary question of in-

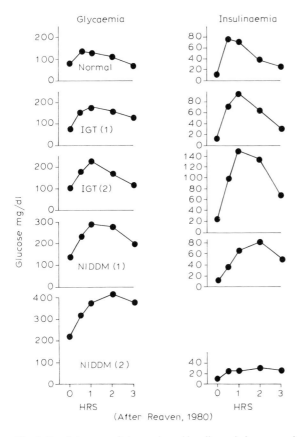

Fig. 5. Parallel curves of glycaemia and insulinaemia in progressively worsening categories of glucose intolerance, showing degrees of insulinaemia, increasing to the level of formal diabetes mellitus, then falling to subnormal values. Drawn from the data of Reaven.

sulin resistance, liability to NIDDM and the link with hypertension and arterial disease risk are provided by preliminary reports of a study of the role of insulinaemia in the excess diabetes and CHD prevalence in Asian Indians in London. McKeigue and his colleagues [25] have recently presented findings in an epidemiologically defined group of more than 700 working men consisting of roughly equal numbers of people of Europid and of S. Asian Indian origin. Examining the hypothesis that insulin resistance underlies the excessive rates of NIDDM and CHD seen in S. Asians in this setting [26, 27], they made a number of anthropometric measurements and estimated glucose, insulin and plasma lipoprotein concentrations fasting and 2 h after a 75 g glucose load in these two ambulant ethnic samples.

Diabetes prevalence was 14.8% in S. Asians, compared with 3.8% in Europeans ($p < 0.01$). Fasting immunoreactive insulin (IRI) was 20% higher and 2 h IRI 66% higher in Asian Indians than in Europeans ($p < 0.05$ and < 0.01 respectively). Plasma triglyceride concentration was 17% higher ($p < 0.02$) and HDL cholesterol 0.1 mmol/l lower ($p < 0.02$) in Asian Indians than in Europids. Systolic and diastolic pressures were both significantly higher in the Asian Indians ($p < 0.05$). There was no difference in weight for height expressed as the body mass index (BMI) between the Indian and Europid samples. However, there were striking differences in fat distributions, with a mean Asian Indian waist–hip ratio (WHR) of 0.97, almost 1 SD higher than the mean of 0.93 for the Europids ($p < 0.01$). Fasting and 2 h IRI correlated strongly with WHR in both ethnic groups, though both were at higher levels in the Indian men. These findings clearly support the notion that NIDDM, dyslipidaemia, raised arterial pressure and increased CHD risk occur in the setting of insulin resistance and centripetal fat distribution but a number of important caveats should be entered.

First, a proportion of the immunoreactivity to insulin on which the notion of the hyperinsulinaemia of insulin resistance is based may arise, not from insulin itself, but from an excess of insulin-like molecules (ILM), notably proinsulin and incompletely split proinsulin in the circulation [28]. These pancreatic islet B-cell products may contribute both directly and indirectly to the manifestation of insulin resistance. They may also exert specific atherogenic effects and contribute to the increased CHD risk in addition to or instead of true hyperinsulinaemia. This explanation clearly cannot be applied to the increased CHD risk of the insulin-dependent diabetic.

Second, the notion that hyperinsulinaemia (or the set of metabolic/hormonal conditions for which it is a marker) is causally related to the increased risk of CHD in NIDDM has been vigorously challenged, principally by Jarrett [29], who is impressed mainly by the difficulty in demonstrating an independent relationship between relative hyperinsulinaemia and the enhancement of CHD risk. He argues that the published findings are inconsistent and that the complex of associated variables – obesity and its distribution, arterial pressure, plasma lipids, sex hormones, physical activity and diet – could account for the relationship between hyperinsulinaemia, glucose intolerance and CHD risk. Finally, the insulin-resistant state and accompanying glucose intolerance are not necessarily associated with dramatically increased rates of CHD. Insulin resistance is very characteristic of the Pima Indian population but their rates of CHD are lower than those of their Europid fellow countrymen [30]. A further notable example of diabetes (mostly NIDDM) with low absolute risk for CHD is to be found in the indigenous Japanese [31]. It seems likely, therefore, that even if 'insulin resistance' (however that is constituted) is the setting in which arterial disease, raised arterial pressure, the diabetic and the dyslipidaemic states arise, other conditions, environmental and/or genetic, must be met before they (singly or multiply) do so.

All of these considerations prompt a further set of questions:
(a) Is arterial disease risk a 'step function' or a 'graduated function' of glucose tolerance/intolerance?
(b) Is the relationship of increased arterial disease risk to glycaemia, arterial presure, insulinaemia, lipidaemia causal or coincident?
(c) What determines absolute (i.e. between population) and relative (i.e. within population) susceptibility to arterial disease in DM?

Risk factors for arterial disease in diabetes

It was largely the apparent anomalous low risk (absolute but not relative) of coronary heart disease in the Japanese diabetic [31] which provoked the WHO Multinational Study of Vascular Disease in Diabetes [32]. Its origins lay in astute clinical observations made by several Japanese colleagues, among whom I would like to highlight my good friend and indefatigable colleague, Dr. Eishi Miki. Having spent some years as a clinical fellow at the Joslin Clinic in the US, he was struck by the much greater frequency with which he encountered coronary heart disease and ischaemic gangrene in diabetic patients in Boston than he did in Tokyo. The relative rarity of these disorders in Japan, as he politely explained to me, was perhaps why my series of talks on arterial disease and diabetes to Japanese clinicians did not arouse quite the enthusiastic interest I had expected!

We agreed to prepare a standardized protocol to compare rates of vascular disease in a London and Tokyo sample of diabetic patients but when we discussed the proposals with the European Diabetes Epidemiology Study Group (EDESG) and elsewhere, many other centres expressed enthusiasm to join and so we sought the sponsorship of WHO. Each participating centre undertook to recruit as representative as possible a sample of about 500 diabetic patients with ages distributed between 35 and 55 years, the sexes equally represented, and stratified for known diabetes duration. Biometric, diabetic, cardiovascular and microvascular status were ascertained using

14

standardized questionnaires and procedures when they existed and constructing them when they did not. A standard resting 12-lead ECG was also included; each record was independently read by our two highly experienced Minnesota Coders [33]. These two invaluable colleagues (Nan Keen and Ceridwen Rose) have coded (and recoded for estimates of observer variation) not only all of the baseline records but also all the follow-up ECGs, establishing a uniquely high standard of quality and consistency for the electrocardiographic information in the WHO Multinational Study.

Comparisons of prevalence of arterial disease among the 14 participating WHO centres, by whatever index it was identified, confirmed significant differences in rates of cardiovascular history and symptoms, ECG abnormalities (Fig. 6) and amputation for limb ischaemia. The Tokyo and Hong Kong diabetic samples (and that from Beijing which later joined the study) demonstrated conspicuously lower atherosclerosis rates than the Europid centres [32].

Mortality follow-up

In 10 of the 14 centres, we have been able to complete a life/death status reascertainment in 95% or more of the original cohort at approximately 8.5 years after the initial

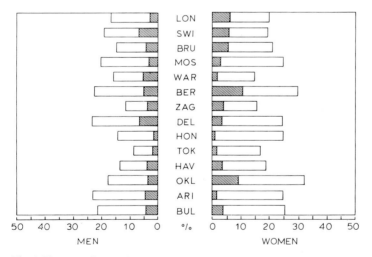

Fig. 6. Electrocardiographic abnormalities in the 14 ethnic/geographic defined diabetic population samples of the WHO multinational study of vascular disease in diabetes at baseline. There were approximately 250 men and 250 women in each sample. Coronary probable (cross-hatched bars) – Minnesota code items 1.1, 1.2, 7.1 (Q-wave abnormalities and L bundle branch block). Coronary possible (open bars) – items 4.1–3, 5.1–3 (ST/T segment/wave abnormalities). The former, more specific indicators of CHD are notably less common in Hong Kong and Tokyo diabetics. They were even lower in Beijing (not shown).

survey [34]. Maximum data on the circumstances of death have been sought for all non-survivors, with a copy of the original death certificate and its English translation as minimum information. Total available information relating to each death has been considered by an independent mortality committee, who assigned an underlying cause of death based upon the application of a rule-set to the information. Subjects were classified as insulin-dependent if they had started insulin injections within one year of diagnosis and continued without break thereafter. All others were classed as non-insulin-dependent. In addition to comparisons of patterns of mortality between the centres, the predictive power for total and circulatory mortality of a number of major risk factors measured at baseline has been explored in the pooled data from these 10 centres. The recognized risk factors for cardiovascular mortality (e.g. 'the big three') function in this diabetic population as in general populations. In simple unvariate analyses systolic and diastolic pressures were strongly predictive for mortality and so, to a lesser extent, were total blood cholesterol and reported smoking habits. ECG abnormalities at baseline were also strongly predictive of circulatory mortality, with the risk of death relating to the type and severity of abnormality at baseline.

Proteinuria and cardiovascular disease

A further predictor of total and cardiovascular mortality also emerged in both IDDM and NIDDM patients in the Multinational Study, namely the presence and degree of clinical proteinuria at baseline. Proteinuria was assessed semi-quantitatively at baseline by a standard salicylsulphonic acid test. Its presence not only strongly predicted circulatory mortality (Table 1), but, in multivariate analysis, did so independently of the other major risk factors in IDDM men and women separately and for NIDDM men and the sexes combined (Table 2). This finding gave additional support to, and further extended, our earlier demonstration that microalbuminuria (i.e.

TABLE 1

Cardiovascular mortality over 8 years in diabetic men and women in the WHO multinational study of vascular disease in diabetes by presence and absence of clinical proteinuria at the baseline ascertainment

| | Men: Proteinuria | | Women: Proteinuria | |
	−ve	+ve	−ve	+ve
Total	1893	180	2028	167
Circulatory death	117 (6.2%)	38 (21.1%)	56 (2.8%)	27 (16.2%)

16

TABLE 2
Baseline factors significantly predicting circulatory disease mortality in Cox multivariate regression analysis of pooled mortality data from the WHO multinational study of vascular disease analysed by sex and diabetes type (IDD, insulin-dependent diabetes; NIDD, non-insulin-dependent diabetes)

	IDD		NIDD	
	Male	Female	Male	Female
Systolic BP	–	–	*	–
Cholesterol	–	–	*	–
Smoking	–	–	*	–
Proteinuria	**	**	–	*
ECG abnormality	***	***	***	***
Duration of DM	–	–	–	***

$*p < 0.05$, $**p < 0.01$, $***p < 0.001$.

rates of albumin excretion exceeding the normal but falling short of clinical proteinuria) in non-insulin-dependent patients was strongly predictive of cardiovascular mortality over the subsequent 15 years [35]. Similar long-term retrospective evidence relating mortality to urinary albumin concentration also came from Mogensen in Denmark [36].

The presence of clinical proteinuria and microalbuminuria might merely be a marker for an added lethality of atherosclerotic disease, an indication, for instance, of a superadded risk of myocardial microangiopathy which might be more likely to determine a fatal outcome in the event of an obstructive coronary episode. Mattock and colleagues [37], however, showed a clear association of urinary albumin excretion in the microalbuminuric range with clinical and electrocardiographic indices of coronary heart disease morbidity in an NIDDM outpatient population. In this study, albumin excretion rate in non-clinically proteinuric patients was significantly correlated with plasma lipids and arterial pressure. The link of albumin excretion with CHD morbidity was, however, independent of these covariables and of a number of other risk factors for atherosclerosis.

Mechanisms

Increased urinary albumin excretion at both macro- and micro-levels thus emerges as a strong and independent risk factor for cardiovascular morbidity and mortality in the non-insulin-dependent diabetic. This is in addition to its predictive power for progressive renal failure and its associated great increase in risk of CHD in the insulin-dependent patient [38].

The association of AER with arterial disease is, at least in part, independent of such associated variables as arterial pressure and dyslipoproteinaemia. The mechanism of the association is uncertain, but there is some evidence, at present indirect and relatively scanty, which supports the explanatory hypothesis that the increased leakage of protein into the urine may be a marker of a generalized increase in vascular permeability. Involving arterioles and small arteries, hyperpermeability may be responsible for so-called plasmatic vasculosis of Lendrum [39]. In larger arteries, increased endothelial permeability may open the way for the entry of atherogenic lipoproteins (especially if they are there at generous 'Western' concentrations) under the driving force of the arterial pressure (especially if it is high) (Fig. 7). Feldt-Rasmussen [40] demonstrated excessive loss of labelled albumin from the circulation in both clinically proteinuric and microalbuminuric insulin-dependent diabetic patients compared with normoalbuminuric diabetics and non-diabetics. Williamson et al. [41] have recently demonstrated that, in the experimental or spontaneously diabetic rat, there is significantly increased permeation of labelled albumin into the aortic wall as well as into other vulnerable tissues.

The determinants of increased permeability in diabetes remain uncertain. It may be by way of enhanced vesicular transport across endothelial cells, through gap junctions between them or due to altered porosity of the intercelllular ground substance/ basement membrane material of the arterial intima. Increased arterial wall permea-

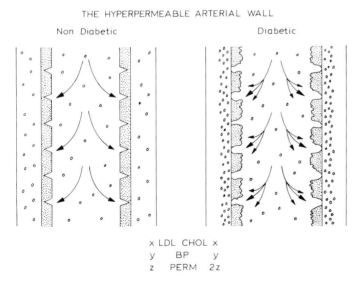

Fig. 7. Diagram of postulated hyperpermeability of arterial wall in diabetes and its implications. At given levels of blood pressure and of dyslipidaemia, more atherogenic particles are admitted to the arterial wall, perhaps explaining the increased susceptibility of the diabetic to atherosclerosis.

18

bility in the diabetic human and the mechanisms responsible for it remain to be directly demonstrated.

Conclusions and implications

It is perhaps fitting to conclude this increasingly speculative discussion with the imagery of a hypothetical, composite, hyperpermeable diabetic blood vessel. At its termination in a glomerular capillary it leaks increased amounts of albumin (though well below the conventional threshold of clinical detection) into the urine. Similar leakiness in its arteriolar and small arterial segment gives rise to plasma seepage into the vessel wall or plasmatic vasculosis: in the larger arteries the hyperpermeability phenomenon expresses itself as enhanced penetration of the intima by atherogenic particles (Fig. 7). Hyperpermeability may be the agency by which the impact of the major arterial disease risk factors are amplified in the diabetic. For a given concentration of atherogenic particles, driven by a given lateral thrust of arterial pressure, more penetration will occur in the diabetic than the non-diabetic artery and more atherosclerotic disease will ensue. If this concept is correct, it follows that although we should, in our therapy, try to reduce the hyperpermeability perhaps by better correction of the diabetic state, it may be even more important and clinically more rewarding to reduce the pathogenic stimuli which have an effect upon it. Our methods for normalizing permeability are at present speculative and experimental; but the arteriopathic risk factors such as dyslipidaemia and hypertension can and should be tackled with particular vigour, even perhaps at lower therapeutic threshold levels in the diabetic, especially in those who exhibit the marker of microalbuminuria. Correction of a hyperpermeability 'amplifier' will perhaps halve the toll of atherosclerotic morbidity and mortality in the 'Western' diabetic; reduction of blood pressure and correction of plasma lipoprotein concentrations will reduce risk by four-fifths or more.

Acknowledgements

In reporting the results of the WHO Multinational Study I, of course, act as spokesman for colleagues and collaborators in all 14 centres and in respect of the mortality follow-up particularly for Dr. John H. Fuller and Ms. Jennie Head, who have coordinated and analysed this phase of the Study. Each centre has found support locally for their local field work. The UK centre, for instance, acknowledges the support of the Medical Research Council and the British Diabetic Association for this study. Thanks are also due to WHO Geneva for funding and supporting the central coordination and analysis of the initial prevalence study and to the U.S. National Institutes of Health and Prof. Elisa Lee of the Biostatistics Department, University of Oklahoma, for funding and undertaking the 8.5-year follow-up of the original cohorts. We acknowledge support through the years from Messrs. Ames/Miles, Servier, Squibb and ICI. Warm thanks are due to Mrs. Nan Keen and Ms. Ceridwen Rose, our two Minnesota Coders, and to Mrs. B. Crowe and Miss V. Nelson for their expert help in the preparation of the manuscript.

References

1. The Joslin Diaries. Personal communication from Dr. Peter Bennett, 1989.
2. Pickering GW. High blood pressure. London: Churchill-Livingstone, 1968.
3. Hamilton M, Pickering GW, Roberts JAF, Sonory GSC. The aetiology of essential hypertension! The arterial pressure in the general population. Clin Sci 1954;13:11–35.
4. Pickering GW. The nature of essential hypertension. Lancet 1959;ii:1027–1028.
5. Sharp CL, Butterfield WJH, Keen H. Diabetes survey in Bedford 1962. Proc R Soc Med 1964;57:193–195,196–200,201–206.
6. Department of Health, Education and Welfare. Blood glucose levels in adults, United States 1960–62. Public Health Service Publication No. 1000, Series 11, No. 18. Washington: US Government Printing Office, 1960–62.
7. Keen H, Jarrett RJ, McCartney P. The ten year follow-up of the Bedford Survey (1962–1972): glucose tolerance and diabetes. Diabetologia 1982;22:73–78.
8. Sasaki A, Suzuki T, Horiuchi N. Development of diabetes in Japanese subjects with impaired glucose tolerance: a seven-year follow-up study. Diabetologia 1982;22:154–157.
9. Rushforth NB, Bennett PH, Steinberg AG, Borch TA, Mier M. Diabetes in the Pima Indians: evidence of bimodality in glucose tolerance distributions. Diabetes 1971;20:756–765.
10. Zimmet P, Whitehouse S. Bimodality of fasting and two-hour glucose tolerance distributions in a Micronesian population. Diabetes 1975;27:793–800.
11. King H, Zimmet P, Bennett P, et al. Glucose tolerance and ancestral genetic admixture in six semi-traditional Pacific populations. Genet Epidemiol 1984;1:315–328.
12. Rosenthal M, McMahon CA, Stern MP, et al. Evidence of bimodality of two hour plasma glucose concentrations in Mexican Americans: results from the San Antonio Heart Study. J Chron Dis 1985;38:5–16.
13. Swales JD (ed). Platt versus Pickering: An episode in recent medical history. The Keynes Press, British Medical Association, 1985.
14. Mather HM, Keen H. The Southall Diabetes Survey: prevalence of known diabetes in Asians and Europeans. Br Med J 1985;291:1081–1084.
15. Verma NPS, Mehta SP, Madhu F, Mather HM, Keen H. Prevalence of known diabetes in an urban Indian environment: the Darya Ganj diabetes survey. Br Med J 1986;293:423–424.
16. Diabetes Mellitus: report of a WHO Study Group. WHO Technical Report Ser 1985;727:1–113.
17. Keen H, Rose GA, Pyke DA, et al. Blood sugar and arterial disease. Lancet 1965;ii:505–509.
18. Jarrett RJ, McCartney P, Keen H. The Bedford Survey: ten year mortality rates in newly diagnosed diabetics, borderline diabetics and normoglycaemic controls and risk indices for coronary heart disease in borderline diabetics. Diabetologia 1982;22:79–84.
19. Reid DD, Brett GZ, Hamilton PJS, et al. Cardiorespiratory disease and diabetes among middle-aged male civil servants; a study of screening and intervention. Lancet 1974;i:469–473.

20. Fuller JH, Shipley MJ, Rose G, Jarrett RJ, Keen H. Mortality from coronary heart disease and stroke in relation to degree of glycaemia: the Whitehall Study. Br Med J 1983;287:867–870.

21. Reaven GM, Olefsky JM. Relationship between heterogeneity of insulin responses and insulin resistance on normal subjects and patients with chemical diabetes. Diabetologia 1977;13:201–206.

22. Reaven GM. Insulin secretion and insulin action in non-insulin-dependent diabetes mellitus; which defect is primary? Diabetes Care 1984;7 (suppl 1):17–24.

23. Ferranini E, Buzzigoli G, Bonadona R, et al. Insulin resistance in essential hypertension. N Engl J Med 1987;317:350–357.

24. Pyorala K, Laakso M, Uusitupa M. Diabetes and atherosclerosis: an epidemiologic view. Diabetes/ Metab Rev 1987;3:463–524.

25. McKeigue PM, Shah B, Marmot MG. Diabetes, insulin resistance and central obesity in South Asians and Europeans. Diabetic Med 1989;6: (Suppl 1):A41–42.

26. McKeigue PM, Marmot MH, Syndercombe Court YD, Cohier DE, Rahman S, Riemersma RA. Diabetes, hyperinsulinaemia and coronary risk factors in Bangladeshi in East London. Br Heart J 1988;60:390–396.

27. McKeigue PM, Mier GC, Marmot MG. Coronary heart disease in South Asians overseas: a review. J Clin Epidemiol 1989;42:597–609.

28. Nagi DK, Hendra TJ, Tempe RC, et al. Split proinsulin and not insulin may be a risk factor for atherogenesis in non-insulin-dependent diabetic subjects. Diabetic Med 1989;6 (Suppl 1):A34.

29. Jarrett RJ. Is insulin atherogenic? Diabetologia 1988;31:71–75.

30. Ingelfinger JA, Bennett PH, Liebow IM, Miller M. Coronary heart disease in the Pima Indians: electrocardiographic findings and post mortem evidence of myocardial infarction in a population with a high prevalence of diabetes mellitus. Diabetes 1976;25:561–565.

31. Jarrett RJ. The epidemiology of coronary heart disease and related factors in the context of diabetes mellitus and impaired glucose tolerance. In: Jarrett RJ, ed. Diabetes and heart disease. Amsterdam: Elsevier, 1984;1–23.

32. Drafting Group, The World Health Organization Multinational Study of Vascular Disease in Diabetes. Prevalence of small vessel and large vessel disease in diabetic patients from 14 centres. Diabetologia 1985;28 (Suppl):615–640.

33. Rose GA, Blackburn H, Gilburn RF, Prineas RJ. Cardiovascular Survey Methods, 2nd Edition. World Health Organization Monograph Series, No. 56, Geneva: WHO, 1982.

34. Fuller JH, Head JA and the WHO Mortality Study Group. Circulatory disease mortality in the WHO Mortality Study. Diabetologia 1987;30:521A.

35. Jarrett RJ, Viberti GC, Argyropoulos A, et al. Microalbuminuria predicts mortality in non-insulin-dependent diabetics. Diabetic Med 1984;1:17–19.

36. Mogensen CE. Microalbuminuria predicts clinical proteinuria and early mortality in maturity onset diabetes. N Engl J Med 1984;6:356–360.

37. Mattock MN, Keen H, Viberti GC, et al. Coronary heart disease and urinary albumin excretion rate in type II (non-insulin-dependent) diabetic patients. Diabetologia 1988;31:82–87.

38. Viberti GC, Hill RD, Jarrett RJ, et al. Microalbuminuria as a predictor of clinical nephropathy in insulin-dependent diabetes mellitus. Lancet 1982;i:1430–1432.

39. Lendrum AC. Deposition of plasmatic substances on vessel walls. Pathol Microbiol 1967;30:681–684.

40. Feldt-Rasmussen B. Increased transcapillary escape rate of albumin in Type I (insulin-dependent) diabetic patients with microalbuminuria. Diabetologia 1986;29:282–286.

41. Williamson JR, Chang K, Titon RG, et al. Increased vascular permeability in spontaneously diabetic BB/W rats and in rats with mild versus severe streptozotocin-induced diabetes. Prevention by aldose reductase inhibitors and castration. Diabetes 1987;36:813–821.

© 1989 Elsevier Science Publishers B.V. (Biomedical Division)
Frontiers of diabetes research: current trends in non-insulin-dependent diabetes mellitus
K.G.M.M. Alberti and R. Mazze, editors

CHAPTER 2

Genetics of NIDDM: pilgrim's progress

S.W. SERJEANTSON[1] and P. ZIMMET[2]

[1]Human Genetics Group, The John Curtin School of Medical Research, Australian National University,
Canberra, Australia, and
[2]Lions-International Diabetes Institute, Royal Southern Memorial Hospital, Caulfield South, Victoria,
Australia

Introduction

Non-insulin-dependent diabetes mellitus (NIDDM) has a strong genetic basis, as evidenced by nearly 100% concordance in monozygotic twins [1] and by abnormal glucose tolerance in more than 30% of siblings of patients with NIDDM [2–4]. Despite the overwhelming evidence for a substantial genetic component, the inherited factors leading to insulin resistance in NIDDM remain unknown.

It is clearly of paramount importance to understand the precise, underlying metabolic defects in NIDDM if therapeutic procedures are to be improved. Currently available procedures can ameliorate glucose intolerance, but NIDDM patients have disturbed lipoprotein metabolism as well as disturbed glucose metabolism. One consequence is development of early atherosclerosis [5] and another is a two- to threefold increase in cardiovascular mortality rates [6].

Traditional biochemical approaches have provided important insights into cellular defects in NIDDM patients [7]. There are metabolic disturbances in the intracellular kinases, for example, including the tyrosine kinase of the β subunit of the insulin receptor [8]. Other reported defects include abnormal stimulation of glucose transport by insulin [9].

The difficulty in biochemical approaches is that there is such a cascade of glucose and lipoprotein metabolic disturbances that the primary defects are obscured by secondary abnormalities. An alternative approach to defining the primary defects in

Correspondence: Professor S.W. Serjeantson, Human Genetics Group, The John Curtin School of Medical Research, Australian National University, PO Box 334, Canberra ACT 2601, Australia.

NIDDM is to identify the specific genes contributing to the disease. Thus the ultimate objectives of genetic studies of NIDDM are to (i) identify and characterize the gene or genes responsible for NIDDM, (ii) determine the precise metabolic functions of those genes in healthy individuals, (iii) identify the specific DNA sequences in defective genes, and (iv) consider the feasibility of replacement therapy.

The first and possibly the most difficult challenge is to identify the major genes contributing to the pathogenesis of NIDDM. In this paper, we shall describe progress made in analysis of candidate genes in NIDDM, discuss why the genetic defects in NIDDM have not yet been identified, and propose strategies that should accelerate our search for the NIDDM genes.

Candidate genes in NIDDM

The complexity of metabolic abnormalities in NIDDM means that there is potentially a large number of genes that are candidates in the search for the primary inherited defect(s). Analysis of these candidate genes has not been ordered by their relative likelihood of contributing to the pathogenesis of the disease but, rather, by the availability of cloned segments of human DNA. Cloned genes include those for insulin [10], the insulin receptor [11,12] and the erythrocyte-type glucose transporter [13]. Generous international collaboration has meant that these clones have been widely distributed for analysis in NIDDM patients.

The insulin gene

The insulin (INS) gene on the short arm of chromosome 11 (11p15.5; Ref. 14) is closely linked with a hyper-variable region of DNA, characterized by variation in the number of tandem repeats 14 base pairs (bp) in length [15]. There are two distinct size classes of alleles, yielding *Bgl*I restriction fragments of 2.7–3.3 kb (small inserts) and of 4.3–5.0 kb (large inserts). The close proximity of this length polymorphism to the 5′ end of the insulin gene has led to speculation that it could be involved in regulation of insulin expression [15].

The distribution of small and large DNA insertions near the insulin gene has been examined in various populations as summarized in Table 1. The preliminary study by Bell et al. [15] was based on a small series and found no evidence for association between NIDDM and insulin gene restriction fragment length polymorphisms (RFLPs). Rotwein et al. [16] suggested that individuals homozygous for the large insert 5′ to the insulin gene were more likely to develop NIDDM, but statistical significance was achieved only by pooling data from different racial groups. The finding was confirmed in Danes by Owerbach and Nerup [17], and in the British by Hitman

TABLE 1

Frequencies of large (L) and small (S) DNA inserts 5' to the insulin gene in NIDDM and controls

Study	Population	'Allele' frequency						χ^2
		NIDDM			Controls			df = 1
		n	L	S	n	L	S	
Bell [15]	Americans	12	0.29	0.71	28	0.30	0.70	0.0
Rotwein [16]	Americans	34	0.23	0.77	33	0.18	0.82	0.5
Owerbach [17]	Danes	47	0.35	0.65	56	0.26	0.74	1.9
Hitman [18]	British	71	0.49	0.51	88	0.33	0.67	8.5*
Rotwein [16]	Am. Africans	35	0.40	0.60	28	0.21	0.79	5.2*
Rotwein [16]	Pima	31	0.30	0.70	26	0.19	0.81	1.8
Serjeantson [19]	Micronesians	58	0.24	0.76	60	0.19	0.81	0.9
Xiang [20]	Am. Chinese	93	0.11	0.89	73	0.12	0.88	0.1

*$P < 0.05$.

et al. [18]. There is clearly no association between NIDDM and insulin gene RFLPs in Micronesians [19] or in Chinese Americans [20].

Pedigree analyses of several NIDDM families (e.g. Refs. 18 and 21) and families [22,23] with maturity-onset diabetes of the young (MODY) have failed to implicate the insulin gene in either NIDDM or MODY. Although mutant insulin molecules have been described in rare instances [24], insulin gene mutations are unlikely to be a significant risk factor in NIDDM [25].

The insulin receptor gene

The insulin receptor (INSR) gene on chromosome 19 (9p13.3-p13.2; Ref. 26) is a large gene with the coding region spanning more than 40 kb although the cDNA is approximately 5 kb [11]. There is a marked absence of linkage disequilibrium in this distal region of the short arm of chromosome 19, as originally described with respect to the serum complement component C3, where there was no population linkage disequilibrium between C3 RFLPs and C3 protein variants [27]. Similarly, INSR polymorphic restriction sites generated with enzymes *Bgl*II and *Rsa*I are randomly associated in Micronesians [28] as well as in Caucasoids, Pima Indians and American Africans [29]. In Micronesians, linkage analysis showed the maximum lod score for linkage between the *Bgl*II and *Rsa*I sites was obtained at a recombination fraction of 0.05.

The absence of strong linkage disequilibrium within the insulin receptor gene suggests that an association between NIDDM and a single RFLP is unlikely to be detected in a random population series. There are two alternative approaches. One is to analyse a number of restriction sites and correlate INSR haplotypes with NIDDM. This analysis has been undertaken by Xiang et al. [20], using *Xba*I, *Rsa*I and *Kpn*I, in Chinese Americans with NIDDM. This repertoire of enzymes generates 12 possible haplotypes, all of which are present in the Chinese population, demonstrating once again the lack of linkage disequilibrium in the INSR gene. Xiang et al. [20] identified two haplotypes that could be protective against NIDDM in Chinese.

In the absence of population linkage disequilibrium, pedigree analysis is clearly a much more powerful approach than comparison of RFLP prevalence data. Our own studies [28] on insulin receptor gene RFLPs in eight extended Micronesian families with a total of 170 family members aged over 20 years failed to implicate the INSR gene in NIDDM. As shown in Table 2, linkage between NIDDM and either the *Bgl*II or *Rsa*I polymorphic sites of the insulin receptor gene could not be demonstrated, irrespective of whether diabetes was considered a dominant trait with complete penetrance or a recessive trait with 90% penetrance. However, since lod scores did not fall below -2, the possibility of some minor contribution of the INSR locus cannot be definitely excluded.

The erythrocyte-type glucose transporter gene

The erythrocyte-type glucose transporter (GLUT) gene on the short arm of chromosome 1 (1p35-p31.3; Ref. 30), first cloned by Mueckler et al. [13] is associated with *Xba*I RFLPs in Caucasoids [30], with an additional *Bgl*II RFLP in Micronesians [31] and in Chinese [20]. In Micronesians, *Bgl*II-digested DNA has allelic fragments of 7.8 kb and 6.2 kb when hybridized with the GLUT clone, whereas the *Bgl*II fragment

TABLE 2

Lod scores for linkage between insulin receptor gene RFLPs and NIDDM

Genetic markers	Recombination fraction (θ)				
	0.0	0.1	0.2	0.3	0.4
*Bgl*II, *Rsa*I	0.70	0.74	0.58	0.34	0.11
NIDDM dominant					
NIDDM, *Bgl*II	-0.34	-0.63	-0.29	-0.12	-0.03
NIDDM, *Rsa*I	0.10	-0.34	-0.12	-0.04	-0.01
NIDDM recessive					
NIDDM, *Bgl*II	-0.99	-0.52	-0.26	-0.10	-0.02
NIDDM, *Rsa*I	-0.48	-0.23	-0.11	-0.04	-0.01

in Caucasoids is invariably 7.8 kb. Micronesians have acquired the extra *Bgl*II site on a chromosome carrying the *Xba*I/6.5 kb fragment, since the *Bgl*II/6.2 kb fragment invariably cosegregated with *Xba*I/6.5 kb, whereas the *Bgl*II/7.8 kb fragment occurred in conjunction with either the *Xba*I/6.5 kb or the *Xba*I/6.3 kb alleles.

Population studies of GLUT RFLPs in NIDDM patients and controls have been undertaken in several laboratories. These studies are summarized in Table 3. Li et al. [32] reported a consistent increase in the GLUT/*Xba*I/6.5 kb (designated 6.3 kb by these authors) allele in North Europeans, South Europeans and Japanese. However, GLUT RFLPs were clearly not associated with NIDDM in Chinese Americans [20], or in the small unrelated Micronesian sample [31].

In Micronesians, our efforts have once again been applied to family analyses [31]. Eight extended families segregating for NIDDM were examined for *Bgl*II and *Xba*I RFLPs. Lod scores were generated using the computer program LIPED, with scores based on *Bgl*II RFLP results for 83 adults and on *Xba*I RFLPs for 43 adults. Linkage analyses were performed with NIDDM accorded several different modes of inheritance, but those generated under the assumption of a dominant trait with 100% penetrance are given in Table 4.

Lod scores for linkage of NIDDM and GLUT RFLPs were negative, but uninformative, when all families were considered (Table 4). Summation across seven families, however, clearly rejected the hypothesis of close linkage ($< 10\%$ recombination) between NIDDM and the GLUT gene. In the eighth extended family, lod scores obtained from analysis of *Bgl*II and *Xba*I RFLPs were consistently positive, although less than 3.0, the minimum value generally required for statistical significance. This

TABLE 3

RFLP allele frequencies at the erythrocyte-type glucose transporter locus in NIDDM and controls

Study	Population	Allele frequency						χ^2
		NIDDM			controls			df = 1
		n	X1[a]	X2	n	X1	X2	
Li [30]	Europeans	142	0.41	0.59	145	0.28	0.72	11.3*
Li [30]	Japanese	45	0.34	0.66	49	0.14	0.86	35.3*
Xiang [19]	Am. Chinese	92	0.27	0.73	73	0.20	0.80	2.2
Serjeantson [29]	Micronesians	18	0.56[b]	0.44[c]	19	0.63[b]	0.37[c]	0.4

[a] X1, *Xba*I/6.5 kb; X2, *Xba*I/6.3 kb.

[b] *Bgl*II/7.8 kb.

[c] *Bgl*II/6.2 kb.

* $P < 0.01$.

TABLE 4

Lod scores for linkage between erythrocyte-type glucose transporter gene RFLPs and NIDDM

Families	Recombination fraction			
	0.1	0.2	0.3	0.4
All families				
BglII	−1.34	−0.40	−0.05	0.03
XbaI	−0.96	−0.18	0.05	0.02
Seven families				
BglII	−1.82	−0.86	−0.35	−0.08
XbaI	−1.98	−0.98	−0.57	−0.04
One family				
BglII	0.48	−0.46	0.30	0.11
XbaI	1.02	0.81	0.53	0.06

positive lod score may have occurred in one of eight families simply by chance, or alternatively could suggest genetic heterogeneity in NIDDM even in the relatively homogeneous population of Nauru. An alternative explanation in this family, which has several members descended from mixed Caucasoid by Micronesian marriages, is that the BglII/6.2 kb fragment is simply a marker for Micronesian ancestry which, on the basis of HLA data [19], is also a marker for predisposition to NIDDM.

Additional GLUT/BamHI fragment in Micronesians

Micronesians, like Caucasoids [30], do not show any polymorphisms in commonly occurring restriction sites when digested DNA is hybridized with a 3′ fragment of the GLUT gene, described elsewhere as the hGT2-1 clone [30]. However, Micronesians invariably show a BamHI/1.1 kb fragment that is absent from all ($n = 38$) Caucasoids tested. BamHI-digested DNA shows two monomorphic bands of 7.2 kb and 1.9 kb on filters washed at high stringency, with an additional 3.0 kb fragment seen at low stringency. Whether this band represents a partial gene duplication capable of affecting glucose transporter gene regulation, or a missing BamHI site in non-coding DNA, or even a second glucose transporter gene, remains to be defined.

Inconsistencies in population analyses of candidate genes

A large number of studies have reported associations between NIDDM and a range of genetic markers that includes not only the candidate genes discussed here but also blood group [33,34], HLA [19,35] and serum protein [34,36] markers. These studies have considerable limitations in that there is a high risk of obtaining evidence of a false association. A spurious result can readily result if patients and controls are not carefully matched for ethnic background. This matching can be extremely difficult, if not impossible to achieve, unless patients are matched with an unaffected sibling. In Micronesia, for example, the frequency of HLA-Bw22 (Bw56) is significantly increased in NIDDM patients compared with controls. However, HLA-Bw56 is a common antigen in Micronesians, with an antigen frequency of 20% in NIDDM patients and 11% in controls, whereas in Caucasoids it is extremely rare, at about 1%. Our HLA studies in Micronesia have shown that people with foreign (mainly Caucasoid) HLA genes are significantly less likely to develop NIDDM than are those people with pure Micronesian ancestry [19]. Thus the increase in HLA-Bw56 in NIDDM may simply reflect an increase in the proportion of Micronesian genes in NIDDM patients compared with controls.

In the examples of Micronesians and Pima Indians, where HLA associations with NIDDM have been found [19,35], the need for concern about possible population stratification is obvious. The same concern, however, is needed in less obvious situations, such as the population of London, where recently a dramatic association between vitamin-D-binding protein Gc markers and HIV1 infection was claimed [37], but could not be supported by other studies [38]. Similarly, reports of strong associations between INS [18] and GLUT [32] RFLPs with NIDDM in the London population must be interpreted with caution.

With recombinant DNA technology, there is the potential for many additional candidate genes to be examined. The laboratory with poorly matched controls is the one most likely to find an apparent association with NIDDM and the one most likely to have its study published. This not only results in wasted efforts in other laboratories, unsuccessfully attempting to confirm spurious results, but diverts energy and expertise from achieving the final goal. We believe that claims of weak population associations should be accompanied by pedigree analyses. The very least requirement should be analysis of another unlinked, highly variable genetic locus, to show that patients and controls are ethnically matched. With recombinant DNA technology it is an easy matter to rehybridize nylon membranes, prepared for analysis of the candidate gene with additional clones, such as those for HLA-DRβ [39] or minisatellites [40].

Other candidate genes

The erythrocyte-type glucose transporter (HepG2 glucose transporter) is only one of a family of glucose transporters that can be translocated from an intracellular membrane pool to the cell surface. The glucose transporters have different tissue distributions. The recent cloning of several mammalian glucose transporter genes [13,41,42], including a rat insulin-regulatable glucose transporter [42] which is expressed in brown and white adipose tissue, heart and skeletal muscle, has provided further candidate genes that could provide the inherited defect contributing to NIDDM. The recent purification of a peptide forming amyloid (islet or insulinoma amyloid polypeptide) in the pancreases of NIDDM patients has also provided another candidate gene [43] for testing in NIDDM.

Why have the inherited defects in NIDDM not yet been found?

In the past five years, recombinant DNA technology has led to chromosomal localization of many genetic disorders. The diseases most amenable to genetic analysis have been those with a clear mode of inheritance, a known inherited biochemical defect and early age of onset, such as haemophilia A or Factor VIII deficiency [44]. However, other single gene disorders, for which no biochemical defect was known, have also been mapped to precise chromosomal regions and candidate genes identified. Diseases in this category include cystic fibrosis [45] and Duchenne muscular dystrophy [46]. Less amenable have been diseases with some age-dependent penetrance, but DNA RFLP linkage markers for polyposis coli [47], polycystic kidney disease [48], multiple endocrine neoplasia [49] and Alzheimer's disease [50] have been found. Definition of markers for these diseases has been possible by linkage analysis of RFLPs and disease in well-defined pedigrees, using random probes.

   Why, then, are there as yet no known RFLP markers for NIDDM? There are two reasons for this. One relates to the direction of the research effort. The second reason for slow progress can be attributed to factors related to NIDDM.

The research effort

For NIDDM, unlike polyposis coli and many other diseases, there has been no shortage of ideas regarding the candidate genes that should be cloned. These genes are increasingly becoming available and already include the apolipoprotein genes (e.g. Ref. 51) as well as the insulin gene [10], the insulin receptor gene [11,12] and the erythrocyte-like glucose transporter gene [13], as already discussed. The continuing availability of candidate probes has meant that much of the research effort has concentrated on quick screening in population-based series, comparing NIDDM patients with controls with respect to the frequency of specific DNA markers associated with candidate genes. In contrast, for diseases with no available candidate gene probes, the approach has been systematic analysis of the human genome, applying random probes in well-defined families. The reliance on population studies has resulted in a rather confused genetic literature on NIDDM, with weak disease associations reported and refuted for every candidate gene yet tested. It is clear, however, that if more than one gene is involved in NIDDM, with susceptibility determined either by different genes in different families or by the summation of effects at two or more loci, then pedigree analyses are mandatory. There is no published study of the distribution of random probes in multiple NIDDM families, although we have analysed random traditional genetic markers in one Australian MODY family [52].

Factors relating to NIDDM that hinder pedigree analysis

NIDDM is a common disorder in developed and developing countries, so that superficially it would seem a relatively easy task to establish a series of well-defined pedigrees for genetic analysis. In many diseases with age-dependent penetrance, such as Huntington's Chorea, those affected can be assumed to have the susceptibility gene. In NIDDM, this is less certain, in that environmental factors such as obesity and inactivity can certainly influence insulin sensitivity [53] and glucose tolerance [54], possibly in people who do not necessarily have a full repertoire of genes for NIDDM susceptibility. The 'over-diagnosis' of NIDDM, to include sporadic cases, is a much more serious error in linkage analysis than under-diagnosis, as discussed by O'Rahilly et al. [55]. Other complexities in the genetic analysis of NIDDM include defining the mode of inheritance, late age of onset, variable penetrance rates and possible genetic heterogeneity.

Mode of transmission of NIDDM
Although it would seem important, if not essential, to define the mode of inheritance of NIDDM before undertaking linkage analyses, the absence of clear-cut transmission of NIDDM need not prevent pedigree analysis. Modern computer programs permit linkage analyses under varying hypotheses of the mode of transmission, accompanied by age-dependent penetrance distributions. That is, even if the mode of inheritance is unknown, lod scores for linkage can be calculated according to dominant, codominant or recessive modes of transmission, with variable penetrance parameters. Nevertheless, an a priori hypothesis regarding the inheritance of NIDDM would be extremely useful in determining the sample sizes required for linkage analyses.

In three populations with a high prevalence of NIDDM, clear bimodality in glucose tolerance has been shown [56–58], strongly implicating a single gene in NIDDM in these groups. Serjeantson et al., in analysis of pedigrees of Micronesians from Nauru, found evidence for a single major gene [4]. In a population where the disease is common, it is often difficult to discriminate the mode of inheritance, and observed family distributions could not differentiate between a dominant gene with 95% penetrance and a recessive gene with 79% penetrance. Subsequent formal segregation analysis, using the computer program POINTER [59] to examine an age-adjusted score based on fasting glucose levels and glucose levels after administration of a 75 g glucose load, favoured a dominant or codominant mode of inheritance, as shown in Table 5.

Table 5 provides the maximum likelihood estimates of segregation parameters using a power transform appropriate for two commingling distributions. The multi-factorial component has heritability H in offspring and HZ in parents. The major gene for hyperglycemia has a frequency q, with the degree of dominance defined as d, where $d = 0$ when the major gene is recessive and $d = 1$ when it is dominant. The parameter t, referred to as displacement, is the distance between the two homozygous genotypes at the major locus and is measured in standard deviations. In fitting the general model, the dominance parameter of the major gene converged to $d = 1$, favouring a dominant mode of inheritance for hyperglycemia. However, for values of d ranging from 50 to 100%, there is little change in the likelihoods and a codominant component fits equally well. As shown in Table 5, the data do not fit a recessive model, with $\chi^2[1] = 7.77$, $P < 0.01$.

Genetic analyses of populations with a high prevalence of diabetes, as seen in Nauruans and in the Pima Indians, have sometimes been dismissed as MODY, rather than as NIDDM, because of a comparatively early age of onset. We would suggest that the clinical and epidemiological profiles of NIDDM in these populations are quite compatible with NIDDM but endorse the conclusions of O'Rahilly et al. [55] that a gene dose effect is operating. That is, patients homozygous for NIDDM susceptibility genes are likely to have an earlier age of onset of NIDDM than those heterozygous for the defective gene. The gene dose effect, supported by the study of Viswanathan et al. [60], may suggest that some apparently MODY families are simply part of the spectrum of NIDDM.

TABLE 5

Results of segregation analyses of hyperglycemia in Micronesians

Model			d	t	q	H	Z	χ^2
								df = 1
General model			1^a	1.474	0.137	0.310	0.096	–
Dominant	$(d = 1)$	(1)		1.474	0.137	0.310	0.096	0.00
Codominant	$(d = 0.5)$	(0.5)		2.627	0.159	0.308	0.095	1.49
Recessive	$(d = 0)$	(0)		1.504	0.498	0.311	0.088	7.77*

[a] Parameter went to this bound.
[b] Parameters in brackets have been fixed.
* $P < 0.01$ for goodness-of-fit.

Late age of onset of NIDDM

The late age of onset of NIDDM means that it is difficult to obtain large two- or three-generation pedigrees. This situation is exacerbated by the premature mortality of those with NIDDM. There is a sharp fall in average 2-hour blood glucose levels in Micronesians aged over 50 years. This fall may in part be attributable to older people with normal genes shifting above the WHO criterion for NIDDM, but is at least in part due to the differential mortality of those with the most severe diabetes.

Variable penetrance rates

An important question in pedigree analysis is whether young people with impaired glucose tolerance, but not 'abnormal' glucose tolerance under WHO criteria for diabetes [61], should be classified as being 'at-risk' and therefore considered to have the diabetogenic genotype. In Nauru, if 2-hour glucose levels are age-adjusted so that the 'cut-off' point for hyperglycemia is age-dependent, then clustering in families is quite clear, as shown in Table 6 and elsewhere [3]. That is, a 2-hour glucose value of 8 mmol/l is considered diabetogenic in a 20-year-old, but not in a 60-year-old.

These data strongly suggest that for pedigree analysis, it is essential to glucose-tolerance test all family members for generation of an age-dependent penetrance function, rather than relying on verbal reports of diabetes in family members.

Genetic heterogeneity

If different loci contribute to NIDDM in different families, then this can easily be missed in population comparisons but should be evident in pedigree analyses. As described by Lander and Botstein [62], the chance that a genetic marker will fail to co-segregate with a trait is the apparent recombination fraction $\theta = \theta\alpha + 1/2(1-\alpha)$. Linkage will appear to be loose if additional loci contribute to disease, even if one has pinpointed one specific locus. Examples are seen in analysis of linkage between

TABLE 6

Familial clustering of hyperglycemia in Micronesians

Parental status in glucose tolerance	Number of offspring	Hyperglycemic (%)
Two parents tested:		
Both abnormal	43	79.1
One abnormal	77	48.1
Both normal	20	5.0
One parent tested:		
Parent abnormal	177	59.3
Parent normal	122	41.0
Neither parent tested:	438	53.2

HLA-DR and insulin-dependent diabetes mellitus (IDDM), where $\theta = 0.04$ [63], suggesting either that the primary susceptibility gene is distant from HLA-DR, or, more likely, that HLA-DR or -DQ is a primary susceptibility locus with influences from additional non-HLA determinants. This should not be a problem, as long as loose linkage can be accepted as evidence for a primary disease-promoting gene plus additional, non-linked effects.

Need to establish well-defined multiplex NIDDM families for genetic analysis

Although the problems in pedigree analysis of NIDDM are formidable, they are not insurmountable. Family studies can detect linkage up to 15 000 kb, compared with about 100 kb in population studies that rely on linkage disequilibrium [64]. This makes it feasible to apply random probes in NIDDM kindreds, but pedigree analysis is clearly the method of choice in examining candidate probes also. An alternative approach is analysis of sib pairs [65], but possible genetic heterogeneity in NIDDM makes this a less attractive strategy than linkage analysis.

Conclusions

There is an urgent need to identify multiplex NIDDM families prepared to participate in an internationally coordinated study of the genetics of NIDDM. In order to avoid possible confusion with MODY and the possible complications of gene-dosage effects, pedigrees would ideally consist of one affected parent and at least three affected children. Lymphocytes from volunteer family members would be immortalized by transformation with Epstein-Barr virus, to produce unlimited quantities of DNA for distribution to interested laboratories. Specific laboratories may choose to undertake in-depth analyses of particular chromosomes with random DNA probes, to avoid duplication of research effort. Analysis of candidate genes is not, of course, precluded by application of random probes, but in our opinion the over-dependence of NIDDM genetics on the promise of candidate molecular clones has (with hindsight) delayed progress in genetic analyses of NIDDM.

Acknowledgements

This work was supported in part by NIH grant AM25446.

References

1. Barnett AH, Eff C, Leslie RDG, Pyke DA. Diabetes in identical twins: a study of 200 pairs. Diabetologia 1981;20:87–93.
2. Köbberling J, Tillil H. Empirical risk figures for first degree relatives of non-insulin dependent diabetics. In: Köbberling J, Tattersall R, eds. The genetics of diabetes mellitus. London: Academic Press, 1982; 201–209.
3. O'Rahilly S, Spivey RS, Holman RR, Nugent Z, Clark A, Turner RC. Type II diabetes of early onset: a distinct clinical and genetic syndrome? Br Med J 1987;294:923–928.
4. Serjeantson S, Zimmet P. Diabetes in the Pacific: evidence for a major gene. In: Baba S, Gould M, Zimmet P, eds. Diabetes mellitus: recent knowledge on aetiology, complications and treatment. Sydney: Academic Press, 1984; 23–40.
5. Sorge F, Schwatzkopff W, Neuhaus GA. Insulin response to oral glucose in patients with previous myocardial infarction and in patients with peripheral vascular disease: Hyperinsulinemia and its relationship to hypertriglyceridemia and overweight. Diabetes 1976;25:586–594.
6. Barrett-Connor E, Orchard T. Diabetes and heart disease. In: Harris, ed. Diabetes in America. NIH Publication No. 85-1468, 1985; XVI:1–41.
7. Samian R, Stansbie D, Dawson A, Galton DJ. Effects of alanine and fructose-1,6-bisphosphate on the activity of human adipose tissue pyruvate kinase. Clin Sci 1980;59:1P.
8. Friedenberg GR, Henry RR, Klein HH, Reichart DR, Olefsky JM. Decreased kinase activity of insulin receptors from adipocytes of non-insulin dependent diabetic subjects. J Clin Invest 1987;79:240–250.
9. Kashiwagi A, Verso MA, Andrews J, Vasquez B, Reaven GM, Foley JE. In vitro insulin resistance of human adipocytes isolated from subjects with non-insulin dependent diabetes mellitus. J Clin Invest 1983;72:1 246–1 254.
10. Bill GI, Picket RL, Rutter WJ, Cordell B, Tischer E, Goodman HM. Sequence of the human insulin gene. Nature 1980;284:26–32.
11. Ullrich A, Bell JR, Chen EY, et al. Human insulin receptor and its relationship to the tyrosine kinase family of oncogenes. Nature 1985;313:756–761.
12. Ebina Y, Ellis L, Jarnagin K, et al. The human insulin receptor cDNA: the structural basis for hormone-activated transmembrane signalling. Cell 1985;40:747–758.
13. Mueckler M, Caruso C, Baldwin SA, et al. Sequence and structure of a human glucose transporter. Science 1985;229:941–945.
14. Human Gene Mapping Workshop 9. Paris. Cytogenet Cell Genet 1987;46:29–77.
15. Bell GI, Karam JH, Rutter WJ. Polymorphic cDNA region adjacent to the 5' end of the human insulin gene. Proc Natl Acad Sci USA 1981;78:5 759–5 763.
16. Rotwein PS, Chirgwin J, Province M, et al. Polymorphism in the 5' flanking region of the human insulin gene: a genetic marker for non-insulin-dependent diabetes. N Engl J Med 1983;308:65–71.
17. Owerbach D, Nerup J. Restriction fragment length polymorphism of the insulin gene in diabetes mellitus. Diabetes 1982;31:275–277.
18. Hitman GA, Jowett NI, Williams LG, Humphries S, Winter RM, Galton DJ. Polymorphisms in the 5'-flanking region of the insulin gene and non-insulin-dependent diabetes. Clin Sci 1984;66:383–388.
19. Serjeantson SW, Owerbach D, Zimmet P, Nerup J, Thoma K. Genetics of diabetes in Nauru: effects of foreign admixture, HLA antigens and the insulin-gene-linked polymorphism. Diabetologia 1983;25:13–17.
20. Xiang K-S, Cox NJ, Sanz N, Huang P, Karam JH, Bell GI. Insulin-receptor and apolipoprotein genes contribute to development of NIDDM in Chinese Americans. Diabetes 1989;38:17–23.

21. Elbein SC, Corsetti L, Goldgar D, Skolnick M, Permutt MA. Insulin gene in familial NIDDM: lack of linkage in Utah Mormon pedigrees. Diabetes 1988;37:569–576.
22. Bell JI, Wainscoat JS, Old JM, et al. Maturity onset diabetes of the young is not linked to the insulin gene. Br Med J 1983;286:590–592.
23. Andreone T, Fajans S, Rotwein P, Skolnick M, Permutt A. Insulin gene analysis in a family with maturity onset diabetes of the young. Diabetes 1985;34:108–112.
24. Haneda M, Polonsky KS, Bergenstal RM, et al. Familial hyperinsulinemia due to a structurally abnormal insulin: definition of an emerging new clinical syndrome. N Engl J Med 1984;310:1 288–1 294.
25. Sanz N, Karam JH, Horita S, Bell GI. Prevalence of insulin gene mutations in non-insulin dependent diabetes mellitus. N Engl J Med 1986;314:1 322–1 323.
26. Yang-Feng TL, Franke U, Ullrich A. Gene for human insulin receptor: localization to site on chromosome 19 involved in pre-B-cell leukemia. Science 1985;228:728–731.
27. Donald JA, Ball SP. Approximate linkage equilibrium between two polymorphic sites within the gene for human complement component 3. Ann Hum Genet 1984;48:269–273.
28. Serjeantson SW, White BS, Bell GI, Zimmet P. RFLPs in the insulin receptor gene and type 2 diabetes in the Pacific. In: Sasazuki T, ed. New approach to genetic disease. Tokyo: Academic Press, 1987; 23–30.
29. Elbein SC, Corsetti L, Ullrich A, Permutt MA. Multiple restriction fragment length polymorphisms at the insulin receptor locus: a highly informative marker for linkage analysis. Proc Natl Acad Sci USA 1986;83:5 223–5 227.
30. Shows TB, Eddy RL, Byers MG, et al. Polymorphic human glucose transporter gene (GLUT) is on chromosome 1p31.3-p35. Diabetes 1987;36:546–549.
31. Serjeantson SW, White B, Bell GI, Zimmet P. The glucose transporter gene and Type 2 diabetes in the Pacific. In: Proc 13th Int Diabetes Fed Congr. Amsterdam: Excerpta Medica (in press).
32. Li SR, Baroni MG, Oelbaum RS, Stock J, Galton DJ. Association of genetic variant of the glucose transporter with non-insulin-dependent diabetes mellitus. Lancet 1988;2:368–370.
33. Mourant AE, Kopec AC, Domaniewska-Sobczak K. Blood groups and diseases. Oxford: Oxford University Press, 1978.
34. Stein MP, Ferrell RE, Rosenthal M, Haffner SM, Hazuda HP. Association between NIDDM, Rh blood group, and haptoglobin phenotype. Diabetes 1986;35:367–391.
35. Williams RC, Knowler WC, Butler WJ, et al. HLA-A2 and Type 2 (insulin independent) diabetes mellitus in Pima Indians: an association of allele frequency with age. Diabetologia 1981;21:460–463.
36. Kirk RL, Serjeantson SW, Zimmet P. Genes and diabetes in the Pacific. In: Mimura G, Baba S, Goto Y, Köbberling J, eds. Clinico-genetic genesis of diabetes mellitus. Amsterdam: Excerpta Medica, 1982;597:34–40.
37. Eales L-J, Nye KE, Parkin JM, et al. Association of different allelic forms of group specific component with susceptibility to and clinical manifestation of human immuno-deficiency virus infection. Lancet 1987;i:999–1 002.
38. Thymann M, Dickmeiss E, Svejgaard A, Pedersen C, Bygbjerg I, Faber V. Aids and the Gc protein. Lancet 1987;1:1 378.
39. Long EO, Wake CT, Strubin M, et al. Isolation of distinct cDNA clones encoding HLA-DRβ chains by use of an expression assay. Proc Natl Acad Sci USA 1982;79:7 465–7 469.
40. Jeffreys AJ, Wilson V, Thein SL. Hypervariable 'minisatellite' regions in human DNA. Nature 1985;314:67–73.
41. Birnbaum MJ, Haspel HC, Rosen OM. Cloning and characterization of a cDNA encoding the rat brain glucose-transporter protein. Proc Natl Acad Sci USA 1986;83:5 784–5 788.
42. James DE, Strube M, Mueckler M. Molecular cloning and characterization of an insulin-regulatable glucose transporter. Nature 1989;338:83–87.

43. Mosselman S, Höppener JWM, Zandberg J, et al. Islet amyloid polypeptide: identification and chromosomal localization of the human gene. FEBS Lett 1988;239:227–232.

44. Gitschier J, Wood WI, Goralka TM, et al. Characterization of the human factor VIII gene. Nature 1984;312:326–330.

45. Knowlton RG, Cohen-Haguenauer O, Van Cong N, et al. A polymorphic DNA marker linked to cystic fibrosis is located on chromosome 7. Nature 1985;318:381–382.

46. Monaco AP, Neve RL, Colletti-Feener C, Bertelson CJ, Kurnit DM, Kunkel LM. Isolation of candidate cDNAs for portions of the Duchenne muscular dystrophy gene. Nature 1986;323:646–650.

47. Bodmer WF, Bailey CJ, Bodmer J, et al. Localization of the gene for familial adenomatous polyposis in chromosome 5. Nature 1987;328:614–616.

48. Reeders ST, Breuning MH, Davies KE, Nicholls RD, Jarman AP, Weatherall DJ. A highly polymorphic DNA marker linked to adult polycystic kidney disease on chromosome 16. Nature 1985;317:542–544.

49. Simpson NE, Kidd KK, Goodfellow PJ, et al. Assignment of multiple endocrine neoplasia Type 2A to chromosome 10 by linkage analysis. Nature 1987;328:528–530.

50. St George-Hyslop PH, Tanzi RE, Polinsky RJ, et al. The genetic defect causing familial Alzheimer's disease maps on chromosome 21. Science 1987;235:885–890.

51. Luo C-C, Li W-H, Moore MN, Chan L. Structure and evolution of the apolipoprotein multigene family. J Mol Biol 1986;187:325–340.

52. Serjeantson SW, Zimmet P. Analysis of linkage relationships in maturity-onset diabetes of young people and independent segregation of C6 and HLA. Hum Genet 1982;62:214–216.

53. Wirth A, Diehm C, Mayor H. Plasma C-peptide and insulin in trained and untrained subjects. J Appl Physiol 1987;50:70–71.

54. Zimmet P. Type 2 (non-insulin-dependent) diabetes – an epidemiological overview. Diabetologia 1982;22:399–411.

55. O'Rahilly S, Wainscoat JS, Turner RC. Type 2 (non-insulin-dependent) diabetes mellitus: new genetics for old nightmares. Diabetologia 1988;31:407–414.

56. Rushforth NB, Bennett PH, Sternberg AG, Burch TA, Miller M. Diabetes in Pima Indians: evidence of bimodality in glucose tolerance distributions. Diabetes 1971;20:756–765.

57. Zimmet P, Whitehouse S. Bimodality of fasting and two-hour glucose tolerance distributions in a Micronesian population. Diabetes 1978;27:793–800.

58. Raper LR, Taylor R, Zimmet P, Milne B, Balkan B. Bimodality in glucose tolerance distributions in the urban Polynesian population of Western Samoa. Diabetes Res 1984;1:19–26.

59. Lalouel JM, Morton NE. Complex segregation analysis with pointers. Hum Hered 1981;31:312–321.

60. Viswanathan M, Mohan V, Snehelatha C, Ramachandran A. High prevalence of Type 2 (non-insulin-dependent) diabetes among the offspring of conjugal Type 2 diabetic parents in India. Diabetologia 1985;28:907–910.

61. WHO expert committee on Diabetes Mellitus Second Report. Technical Report Series No. 646, 1980.

62. Lander ES, Botstein D. Strategies for studying heterogeneous genetic trait in humans by using a linkage map of restriction fragment length polymorphisms. Proc Natl Acad Sci USA 1986;83:7353–7357.

63. Green A, Morton NE, Iselius L, et al. Genetic studies of insulin-dependent diabetes mellitus: segregation and linkage analyses. Tissue Antigens 1982;19:213–221.

64. Lander E, Botstein D. Mapping complex genetic traits in humans: new methods using a complete RFLP linkage map. Cold Spring Harbor Symp Quant Biol 1986;LI:49–62.

65. Suarez BK. A sib-pair strategy for the use of restriction fragment length polymorphisms to study the mode of transmission of Type II diabetes. Am J Hum Genet 1983;35:34–48.

CHAPTER 3

The prevalence and incidence of non-insulin-dependent diabetes mellitus

GARY K. DOWSE and PAUL Z. ZIMMET

WHO Collaborating Centre for Epidemiology of Diabetes Mellitus and Health Promotion for Non-communicable Disease Control, Lions-International Diabetes Institute, PO Box 185, Caulfield South, Victoria 3162, Australia

Introduction

Non-insulin-dependent diabetes mellitus (NIDDM) accounts for approximately 80–90% of the total burden of diabetes in developed countries, and almost 100% in many developing populations [1,2]. It also contributes a substantial proportion of the total morbidity, mortality and associated economic costs attributable to all cases of diabetes [3,4]. Therefore, descriptive and analytical epidemiological studies of NIDDM are of profound importance with regard to health care planning, aetiological research and hopes for prevention of this disease.

Diabetes has been recognized since antiquity, and Hindu physicians of the 6th century AD are credited with describing an association with affluence [5,6]. European physicians in Asian and African colonies became increasingly aware of geographic and ethnic differences in the occurrence of diabetes towards the end of the 19th century [7]. Substantive documentation of differences in the prevalence of diabetes between ethnic groups, and variations dependent on factors such as age, sex, socio-economic status and body mass have only become available since the 1960s. By this time, oral glucose tolerance testing (OGTT) had become generally accepted as a tool for diagnosis of diabetes, but blood glucose cut-off levels were defined either arbitrarily or based on statistical grounds [8,9]. Pioneering cross-population studies using standardized criteria, such as those of West and Kalbfleisch [7,10], clearly established that there was considerable variation in the prevalence of diabetes between populations.

Development of standardized criteria

The need to screen asymptomatic persons with some form of glucose tolerance test so as to derive 'true' prevalence estimates for what was to become known as NIDDM became accepted practice during the 1960s and 1970s. However, direct comparison of results was hampered by different glucose loads and various diagnostic cut-off points, as well as differences in population age-distributions and sampling methods [2,11].

Recognition of these and more clinically-based problems led to calls for internationally standardized criteria for classification and diagnosis of diabetes, and for reporting of epidemiological studies [12,13]. Coinciding with this, two critical types of information became available which allowed a more scientific basis for defining the disease. These were:

1. Longitudinal data relating baseline glucose levels to risk of micro- and macro-vascular complications and progress to 'overt' diabetes [14–20].
2. Demonstration in the high-diabetes-prevalence Pima Indian [21,22] and Nauruan [23] populations of bimodality of plasma glucose distributions.

Fortunately the cut-off levels for fasting and 2-hour glucose suggested by the longitudinal 'risk' studies [14–20] closely approximated the mid-points separating the 'diabetic' and 'normal' modes in the Nauruans and Pimas [21–23]. This fact allowed two international panels of experts, the US National Diabetes Data Group (NDDG) in 1979 and the World Health Organization (WHO) Expert Committee on Diabetes Mellitus in 1980, to propose similar (but unfortunately not identical) criteria for classification and diagnosis of diabetes and related disorders [11,24].

In 1985, the WHO recommendations were further refined and some ambiguities clarified [25]. At this time it was also suggested that for the purpose of epidemiological studies a single blood glucose concentration measured 2 h after a 75 g oral glucose load was sufficient for classifying a subject's glucose tolerance status [25–27]. The acceptance by the international community of the NDDG and WHO recommended criteria coincided with increasing concern over apparent epidemics of NIDDM in many populations experiencing rapid socio-economic development and Westernization. Consequently, there is now much more information available on the epidemiology of NIDDM in developing than already-developed populations [28].

Harris et al. [27] have considered the differences in prevalence estimates derived through use of either the NDDG or the WHO criteria and recommended use of the latter, largely because they are simpler to apply. The WHO criteria result in a relative over-estimate of IGT prevalence, because of the NDDG requirement for an additional elevated blood glucose level during the OGTT [11,25]. Popular usage appears to have decided in favour of the WHO criteria: of the many prevalence studies conducted around the world (including studies in the US) in the last decade, the majority have reported results using the simpler WHO criteria.

Problems with current criteria

Whilst undoubtedly the NDDG and WHO recommendations provided a rational and scientific consensus for diagnostic criteria of NIDDM, and spawned a large number of epidemiological investigations, there remain several problems when studies are compared.

1. *Size of glucose load:* Unfortunately the NDDG and WHO guidelines were not sufficiently clear in emphasizing that 75 g of glucose meant 75 g of anhydrous glucose or equivalent. As glucose monohydrate is the cheapest and most readily available form of glucose, it has been used in many epidemiological studies, particularly large population surveys, with the result that an amount equivalent to 68 g of anhydrous glucose has been used as the loading dose [29]. It is now impossible to tell from the majority of published papers whether '75 g of glucose' refers to glucose monohydrate or another form. Hence one is also unable to determine which load has actually been used most often. Studies are currently under way to clarify the resultant effect of such small differences (average 3 mmol/l) in size of glucose load on blood glucose levels and prevalence estimates for diabetes and IGT. It has previously been demonstrated that there are large differences (mean 3 mmol/l) in 2-hour blood glucose levels when 50- and 100-g glucose loads are given to subjects with glucose intolerance [30].

2. *Timing of blood tests:* Remarkably, it is difficult to find reference in all but a very few published studies to standards by which investigators have included/excluded subjects from analyses related to the timing of the 2-hour post-load test [1,31]. Given the vagaries of field survey conditions, it is most unlikely that all subjects will have their 2-hour blood test taken precisely on time. It is probable, therefore, that each group of investigators has made a different decision regarding what is acceptable.

3. *Reporting of results:* Bennett [13] presented rational arguments for standardized reporting of results from epidemiological studies of diabetes. One of the simplest recommendations concerned the break-down of data by 5- or 10-year age-groups such as 25–34, 35–44, ... rather than 20–29, 30–39, etc. Unfortunately, this has not yet been adopted by all investigators, which unnecessarily complicates comparison of results from different studies, whether by age-specific or age-adjusted frequencies or mean values. Similarly, glucose distributions are rarely reported, although this may often reflect editorial censure.

4. *Screening tests prior to OGTT:* In an attempt to lessen expense and avoid logistic problems, a number of studies conducted since the appearance of the WHO and NDDG criteria have attempted to limit the population to whom they give full diagnostic OGTTs by various means, including first performing screening tests based on random or fasting blood glucose values, using various cut-offs [32–34]. By such

means the 'true' prevalence of NIDDM and IGT (given that they are defined by the standard OGTT) will always be under-estimated to some degree, depending on the cut-off level chosen [26]. The simplest way to obtain more accurate prevalence estimates in such circumstances would be to perform OGTTs on a sample of the subjects undergoing screening tests and to correct the final prevalence figures.

Do we need the OGTT?

There is also, however, a more fundamental question regarding the current criteria: whether asymptomatic subjects found to have abnormal glucose tolerance in the 'diabetic range' (≥ 11.1 mmol/l) but with normal fasting glucose levels (< 7.8 mmol/l) should indeed be classed as having 'diabetes'. At present, in epidemiological investigations, this is certainly the case. In clinical practice, of course, it is not, as glucose tolerance tests are very rarely performed on asymptomatic individuals and hence the question does not arise. The Bedford [14] and Whitehall [15] surveys from which the 2-hour levels of 11.1 mmol/l were derived, as indicating risk of microvascular complications, did not examine the question of whether the 2-hour level acted independently of the level of fasting glycaemia. It is known from a number of studies that almost 100% of subjects with a fasting plasma glucose level of 7.8 mmol/l or higher will also have a 2-hour plasma glucose level of at least 11.1 mmol/l [26,27]. The question immediately arises, therefore, whether the microvascular complication rates associated with abnormal glucose tolerance in reality reflected the fasting glucose.

The only published data which can shed some light on this issue come from the Pima studies. In cross-sectional data Rushforth et al. [22] found that 'diabetes-specific' complications (retinopathy and/or nephropathy) occurred only in subjects with either fasting plasma glucose levels ≥ 8 mmol/l or 2-hour glucose levels ≥ 14 mmol/l. The fasting level alone conveniently identified those at risk. Similarly, in longitudinal data (over 3 years), proteinuria did not appear in subjects with low fasting plasma glucose (< 7.8 mmol/l), but retinopathy did develop in 2 of 22 subjects who had fasting levels < 7.8 mmol/l and 2-hour levels ≥ 11.1 mmol/l [16]. If the legitimacy of 2-hour levels for diagnosis of NIDDM rests on these 2 cases, then this would seem rather insubstantial evidence, as these subjects could indeed have had high fasting levels in the past and/or soon after their initial OGTT.

Evidence from longitudinal studies in Nauruans suggests that subjects with high 2-hour plasma glucose levels, but normal fasting glycaemia, suffer microvascular complication rates more compatible with the IGT category than with diabetic subjects who have fasting hyperglycaemia (≥ 7.8 mmol/l). As depicted in Fig. 1, there was little difference in occurrence rates (a mixture of prevalent and incident cases, relative to baseline) at follow-up of both retinopathy and macroalbuminuria when

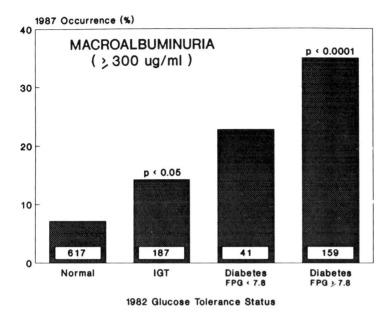

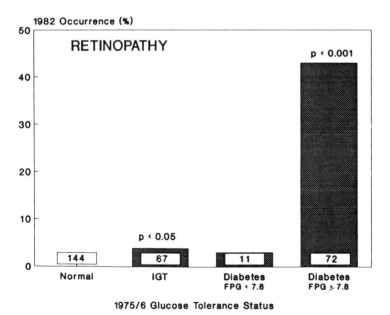

Fig. 1. Relationship of base-line glucose tolerance and fasting plasma glucose levels to occurrence (mixed prevalent and incident cases) of retinopathy (1975/6–82) and macroalbuminuria (1982–87) at follow-up. Occurrence rates are age-standardized. Significance tests versus normal group

fasting normoglycaemic 'diabetic' subjects were compared with those with IGT. This has also been demonstrated for mortality and other indices of morbidity in this population [35]. One of the problems with these studies relates to the association of outcome events with unstable baseline information. The short- and long-term variability of glucose tolerance tests is well recognized [36,37], and mis-classification of subjects may have a critical effect on outcome associations.

The above discussion serves to indicate that while the current diagnostic criteria are a considerable improvement over previous versions, they should not be seen as immutable. It does not yet appear sufficiently clear that a glucose tolerance test is necessary to define 'diabetes' for either epidemiological studies or the clinical setting. These doubts have been expressed in the past [7,38]. However, for the present and immediate future, at least, the 2-hour 75 g oral glucose (monohydrate or anhydrous!) tolerance test must remain the international standard for comparison of prevalence and incidence data. Notwithstanding the reservations considered above, it is reassuring that the findings of the pioneering longitudinal risk [14–20] and bimodality [21–23] studies have in general been supported by results from other populations [39–42]. This suggests that the fasting and 2-hour blood glucose cut-off points derived from those early studies, and hence also the diagnostic criteria, are applicable across populations.

Study design

Whilst many studies conducted in adult populations report the prevalence of 'diabetes', and do not clearly distinguish between cases of insulin-dependent diabetes mellitus (IDDM) and NIDDM, it is reasonable (particularly so for developing countries, where IDDM appears to be rare) and common practice to equate the prevalence of all classifications of diabetes to that of NIDDM [28].

This review will primarily consider studies which have based their diagnosis on WHO criteria [24,25], while recognizing that there remain differences in the way those criteria have been applied. There are as yet few incidence estimates available using the new criteria, although a number of longitudinal studies are now in progress and may be expected to report over the next few years.

The following sampling strategies have been used to derive estimates of NIDDM occurrence.

1. *Selected community samples:* The communities are usually selected because of convenience, and/or because they are judged to be 'typical' given the a priori objectives of the investigators (e.g. comparing rural vs. urban dwellers) [1,43–45]. Randomization within the sample (e.g. by household) is possible, but is not usually performed.

2. *Random cluster sampling:* This technique has been used to advantage in a recent national prevalence survey conducted in Mauritius [48]. All adults resident within the randomly selected clusters were surveyed.

3. *Random sampling (individual level):* A recent estimate of diabetes prevalence in Australia was derived from a national population sample based on electoral rolls [49]. However, the study was limited to residents of large cities and did not use an OGTT. The closest to a true national estimate using the OGTT is probably that based on a stratified sampling scheme in the US population [31].

4. *Whole populations:* Few defined groups are small enough to allow this luxury, but prime examples are the studies in Nauruans [40,46] and Pima Indians [47]. Because of their size, uniquely high prevalence of NIDDM, relative isolation, and stability, these particular populations have also been subject to longitudinal study.

Investigators and reviewers alike have found it convenient to accept estimates derived from these various sampling strategies as being representative of a particular country, ethnic group or stage of development [2,28]. It is important to recognize the potential danger of this approach, particularly where estimates are based on small sample size. In general, the first and second of the study designs described above are the most practical to apply in epidemiological investigations of NIDDM.

Factors influencing prevalence and incidence

Ethnic variation

The prevalence of NIDDM varies extremely widely, from a low of zero in a small community of Melanesians studied in the Highlands of Papua New Guinea (PNG) [50] to the extreme high of 39% and 45%, respectively, in male and female Pima Indians aged 25 years and over [51]. A number of more exhaustive reviews are available to interested readers [2,3,7,28,52]. The Western Pacific region, home to populations diverse in both genetic background and stage of socio-economic development, provides a dramatic example of the variation in prevalence of NIDDM (Fig. 2). Nauruans have an age-standardized prevalence 13 times that of European Australians.

Evidence for the interaction between genes and environment in determining NIDDM occurrence has come from the following observations:

1. *Increase in prevalence over time:* Although there may not be historical data on glucose tolerance, there is sufficient anecdotal and documentary evidence from early medical records and local sources to show that NIDDM either did not occur or was extremely unusual in traditional populations which now experience particularly high rates of the disease [51,53]. A rise in prevalence based on OGTT results

44

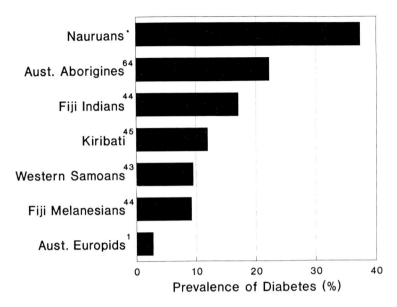

Fig. 2. Age-standardized prevalence of diabetes in adults aged 25–74 years in various Western Pacific populations. (Numbers indicate reference;* 1987 follow-up, unpublished; all studies used WHO Criteria (1985).)

has been documented in recent times in the Pima Indians [47,51] and has been inferred for the lower-prevalence US population based on the results of health interview surveys [54].

2. *Rural–urban differences:* Studies conducted in the Western Pacific region in the Polynesians of Western Samoa [43], Micronesians of Kiribati [45] and Melanesians of Fiji [44] have shown higher prevalence in subjects of the same genetic background living in more modernized urban environments than in their counterparts who maintain relatively traditional lifestyles.

3. *Increase in migrants:* Increased prevalence and incidence of NIDDM have been demonstrated in Polynesians from Tokelau who have migrated to New Zealand relative to those who have remained in the home islands [55]. A similar phenomenon has been documented in Wallis Islanders who have taken up residence in New Caledonia [56], and Japanese who have migrated from Hiroshima to Hawaii appear to be much more susceptible to NIDDM than their contemporaries in Japan [57].

Asian Indians who have migrated to diverse locations such as South Africa [58], Fiji [44], Mauritius [48] and the United Kingdom [59] experience an exceptionally high prevalence of NIDDM. Whilst there are no direct studies comparing prevalence in genetically similar groups who have remained in India, it has been inferred from other data that the prevalence in India is much lower [60]. These facts have always been a little difficult to reconcile, however, as Indian migrants characteristically maintain their traditional culture (as reflected in religion, dress, diet) even several generations after migration, although it is granted that in general they become more affluent and less subject to the vicissitudes of the Indian weather and its effect on nutrition. A recent study in an urban population in South India has found the prevalence to be similar to that of migrant Indians [61]. This suggests that with continuing development India may face a potentially enormous epidemic of NIDDM, presuming that the prevalence is indeed currently lower in less affluent rural areas.

4. *Differences between ethnic cohabitants:* There are numerous examples of striking differences in prevalence between ethnic groups residing in the same country. Data from a number of studies highlight differences between American Indians, Hispanics and the European and African populations of the USA [31,47,62]. Migrant Asian Indians have been found to have much higher prevalence than their cohabitants in studies in many countries [60], including Fiji [44], South Africa [58] and Singapore [63]. Australian Aborigines living in an urban environment have an age-adjusted prevalence of NIDDM 8 times that of European-origin Australians [1,64] (Fig. 2).

5. *Differences related to genetic mixing:* Studies of genetic admixture in high-prevalence populations such as Nauruans [65] and Mexican-Americans [62] have suggested that the prevalence of NIDDM declines as the proportion of foreign genes increases. Similarly, a series of studies in Melanesian populations in the Western Pacific have demonstrated that the prevalence of NIDDM rises dependent on the proportion of Austronesian (Polynesian and Micronesian) genes present [66]. To date, it appears that Melanesians of predominantly non-Austronesian ancestry (descended from early waves of migration into the area) experience a very low frequency of NIDDM and IGT [33,50]. However, these populations have also not yet been exposed to the degree of modernization of other Pacific populations, and hence it may still be too early to judge their position.

The epidemiological observations described above, plus other evidence such as high concordance for NIDDM in monozygotic twins [67] and a possibly autosomal dominant inheritance pattern in Nauruans [68] and Pima Indians [69], have firmly established the concept of genetic factors interacting with environment in the pathogenesis of NIDDM [70]. North American Indians [7,47], Micronesian and Polynesian Pacific islanders [43,45,46], Australian Aborigines [64] and Asian Indians [44,58–61] are particularly susceptible. European-origin populations would appear to occupy the lower end of the susceptibility scale [1,28,31]. The position of South-East Asian populations, Chinese, Japanese, African and other groups is not altogether clear. Studies

46

to date from mainland China [71], although not compatible with WHO criteria, have suggested a low susceptibility to NIDDM, but recent data from Taiwan [72], Singapore [63] and Mauritius [48] suggest a moderate susceptibility in Chinese populations. Similarly, although NIDDM seems to be infrequent in rural Africans [32], it is common in African-origin Creole populations in Surinam [73] and Mauritius [48] as well as in US Blacks [31]. Studies in Sumo wrestlers and migrant Japanese in Hawaii serve to indicate that given a sufficiently adverse environment, Japanese are also susceptible [52,57].

Of some interest is a recent study from the Indian Ocean island of Mauritius [48] which has demonstrated similar age-sex-standardized prevalence of both IGT and NIDDM in Hindu and Muslim Indians, Chinese and Creole (mixed-race African, European and Indian) ethnic groups (Table 1). These data may serve to indicate that, certainly outside the very high-prevalence populations, the importance of environment in explaining differences in prevalence may have been under-estimated in the past. For instance, Indian cooking and dietary habits have been adapted in large measure by the Chinese and Creoles in Mauritius. It is possible that factors such as this, closely associated with a culture and lifestyle, but also with a disease, could give an incorrect impression of strong genetic association.

'Thrifty genotype' hypothesis extended

The marked susceptibility to NIDDM of traditional populations has been explained in terms of the 'thrifty genotype', first proposed in 1962 by Neel [74,75]. This hypothesis suggests that in traditional populations subject to periods of 'feast and famine' (e.g. droughts, hurricanes, long canoe voyages) there was a selective advantage fa-

TABLE 1

Age-sex-standardized* prevalence of IGT and NIDDM in adults aged 25–74 years in four ethnic groups in Mauritius

	n	Prevalence (%)	
		IGT	NIDDM
Indians			
Hindu	2543	16.2	12.4
Muslim	671	15.3	13.3
Creoles	1306	17.5	10.4
Chinese	409	16.4	11.5
Combined	4929	16.6	11.9

* Direct method to total Mauritius population, 1986 [48].

vouring those with a metabolism which stored energy with maximum efficiency. In today's situation of an assured supply of highly refined calories, coupled with sedentary lifestyle, the thrifty genotype becomes disadvantageous, leading to hyperinsulinaemia, and insulin resistance (potentiated by obesity), and eventually to beta cell decompensation and NIDDM [70]. This occurs with much higher frequency than in populations where the genotype has not achieved a similar penetration.

Supportive evidence for the concept of a thrifty genotype (and perhaps an extension of the hypothesis) has come from a recent follow-up study in Nauru which has shown a dramatic fall in the prevalence of IGT from 18.5% to 8.7%, and a stabilization in the prevalence and incidence of NIDDM over the period 1982–1987 compared with the period 1975/6–1982 (unpublished data). More particularly, however, the incidence of progression from normal glucose tolerance to either IGT or NIDDM fell by more than 50% between the two periods (Fig. 3). Occurrence rates for NIDDM remained stable largely because of an increase in the incidence of progression from IGT to NIDDM. The decline in incidence of glucose intolerance in persons with normal glucose tolerance suggests an exhaustion of susceptible individuals carrying the gene(s) for NIDDM, as there were no changes in the frequency of risk factors such as obesity.

Speculatively, this may be the vanguard of a decline in total incidence, and eventu-

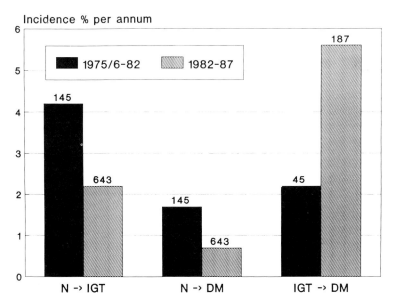

Fig. 3. Trends in cumulative incidence rates for development and progression of glucose intolerance in Nauruans aged 20 years and above. N = normal; IGT = impaired glucose tolerance; DM = diabetes mellitus; arrows indicate progression.

48

ally prevalence, of NIDDM in Nauru. The prevalence in susceptible populations such as the Nauruans [46] and Pimas [47] is high even in teenagers and young adults (see Fig. 5), who already experience the full range of diabetic complications [76], and it is likely that such individuals will tend to have fewer off-spring than their non-diabetic peers [77]. The decline in the frequency of the diabetic genotype will be slow, however, and be dependent on an interaction with primary prevention (lifestyle-related) measures and the medical care system. Whether the 'thrifty genotype' ever occurred with such high frequency in now-developed European and Asian populations, for instance, is unknown. If it did, then it may well have been gradually selected out over the last two millennia until the genes(s) reached a steady rate of transmission at a relatively low frequency and potency, consistent with disease onset in middle and older age, after completion of the reproductive phase.

IGT as a proportion of total glucose intolerance (IGT/TGI)
The prevalence of IGT varies widely between populations [28,78]. Although often of a magnitude in proportion to that of NIDDM, this is by no means consistent. For instance, a community survey of Australian Aborigines found a high prevalence of NIDDM (16.7% and 14.6% in males and females, respectively), but a remarkably low prevalence of IGT (0.7% and 4.2%) [64].

The recent decline in the prevalence and incidence of IGT and stabilization in the

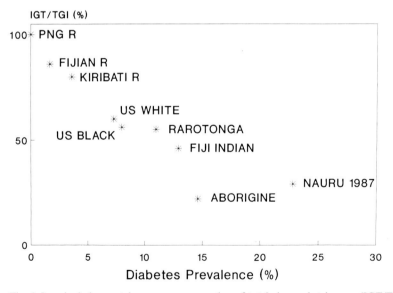

Fig. 4. Impaired glucose tolerance as a proportion of total glucose intolerance (IGT/TGI) versus prevalence of diabetes in adult females in various populations (r = −0.92). R = rural; references to various studies appear in text; all used WHO Criteria (1985).

prevalence and incidence of NIDDM in Nauruans (see above) suggests that an index such as IGT/TGI may serve as an indicator of the 'epidemicity' or potentiality for NIDDM to increase in incidence and prevalence. The IGT/TGI proportion is plotted against crude prevalence of diabetes for a number of populations in Fig. 4, and shows an almost linear relationship. Notably, the less developed rural populations of the PNG Highlands, Fiji and Kiribati show the highest epidemicity, whilst it is lowest for the high-NIDDM-prevalence Aborigines and Nauruans. The IGT/TGI index may serve as a rough public health indicator of a population's susceptibility to higher NIDDM prevalence, although further longitudinal studies will be required to confirm the relationship.

Age

Both the prevalence [1,46,47] and the incidence [47,51] of NIDDM (and IGT) increase with age. In developed populations, the rise in prevalence is initially slow but increases more steeply with advancing age [1,31]. However, the pattern in highly susceptible developing populations such as Nauruans is different (Fig. 5). The prevalence tends to rise linearly from an already high level in young adults, and peaks around the age of 60, after which it declines [46,47]. This fall may be indicative of a survival effect, but may also be a reflection of the recency of epidemic glucose intoler-

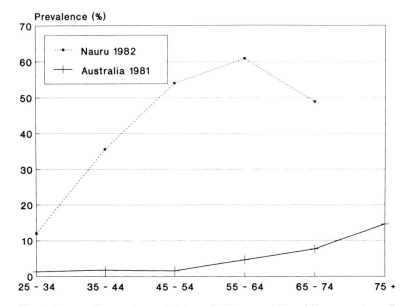

Fig. 5. Age-specific prevalence of diabetes in Nauruans [46] and European Australians (estimate based on the Busselton Survey [1]).

ance in these populations. The older age group probably represent a cohort of individuals less subject to modernization, particularly in their younger days. More recent prevalence data from the Pima Indians [51] and the Nauruans (unpublished data) have not demonstrated the same decline in diabetes prevalence in the upper age groups, suggesting that the 'resistant' cohort may be disappearing.

Sex, parity and pregnancy

Based on his own and other studies West [7] concluded in 1978 that there was little difference between the sexes in susceptibility to NIDDM that could not be explained by other factors. Reviews of published prevalence estimates based on WHO criteria support this assertion: there appear to be an equal number of studies which find higher prevalence in males and which find an excess in females [28,78].

However, there does seem to be an increased prevalence of IGT in females in a majority of population-based studies [28,78]. Incidence data for NIDDM from the Pima Indian studies show a similar rate in males and females only until the time of the menopause, after which the rate is higher in the latter [47,51], but this relationship is not seen in Nauruans (unpublished data). It is yet to be determined whether the apparent sex difference in IGT prevalence is related to differences in risk-factor levels (such as obesity or physical activity), or a more fundamental difference related to hormonal or similar factors, or simply the result of females receiving a relatively larger quantity of glucose in proportion to body size when a fixed-sized glucose load is given [7].

Despite some conflicting evidence, most population-based studies support the view that parity has little direct bearing on the prevalence of NIDDM [7,77]. This is not surprising given the fact that there is little difference in NIDDM prevalence between the sexes. Further confirmatory evidence is available from longitudinal studies in Nauruan women, which have not shown any relationship of parity with subsequent incidence of NIDDM (unpublished data).

Of a different nature, it appears that the intra-uterine environment may have a profound effect on the risk of subsequent development of NIDDM in offspring. Studies in Pima Indians have shown that offspring of pregnant known diabetic women have a much higher incidence of the disease than those of women who develop diabetes only following the pregnancy [79]. These data indicate that control of blood glucose (or other parameters?) during pregnancy may have ramifications beyond those of avoiding maternal and perinatal complications.

Does GDM exist?

It is tacitly assumed in clinical circles that pregnancy either causes, or at least uncovers a predisposition to, glucose intolerance, which is called gestational diabetes mellitus (GDM). Surprisingly, there do not appear to be any population-based data to confirm that glucose intolerance is more common in pregnant than non-pregnant women. Harris [80] has recently reviewed available data for the USA, and found that the prevalence of 'GDM' seems to be no higher than that of glucose intolerance in the general female population.

An analysis of pooled data from representative samples of women from 7 Pacific and Indian Ocean countries (including 558 pregnant women) has shown the prevalence of IGT to be almost identical, and of both newly and previously diagnosed diabetes to actually be lower in pregnant than non-pregnant age-matched women (unpublished data). This suggests that 'GDM' probably represents glucose intolerance which pre-dates pregnancy, and is detected during the antenatal period only because it is sought. These findings require confirmation in other population-based studies, but challenge popular conceptions regarding pregnancy and its effect on glucose tolerance.

Glucose and insulin levels

Longitudinal studies conducted in several populations show that, after controlling for age, the strongest independent risk factor for deterioration to diabetes, either for all subjects or for those with IGT alone, is the base-line blood glucose itself – either the fasting and/or the post-glucose-load level [20,39,81–84].

Data from Nauru have shown that subjects with higher post-load serum insulin levels (presumably indicative of insulin resistance) at base-line were more likely to progress to either IGT or diabetes over a six-year period [83]. Conversely, amongst subjects with IGT, progression to NIDDM was predicted by lower base-line insulin responsiveness. Similar results for subjects with IGT have been described in Japanese [81] and in Pima Indians [84]. These results suggest a teleological sequence leading from compensated hyperinsulinaemia and insulin resistance, through moderate hyperglycaemia and hyperinsulinaemia, to increasing hyperglycaemia and decreasing insulin response, and ultimately to beta cell decompensation and diabetes [70,84]. The tendency to hyperinsulinaemia/insulin resistance may be the modern expression of the 'thrifty genotype' [70].

Obesity

Both clinical and epidemiological data (cross-sectional and longitudinal) support the assertion that obesity is the most powerful and consistently demonstrated modifiable risk factor known for NIDDM [2,7,31,45,51,55,81,83]. West [7] found a strong correlation between 'average fatness' and the prevalence of diabetes in an international comparative study. He remained firmly convinced, after an extensive review of the literature, that differences in body mass explained most of the variability in prevalence of diabetes seen both within and between populations.

More recent work, while not entirely refuting this view, suggests that other risk factors which either interact with or are closely associated with overall body mass may be of fundamental importance. The fact that genetic factors make a large contribution is suggested by findings in Pima Indians of a marked interaction between obesity and parental history of diabetes [51], and observations from twin studies that NIDDM occurs independently of obesity [85].

Similarly, studies in the Pacific and elsewhere have shown that differences in NIDDM prevalence between rural (traditional) and urban (modernized) residents, and between migrants and their peers who remain at home, cannot be explained solely by differences in obesity [2]. There are also data which suggest that the duration and possibly the age at onset of obesity may be important in determining future risk of NIDDM [7,86]. This requires confirmation, but, if it is so, then it may help to explain in part the fact that cross-sectional studies find considerable heterogeneity in the effect of obesity on NIDDM prevalence [87].

A recent analysis of longitudinal data from the Pima Indians found that obesity was not an independent predictor of progression from IGT to NIDDM, after controlling for glucose and insulin levels [84]. The authors interpreted this finding as indicating that the effect of obesity was mediated through its relation to insulin resistance. However, body mass was an independent predictor, along with glucose and insulin levels, in similar studies in Japanese [81] and Nauruans [83], so the mechanism(s) by which obesity may influence the incidence of NIDDM remain unclear.

Cross-sectional and longitudinal data have now established that fat distribution (in particular, in the abdominal area) is an important risk factor for both NIDDM [88,89] and cardiovascular disease [90]. Moreover, centrally-distributed fat seems to act independently of the overall body mass in determining risk of NIDDM [88,89]. Thus far, it appears that differences in fat distribution probably do not explain ethnic differences in NIDDM prevalence [88]. Björntorp [91] has proposed that intra-abdominal fat cells (reflected by measurements of central obesity, such as the waist–hip ratio) are uniquely involved in the pathogenesis of NIDDM, and that the ultimate defect may lie even within the pituitary–adrenal axis. Much work is required to test this hypothesis, but there can be no doubt that the 're-discovery' [92] of centrally distributed fat has provided new impetus to epidemiological research into the determinants of glucose intolerance.

Physical activity

Popular opinion, plus circumstantial evidence, supports the importance of physical activity in determining risk of NIDDM. However, the difficulty of measurement and the close association with other factors such as obesity and nutrition have made direct proof difficult to gather [2,7].

Nonetheless, ecological comparisons of activity levels and NIDDM occurrence between rural and urban populations in the Pacific and elsewhere provide supportive evidence for a beneficial effect of physical activity [2]. More substantively, cross-sectional studies in Fiji [93], Kiribati [45] and Wallis Island [94] have found a lower prevalence of NIDDM in those who were more active. Furthermore, Frisch et al. [95] showed in a retrospective longitudinal study that women college athletes had a lower subsequent risk of developing diabetes than their non-athletic peers.

The probable mechanism by which physical activity might modulate risk of NIDDM is suggested by studies which have demonstrated that exercise results in lower plasma insulin levels and improved insulin sensitivity and glucose tolerance in both normal and NIDDM subjects [96,97]. O'Dea [98] found similar changes in a group of Australian Aboriginal subjects who reverted from a 'modern' to a more 'traditional' lifestyle, in terms of their activity level and diet.

Dietary factors, socio-economic status and stress

These have been extensively reviewed by West [7]. He concluded that there was little evidence to suggest that any specific dietary factor had an effect which was not explainable by a tendency to promote obesity. Similarly, associations with socio-economic status are probably modulated by differences in obesity and physical activity levels.

The role of 'stress' in disease causation remains elusive, and diabetes is no exception in this regard. Despite speculation about central nervous system involvement in the aetiology of NIDDM by some workers there are as yet few supportive data for such a view [2,91,99].

Conclusions

The promulgation by the NDDG and WHO of scientifically derived criteria for classification and diagnosis of diabetes has stimulated new studies of both the occurrence and the determinants of the disease. This has coincided with increased concern regarding apparent epidemics of NIDDM in developing populations. However, there remain differences in the way the new criteria are interpreted, and in the presentation of data, which continue to make comparison of results from different studies frustrating. Although the diagnostic cut-off levels were soundly based on demonstrated risk for development of typical complications of diabetes, results from longitudinal studies in Nauruans suggest that glucose tolerance testing may not be necessary to distinguish those most at risk, and that demonstration of fasting hyperglycaemia may be sufficient.

There can be little doubt that ethnic groups such as Micronesian and Polynesian Pacific islanders, North American Indians, Australian Aborigines and Asian Indians have a genetic susceptibility to developing NIDDM which is exposed when their life-style changes from its traditional form to a modern one, characterized by decreased physical activity, qualitative and quantitative changes in diet, and obesity. For other populations it is more difficult to determine whether apparent differences in preva-lence of NIDDM are genetically or environmentally based. The IGT/TGI proportion in a population may be a rough index of the 'epidemicity' or potential for the inci-dence and prevalence of NIDDM to increase in the future.

The 'thrifty genotype' hypothesis continues to conveniently explain the inherent susceptibility of some populations. Recent evidence for a decline in the incidence of glucose intolerance in Nauru probably indicates a decreasing pool of susceptible indi-viduals. Given the relatively early age-of-onset of NIDDM in such high-prevalence populations, the gene(s) may well decrease in frequency over future generations. It is possible that developed European and Asian populations may have already experi-enced such a selective process, with the result that the diabetic gene(s) have reached a steady frequency and potency consistent in the main with disease onset after com-pletion of the reproductive phase.

In longitudinal studies, age, baseline glucose and insulin levels (fasting and 2-hour) and obesity (as reflected by body mass index) are the most consistent independent predictors for development or progression of IGT and NIDDM. Recent data suggest that a central distribution of fat may be at least as important in determining risk as overall body mass. There is also new evidence that the intra-uterine environment may play a crucial role in determining susceptibility to NIDDM. Despite much popular support there is as yet little direct epidemiological evidence for the importance of physical inactivity in the pathogenesis of NIDDM. It is hoped that future investiga-tors will attempt to refine and develop methods for assessing the relative importance of obesity and fat distribution, and physical activity and fitness as inherited and/or environmentally determined risk factors for incidence of NIDDM.

Acknowledgement

This work was supported by NIH Grant No. DK 25446.

References

1. Glatthaar C, Welborn TA, Stenhouse NS, Garcia-Webb P. Diabetes and impaired glucose tolerance. A prevalence estimate based on the Busselton 1981 survey. Med J Aust 1985;143:436–440.
2. Zimmet P. Type 2 (non-insulin-dependent) diabetes – an epidemiological overview. Diabetologia 1982;22:339–411.
3. Jarrett RJ. Diabetes mellitus. London: Croom Helm, 1986.
4. Gerard K, Donaldson C, Maynard AK. The cost of diabetes. Diabetic Med 1989;6:164–170.
5. Mann RJ. 'Honey urine' to pancreatic diabetes. Mayo Clin Proc 1971;46:56–58.
6. Barach JH. Diabetes and its treatment. New York: Oxford University Press, 1940.
7. West KM. Epidemiology of diabetes and its vascular lesions. New York: Elsevier, 1978.
8. Mayer JH, Womack CR. Glucose tolerance 1. A comparison of four types of diagnostic tests in 103 control subjects and 26 patients with diabetes. Am J Med Sci 1950;219:161–173.
9. Fajans SS, Conn JW. The early recognition of diabetes mellitus. Ann N Y Acad Sci 1959;82:208–218.
10. West KM, Kalbfleisch JM. Influence of nutritional factors on prevalence of diabetes. Diabetes 1971;20:99–108.
11. National Diabetes Data Group. Classification and diagnosis of diabetes mellitus and other categories of glucose intolerance. Diabetes 1979;28:1 039–1 057.
12. West KM. Standardization of definition, classification, and reporting in diabetes-related epidemiologic studies. Diabetes Care 1979;2:65–76.
13. Bennett PH. Recommendations on the standardization of methods and reporting of tests for diabetes and its microvascular complications in epidemiologic studies. Diabetes Care 1979;2:98–104.
14. Jarrett RJ, Keen H. Hyperglycaemia and diabetes mellitus. Lancet 1976;ii:1 009–1 012.
15. Al Sayegh H, Jarrett RJ. Oral glucose tolerance tests and the diagnosis of diabetes: results of a prospective study based on the Whitehall Survey. Lancet 1979;ii:431–433.
16. Pettitt DJ, Knowler WC, Lisse JR, Bennett PH. Development of retinopathy and proteinuria in relation to plasma glucose concentrations in Pima Indians. Lancet 1980;ii:1 050–1 052.
17. Fuller JH, Shipley MJ, Rose G, Jarrett RJ, Keen H. Coronary heart disease risk and impaired glucose tolerance. Lancet 1980;i:1 373–1 376.
18. Jarrett RJ, McCartney P, Keen H. The Bedford survey: ten year mortality rates in newly diagnosed diabetics, borderline diabetics and normoglycaemic controls and risk indices for coronary heart disease in borderline diabetics. Diabetologia 1982;22:79–84.
19. Diabetes Survey Working Party. Ten-year follow-up report on the Birmingham Diabetes Survey of 1961. Br Med J 1976;II:35–37.
20. Jarrett RJ, Keen H, Fuller JH, McCartney M. Worsening to diabetes in men with impaired glucose tolerance ('borderline diabetes'). Diabetologia 1979;16:25–30.
21. Rushforth NB, Bennett PH, Steinberg AG, Burch TA, Miller M. Diabetes in the Pima Indians: Evidence of bimodality in glucose tolerance distributions. Diabetes 1971;20:756–765.
22. Rushforth NB, Miller M, Bennett PH. Fasting and two-hour post-load glucose levels for the diagnosis of diabetes. The relationship between glucose levels and complications of diabetes in Pima Indians. Diabetologia 1979;16:373–379.
23. Zimmet P, Whitehouse S. Bimodality of fasting and two-hour glucose tolerance distributions in a Micronesian population. Diabetes 1978;27:793–800.
24. WHO Expert Committee on Diabetes Mellitus. Second report. Technical Report Series 646. Geneva: WHO, 1980.
25. WHO Study Group. Diabetes mellitus. Technical Report Series 727. Geneva: WHO, 1985.
26. Taylor R, Zimmet P. Limitation of fasting plasma glucose for the diagnosis of diabetes mellitus. Diabetes Care 1981;4:556–558.

56

27. Harris MI, Hadden WC, Knowler WC, Bennett PH. International criteria for the diagnosis of diabetes and impaired glucose tolerance. Diabetes Care 1985;8:562–567.

28. King H, Zimmet P. Trends in the prevalence and incidence of diabetes: non-insulin-dependent diabetes mellitus. Wld Hlth Statist Quart 1988;41:190–196.

29. Alberti KGMM. Diagnostic tools for diabetes mellitus. In: Krall LP, Alberti KGMM, Turtle JR, eds. World book of diabetes in practice. Volume 3. Amsterdam: Elsevier, 1988;12–15.

30. DeNobel E, Van 't Laar A. The size of the loading dose as an important determinant of the oral glucose tolerance test. A study in subjects with slightly impaired glucose tolerance. Diabetes 1978;27:42–48.

31. Harris MI, Hadden WC, Knowler WC, Bennett PH. Prevalence of diabetes and impaired glucose tolerance and plasma glucose levels in US population aged 20–74 yr. Diabetes 1987;36:523–534.

32. Ahren B, Corrigan CB. prevalence of diabetes mellitus in north-western Tanzania. Diabetologia 1984;26:333–336.

33. Eason RJ, Pada J, Wallace R, Henry A, Thornton R. Changing patterns of hypertension, obesity and diet among Melanesians and Micronesians in the Solomon Islands. Med J Aust 1987;146: 465–473.

34. Woo J, Swaminathan R, Cockram C, et al. The prevalence of diabetes mellitus and an assessment of methods of detection among a community of elderly Chinese in Hong Kong. Diabetologia 1987;30:863–868.

35. Dowse GK, Zimmet P, Alberti KGMM. Screening for diabetes and other categories of glucose intolerance. In: Alberti KGMM, Keen H, DeFronzo RA, Zimmet P, eds. International textbook of diabetes mellitus. Chichester: John Wiley, in press.

36. Riccardi G, Vaccaro O, Rivellese A, Pignalosa S, Tutino L, Mancini M. Reproducibility of the new diagnostic criteria for impaired glucose tolerance. Am J Epidemiol 1985;121:422–429.

37. Forrest RD, Jackson CA, Yudkin JS. The glycohaemoglobin assay as a screening test for diabetes mellitus: the Islington diabetes survey. Diabetic Med 1987;4:254–259.

38. Siperstein MD. The glucose tolerance test: A pitfall in the diagnosis of diabetes mellitus. Adv Intern Med 1975;20:297–323.

39. Sasaki A, Suzuki T, Horiuchi N. Development of diabetes in Japanese subjects with impaired glucose tolerance: a seven year follow-up study. Diabetologia 1982;22:154–157.

40. King H, Zimmet P, Raper LR, Balkau B. The natural history of impaired glucose tolerance in the Micronesian population of Nauru: a six-year follow-up study. Diabetologia 1984;26:39–43.

41. Raper LR, Taylor R, Zimmet P, Milne B, Balkau B. Bimodality in glucose tolerance distributions in the urban Polynesian population of Western Samoa. Diabetes Res 1984;1:19–26.

42. Rosenthal M, McMahon CA, Stern MP, et al. Evidence of bimodality of two hour plasma glucose concentrations in Mexican Americans: results from the San Antonio heart study. J Chron Dis 1985;38:5–16.

43. Zimmet P, Faaiuso S, Ainuu J, Whitehouse S, Milne B, DeBoer W. The prevalence of diabetes in the rural and urban Polynesian population of Western Samoa. Diabetes 1981;30:45–51.

44. Zimmet P, Taylor R, Ram P, et al. Prevalence of diabetes and impaired glucose tolerance in the biracial (Melanesian and Indian) population of Fiji: a rural-urban comparison. Am J Epidemiol 1983;118:673–688.

45. King H, Taylor R, Zimmet P, et al. Noninsulin-dependent diabetes (NIDDM) in a newly independent Pacific nation – the Republic of Kiribati. Diabetes Care 1984;7:1 002–1 007.

46. Zimmet P, King H, Taylor R, et al. The high prevalence of diabetes mellitus, impaired glucose tolerance and diabetic retinopathy in Nauru – the 1982 survey. Diabetes Res 1984;1:13–18.

47. Knowler WC, Bennett PH, Hamman RF, Miller M. Diabetes incidence and prevalence in Pima Indians: a 19 fold greater incidence than in Rochester, Minnesota. Am J Epidemiol 1978;108:497–505.

48. Mauritius Non-communicable Disease Study Group. Disease and risk factor prevalence survey. Final Report. Port Louis: Mauritius Ministry of Health, 1989.

49. Welborn TA, Glatthaar C, Whittall D, Bennett S. An estimate of diabetes prevalence from a national population sample: a male excess. Med J Aust 1989;150:78–81.

50. King H, Heywood P, Zimmet P, et al. Glucose tolerance in a highland population in Papua New Guinea. Diabetes Res 1984;1:45–51.

51. Knowler WC, Pettitt DJ, Savage PJ, Bennett PH. Diabetes incidence in Pima Indians: contributions of obesity and parental diabetes. Am J Epidemiol 1981;113:144–156.

52. Ekoe J-M. Diabetes mellitus. Aspects of the world-wide epidemiology of diabetes mellitus and its long-term complications. Amsterdam: Elsevier, 1988.

53. Taylor R, Thoma K. Mortality patterns in the modernized Pacific island nation of Nauru. Am J Public Health 1985;75:149–155.

54. Harris M. The prevalence of diagnosed diabetes, undiagnosed diabetes and impaired glucose tolerance in the United States. In: Melish JS, Hanna J, Baba S, eds. Genetic-environmental interactions in diabetes mellitus. Amsterdam: Excerpta Medica, 1982;70–76.

55. Stanhope JM, Prior IAM. The Tokelau island migrant study: prevalence and incidence of diabetes mellitus. NZ Med J 1980;92:417–421.

56. Taylor R, Bennett P, Uili R, et al. Diabetes in Wallis Polynesians: a comparison of residents of Wallis Island and first generation migrants to Noumea, New Caledonia. Diabetes Res Clin Practice 1985;1:169–178.

57. Kawate R, Yamakido M, Nishimoto Y, Bennett PH, Knowler WC. Diabetes mellitus and its vascular complications in Japanese migrants on the island of Hawaii. Diabetes Care 1979;2:161–170.

58. Omar MAK, Seedat MA, Dyer RB, Rajput MC, Motala AA, Jourbert SM. The prevalence of diabetes mellitus in a large group of South African Indians. S Afr Med J 1985;67:924–926.

59. Mather HM, Keen H. The Southall diabetes survey: prevalence of known diabetes in Asians and Europeans. Br Med J 1985;291:1 081–1 084.

60. Taylor R, Zimmet P. Migrant studies in diabetes epidemiology. In: Mann JI, Pyorala K, Teuscher A, eds. Diabetes in epidemiological perspective. Edinburgh: Churchill Livingstone, 1983;58–77.

61. Ramachandran A, Jali MV, Mohan V, Snehalatha C, Viswanathan M. High prevalence of diabetes in an urban population in south India. Br Med J 1988;297:587–590.

62. Gardner LI, Stern MP, Haffner SM, et al. Prevalence of diabetes in Mexican Americans: relationship to percent of gene pool derived from native American sources. Diabetes 1984;33:86–92.

63. Thai C, Yeo PPB, Lun KC, et al. Changing prevalence of diabetes mellitus in Singapore over a ten-year period. In: Vannasaeng S, Nitianant W, Chandraprasert S, eds. Epidemiology of diabetes mellitus: proceedings of the International Symposium on Epidemiology of Diabetes Mellitus. Bangkok: Crystal House Press, 1987;63–67.

64. Cameron WI, Moffitt PS, Williams DRR. Diabetes mellitus in the Australian Aborigines of Bourke, New South Wales. Diabetes Res Clin Practice 1986;2:307–314.

65. Serjeantson SW, Owerbach D, Zimmet P, Nerup J, Thoma K. Genetics of diabetes in Nauru: effects of foreign admixture, HLA antigens and the insulin-gene-linked polymorphism. Diabetologia 1983;25:13–17.

66. King H, Zimmet P, Bennett P, Taylor R, Raper LR. Glucose tolerance and ancestral genetic admixture in six semitraditional Pacific populations. Genet Epidemiol 1984;1:315–328.

67. Pyke DA. The genetic connection. Diabetologia 1979;17:333–343.

68. Serjeantson S, Zimmet P. Diabetes in the Pacific: evidence of a major gene. In: Baba S, Gould M, Zimmet P, eds. Diabetes mellitus: recent knowledge of aetiology, complications and treatment. Sydney: Academic Press, 1984;23–30.

58

69. Yamashita TS, Mackay W, Rushforth NB, Bennett PH, Houser H. Pedigree analysis of non-insulin-dependent diabetes in the Pima Indians suggest dominant mode of inheritance. Am J Hum Genet 1985;36:1 835.

70. Zimmet P, Dowse G, LaPorte R, Finch C, Moy C. Epidemiology – its contribution to understanding of the etiology, pathogenesis, and prevention of diabetes mellitus. In: Creutzfeldt W, Lefebvre P, eds. Diabetes mellitus: pathophysiology and therapy. Berlin: Springer-Verlag, 1989;5–26.

71. Shanghai Diabetes Research Cooperative Group. Diabetes mellitus survey in Shanghai. Chinese Med J 1980;93:663–672.

72. Tai TY, Yang CL, Chang CJ, et al. Epidemiology of diabetes mellitus among adults in Taiwan, R.O.C. In: Vannasaeng S, Nitianant W, Chandraprasert S, eds. Epidemiology of diabetes mellitus: proceedings of the International Symposium on Epidemiology of Diabetes Mellitus. Bangkok: Crystal House Press, 1987;42–48.

73. Schaad JDG, Terpstra J, Oemrawsingh I, Nieuwenhuijzen Kruseman AC, Bouwhuis-Hoogerwerf ML. Diabetes prevalence in the three main ethnic groups in Surinam (South America): a population survey. Neth Med J 1985;28:17–22.

74. Neel JV. Diabetes mellitus: a thrifty genotype rendered detrimental by 'progress'? Am J Hum Genet 1962;14:353–362.

75. Neel JV. The thrifty genotype revisited. In: Kobberling J, Tattersal R, eds. The genetics of diabetes mellitus. Proceedings of the Serono Symposium. London: Academic Press, 1982;283–293.

76. King H, Balkau B, Zimmet P, et al. Diabetic retinopathy in Nauruans. Am J Epidemiol 1983;117:659–667.

77. Sicree RA, Hoet JJ, Zimmet P, King HOM, Coventry JS. The association of non-insulin-dependent diabetes with parity and still-birth occurrence amongst five Pacific populations. Diabetes Res Clin Practice 1986;2:113–122.

78. Zimmet P, Taylor R, Whitehouse S. Prevalence rates of impaired glucose tolerance and diabetes mellitus in various Pacific populations according to the new criteria. Bull WHO 1982;60:279–282.

79. Pettitt DJ, Aleck KA, Baird HR, Carraher MJ, Bennett PH, Knowler WC. Congenital susceptibility to NIDDM. Role of intrauterine environment. Diabetes 1988;37:622–628.

80. Harris MI. Gestational diabetes may represent discovery of pre-existing glucose intolerance. Diabetes Care 1988;11:402–411.

81. Kadowaki T, Miyake Y, Hagura R, et al. Risk factors for worsening to diabetes in subjects with impaired glucose tolerance. Diabetologia 1984;26:44–49.

82. Balkau B, King H, Zimmet P, Raper LR. Factors associated with the development of diabetes in the Micronesian population of Nauru. Am J Epidemiol 1985;122:594–605.

83. Sicree RA, Zimmet PZ, King HOM, Coventry JS. Plasma insulin response among Nauruans. Prediction of deterioration in glucose tolerance over 6 yr. Diabetes 1987;36:179–186.

84. Saad MF, Knowler WC, Pettitt DJ, Nelson RG, Mott DM, Bennett PH. The natural history of impaired glucose tolerance in the Pima Indians. N Engl J Med 1988;319:1 500–1 506.

85. Barnett AH, Eff C, Leslie RDG, Pyke DA. Diabetes in identical twins. A study in 200 pairs. Diabetologia 1981;20:87–93.

86. Modan M, Karasik A, Halkin H. Effect of past and concurrent body mass index on prevalence of glucose intolerance and type 2 (non-insulin-dependent) diabetes and on insulin response; the Israeli study of glucose intolerance, obesity and hypertension. Diabetologia 1986;29:82–89.

87. King H, Zimmet P, Raper LR, Balkau B. Risk factors for diabetes in three Pacific populations. Am J Epidemiol 1984;199:396–409.

88. Haffner SM, Stern MP, Hazuda HP, Rosenthal M, Knapp JA, Malina RM. Role of obesity and fat distribution in non-insulin dependent diabetes mellitus in Mexican-Americans and non-Hispanic whites. Diabetes Care 1986;9:153–161.

89. Ohlson LO, Larsson B, Svardsudd K, et al. The influence of body fat distribution on the incidence of diabetes mellitus. 13.5 years of follow-up of the participants in the study of men born in 1913. Diabetes 1985;34:1 055–1 058.

90. Larsson B, Svardsudd D, Welin L, Wilhelmsen L, Björntorp P, Tibblin G. Abdominal adipose tissue distribution, obesity, and risk of cardiovascular disease and death. 13-year follow-up of participants in the study of men born in 1913. Br Med J 1984;288:1 401–1 404.

91. Björntorp P. Abdominal obesity and the development of non-insulin-dependent diabetes mellitus. Diabetes/Metab Rev. 1988;4:615–622.

92. Vague J. The degree of masculine differentiation of obesities: a factor determining predisposition to diabetes, atherosclerosis, gout and uric calculus disease. Am J Clin Nutr 1956;4:20–34.

93. Taylor R, Ram P, Zimmet P, Raper LR, Ringrose H. Physical activity and prevalence of diabetes in Melanesian and Indian men in Fiji. Diabetologia 1984;27:578–582.

94. Taylor RJ, Bennett PH, LeGonidec G, et al. The prevalence of diabetes mellitus in a traditional-living Polynesian population: the Wallis Island survey. Diabetes Care 1983;6:334–340.

95. Frisch RE, Wyshak G, Albright TE, Albright NL, Schiff I. Lower prevalence of diabetes in female former college athletes compared with nonathletes. Diabetes 1986;35:1 101–1 105.

96. Trovati M, Carta Q, Cavalot F, et al. Influence of physical training on blood glucose control, glucose tolerance, insulin secretion and insulin action in non-insulin-dependent diabetic patients. Diabetes Care 1984;7:416–420.

97. Devlin JT, Horton ES. Effects of prior high-intensity exercise on glucose metabolism in normal and insulin-resistant men. Diabetes 1985;34:973–979.

98. O'Dea K. Marked improvement in carbohydrate and lipid metabolism in diabetic Australian Aborigines after temporary reversion to traditional lifestyle. Diabetes 1984;33:596–603.

99. Surwit RS, Feinglos MN. Stress and autonomic nervous system in type II diabetes. A hypothesis. Diabetes Care 1988;11:83–85.

CHAPTER 4

Hyperandrogenicity and insulin resistance as predictors for non-insulin-dependent diabetes mellitus in women

PER BJÖRNTORP

Department of Medicine I, Sahlgren's Hospital, S-413 45 Göteborg, Sweden

Introduction

Hyperandrogenicity in women has for some time been connected with the development of NIDDM. This field has attracted much interest recently, because strong statistical associations have been repeatedly found between androgens and insulin in women with conditions characterized by hyperandrogenicity such as the polycystic ovary syndrome. It is not clear, however, which is the primary factor: the hyperandrogenicity or the hyperinsulinemia.

'Diabetes in women with beard' was described in 1921 [1]. This condition was shown to be associated with polycystic ovaries, increased levels of circulating, active androgens and signs of hyperandrogenicity [2]. This polycystic ovarian syndrome (PCO) is often followed by obesity and signs of insulin resistance, and non-insulin-dependent diabetes mellitus (NIDDM). Since obesity, insulin resistance and NIDDM are closely associated in general, this coupling is also an expected finding in the PCO syndrome.

Recent studies have shown, however, that women with PCO without obesity are also markedly insulin-resistant [3–5]. Such women are further characterized by elevation of blood pressure and plasma lipids. Although they do not have an increased body fat mass their body fat seems to be distributed mainly to the abdominal adipose tissue regions. Furthermore, adipose tissue morphology and metabolism also have male characteristics [5].

62

Correlations between hyperandrogenicity and insulin

In several reports, various signs of insulin resistance have now been found to correlate strongly with the hyperandrogenicity of PCO women, including those who are not obese [3–7]. This is also found in women with abdominal obesity who have signs of moderate hyperandrogenicity clinically and in terms of elevated free testosterone and low sex hormone binding globulin (SHBG) [8]. A picture then seems to emerge where hyperandrogenicity, insulin resistance and abdominal distribution of body fat are closely statistically connected in cross-sectional studies.

The cause-effect relationships are, however, far from clear. Although there appears to be a consistent picture with regard to the statistical correlations between various measurements of hyperandrogenicity and insulin resistance or hyperinsulinemia, the information from case-control or cross-sectional epidemiological studies does not allow a conclusion as to which is the primary and which the secondary of these two phenomena. Intervention studies are more helpful in this regard. Treatment of PCO women with anti-androgens [9] or spironolactone [10] decreased hyperinsulinemia, while treatment with female sex hormones did not, despite the normalization of serum concentrations of androgens and the disappearance of clinical symptoms of hyperandrogenicity [5]. Administration of androgens to women [11,12] and in excess to men [13] is followed by marked insulin resistance. On the other hand, long-term administration of androstendione to female monkeys, followed by markedly elevated testosterone values in plasma, is not associated with signs of insulin resistance [14].

There is evidence that hyperinsulinemia is followed by increased androgen production [15]. Insulin causes increased androgen secretion at a cellular level in in vitro systems [16,17]. Hyperinsulinemia persists after suppression of ovarian overproduction of androgens in the PCO syndrome [18]. Furthermore, androgens decrease rapidly after insulin treatment withdrawal in diabetes [19], and insulin has effects at the gonadotropin level [20,21]. On the other hand, induction of relatively short-term hyperinsulinemia (< 24 h) in normal women is not followed by increased androgen production [22], and the hyperandrogenicity of the PCO syndrome has been reported to be independent of hyperinsulinemia [23]. To add to the confusion, androgens other than testosterone, such as dihydroepiandrosterone sulfate, are elevated in hyperandrogenic syndromes in women, and levels are inversely correlated with insulin concentrations [24,25]. It is thus not possible to conclude from these data how hyperinsulinemia and hyperandrogenicity in women are related. Recently, however, additional information has emerged which has elucidated this question further, as will be reviewed below.

Correlations between insulin, hyperandrogenicity and abdominal distribution of adipose tissue in population studies

Recently, cross-sectional data from population studies have suggested that not only are obesity and sex hormones related to insulin concentrations, but also body fat distribution as measured by the waist/hip ratio (WHR). In studies of Swedish and Mexican-American women it has been reported that these factors are closely interrelated, and a low sex hormone binding globulin (SHBG) concentration and a high WHR were both correlated with insulin independently of obesity [26,27]. This has also been reported recently in cohorts of women from different European countries [28]. Whereas body mass index (BMI) could be sorted out from the interrelationships in these studies, it is less clear which of the two factors, WHR and hyperandrogenicity, was most tightly coupled to insulin. In the Swedish study [26] both factors seemed to be equally closely associated with insulin. In the study of Mexican-American women [27] a low SHBG remained significant after adjusting for BMI and WHR. Whether WHR remained an independent variable was not stated. It seems clear, however, from these three population studies that insulin, WHR and a low SHBG are closely interrelated. This has also been reported in case-control studies including obese subjects with different adipose tissue distribution [8].

Causes of hyperinsulinemia

Hyperinsulinemia might be due to several causes. The most obvious is increased insulin secretion. A decreased uptake of insulin in the liver might also cause peripheral hyperinsulinemia. Furthermore, decreased insulin effectiveness in the periphery could result in a compensatory hyperinsulinemia. These three factors are thus interconnected and may in fact amplify each other. Hypersecretion of insulin might thus cause both decreased hepatic insulin clearance and peripheral hyperinsulinemia and insulin resistance. A decreased hepatic insulin clearance produces peripheral hyperinsulinemia and insulin resistance. Primary peripheral insulin resistance might trigger increased insulin secretion: A cycle is thus created.

That increased insulin secretion is connected with obesity, has been well established, and it is apparently independent of adipose tissue distribution [30]. The potential connections between hepatic insulin clearance and peripheral insulin resistance with low SHBG and high WHR will be discussed in the following section.

Insulin resistance in muscle in relation to hyperandrogenicity

Insulin resistance is a marked feature of a high WHR and a low SHBG, when meas-

ured with the euglycemic clamp technique [9,29,31]. This method principally estimates the insulin resistance of muscle tissue, which then becomes of primary importance. It is of interest that women with high WHR and low SHBG have muscle tissue
which is characterized by a low number of red, slow-twitch, type I fibers, compensated for by more white, fast-twitch, type IIb fibers. The insulin resistance seen in this
condition is correlated with these morphology characteristics of muscle, which indeed
might be the cause of the insulin resistance [31]. Other studies have shown that type
I fibers are more insulin-sensitive and contain more insulin receptors than white
fibers [32,33]. Similar observations have been made in men [34].

In addition, a low capillary density is associated with insulin resistance in normal
as well as obese men and women and is correlated with WHR [34–36]. It is not clear
how this might be causally associated with insulin resistance. It is, however, remarkable that the transport of glucose through these capillaries to the site of uptake is
in principle instantaneous, while the time for insulin transport to its receptor might
well be much longer.

Although muscle fiber composition is considered to be regulated by genetic factors
[37], it is clear that environmental factors also play important roles. Thus, steroid
hormones have been reported to influence muscle fiber composition in man, including both corticosteroids and sex steroid hormones [38–42].

The relationship between androgens, muscle fiber composition and insulin resistance has recently been studied in the rat. Female rats were given testosterone for 3
months to produce serum concentrations seen in hyperandrogenic women. This was
followed by a dramatic increase in insulin resistance, as measured by the euglycemic
clamp. In this study it was also possible to examine in which tissue insulin resistance
was increased at the cellular level. The three main metabolic tissues, muscle, liver and
adipose tissue, were examined. Muscle showed a marked insulin resistance, when examined in individual muscles with different muscle fiber composition. The most
marked insulin resistance occurred in those muscles which were most insulin-sensitive
from the outset, i.e., the muscles with mainly red, slow-twitch, type I fibers. These
muscles had also markedly changed their morphology after testosterone treatment.
The previously red muscle fibers were now to a large extent replaced by white, fast-
twitch, type II fibers, particularly the glycolytic subgroup type IIb. Furthermore, capillarization of muscle was less dense after treatment [42]. There was not much
change in adipose tissue insulin sensitivity in terms of the inhibitory power of insulin
on lipolysis (personal observation). There were no signs of insulin resistance in the
liver measured as stimulation of amino acid transport in isolated hepatocytes. It was
also noted that insulin uptake and degradation were actually higher than in controls
(personal observation).

This study clearly shows that administration of testosterone to female rats is followed by a marked insulin resistance due to alterations in muscle tissue. These

changes include a rather marked change of fiber distribution towards fewer red and more white fibers. The former are known to be more insulin-sensitive, owing to a higher density of insulin receptors [32]. A replacement of red by white fibers would then presumably mean a diminished insulin sensitivity because of the reduced number of insulin receptors in such muscle. The diminished capillarization might also be followed by a decreased insulin sensitivity due to diffusion problems from the capillary to the cellular site of action of insulin.

A recent study [14] did not show an effect on insulin resistance of long-term administration of androgens to female monkeys. The reason for the discrepancy between this study and that in rats [42] is not clear. Insulin resistance and the morphological characteristics of muscle were, however, not directly measured in the monkeys.

The study in rats referred to [42] and previous studies in humans [11–13] are in agreement, showing a clear increase in insulin resistance after administration of androgens. Furthermore, other studies have previously shown that androgens tend to shift muscle fiber composition from red insulin-sensitive to white less insulin-sensitive fibers [40,41].

It therefore seems to be a realistic possibility that androgens actually produce insulin resistance by decreasing the muscle potential for responding to insulin. This does not of course, rule out the possibility that the reverse can also be the case, i.e. that hyperinsulinemia causes or aggravates the hyperandrogenicity in the women in question.

The association between hepatic insulin clearance and elevated WHR and low SHBG

The least complicated way to approach this problem seems to be by discussing the potential correlation between a low SHBG and hepatic insulin clearance.

There is a report that insulin clearance in the liver is decreased in rats treated with testosterone [9]. We have, however, been unable to confirm this. In the in situ perfused rat liver no effects of testosterone administration were found (Strömblad and Björntorp, unpublished results). In isolated hepatocytes from female rats treated with testosterone, insulin uptake was rather higher than in controls and insulin effects were unaffected. In obese women both WHR and low SHBG have been found to be closely associated with a low hepatic clearance of insulin [29].

Statistical approaches to this problem might not be sensitive enough to separate the effects of these two closely connected factors on hepatic insulin clearance, in analogy with the results in epidemiological studies referred to above, where the correlations between insulin and WHR or SHBG could not be separated with certainty.

Intraabdominal adipose tissue and hepatic clearance of insulin

Before discussing the potential cause-effect relationships between hepatic insulin clearance and the WHR, it is necessary to consider the significance of an elevated WHR. This has recently been reviewed [43] and will be briefly summarized in the following.

Although a high WHR indicates an increased abdominal fat mass [43], it is increasingly clear that the intraabdominal fat mass, measured by computerized tomography, is most important for the associations in question, including, for example, peripheral insulin concentrations and glucose intolerance. The question then arises whether intraabdominal adipose tissue might cause a decreased hepatic clearance of insulin.

Intraabdominal adipose tissues, particularly those drained by the portal vein ('portal tissues'), have specific characteristics. These tissues are excessively sensitive to lipolytic stimuli, probably because of a high density of β-adrenergic receptors. This is the case in men, non-obese or obese, and in abdominally obese women. This would be expected to result in very high concentrations of free fatty acids (FFA) in the portal vein. This means that the liver would be heavily exposed to FFA in these conditions. Recent evidence shows that this would have a number of unwanted consequences.

Recent studies have shown that insulin uptake is influenced in a sensitive, dose-dependent manner by FFA. This has been seen both in the in situ perfused rat liver and in isolated hepatocytes. In the latter system this is found as an inhibition in parallel of insulin binding, due to a decreased number of insulin receptors, and of insulin degradation and insulin function. In addition, portal FFAs are thus expected to influence hepatic gluconeogenesis by decreasing its inhibition by insulin. FFAs are also known to stimulate hepatic gluconeogenesis through activation of key gluconeogenetic enzymes.

The end result of this would be peripheral hyperinsulinemia as well as hyperglycemia, conditions close to clinically overt NIDDM. In addition, FFA seem to drive VLDL synthesis, resulting in elevated VLDL, LDL and apoB 100 concentrations in the circulation. Furthermore, hyperinsulinemia has been suggested to be a cause of hypertension. Portal FFA might therefore be a generator of a number of risk factors not only for NIDDM, but also for cardiovascular disease. This problem has recently been reviewed in detail [43].

It should be noted that androgens might play a role in this chain of events. One of the main effects of testosterone on adipose tissue is to increase the number of β-adrenergic receptors, characteristic of portal adipose tissues in men and women with hyperandrogenicity. It might be speculated that testosterone has actually caused this specifically in the portal adipose tissues.

Summary of possible pathogenetic mechanisms linking insulin resistance and hepatic clearance of insulin to hyperandrogenicity and intraabdominal adipose tissue

In summary, it is clear that the statistical associations between androgenicity, elevated WHR and hyperinsulinemia might have different explanations. Further, they may affect each other by separate mechanisms elevating insulin concentrations in plasma. The hyperandrogenicity might be active primarily via an effect on peripheral muscular insulin sensitivity, while a high WHR might show its effect mainly by producing excess portal FFA inhibiting hepatic clearance of insulin, and increasing hepatic gluconeogenesis. These two mechanisms combined would be efficient in creating hyperinsulinemia, insulin resistance, hyperglycemia and subsequently clinically overt NIDDM.

An interesting remaining point is the possibility that WHR and hyperandrogenicity in women might be causally interrelated. One obvious way, discussed above, is that hyperinsulinemia is caused by the effects of FFA on hepatic insulin clearance, which in turn results in hyperandrogenicity. It seems at least equally possible that the hyperandrogenicity is the primary factor, causing accumulation of intraabdominal fat, a typical male feature. Potential mechanisms for this are, however, currently not known.

Prospective studies of development of NIDDM in relation to hyperandrogenicity and abdominal body fat distribution

Prospective studies of the development of NIDDM where hyperandrogenicity, insulin and WHR have been examined separately and together as risk factors have now been performed. In randomly selected women in Gothenburg, Sweden, the main independent risk factors for the development of NIDDM were obesity, high WHR, low SHBG and fasting insulin (Refs. 27,44, unpublished observations). It is of interest that it is not possible to statistically separate these risk factors, except obesity. Just as in the case of the cross-sectional studies referred to above, they each seem to be equally powerful, suggesting a close association with each other.

A low SHBG as risk factor for NIDDM seemed to show several unique characteristics (unpublished observations). First, the strength of this risk increased abruptly and steeply within the lowest quintile of values, showing no gradual increase. Second, the degree of risk increase in the lowest quintile was quite remarkable, being about 20-fold in comparisons between the lowest 10% of the SHBG distribution and the upper 80% of the population. Some of these characteristics are also found for the WHR as a risk factor [27].

68

These observations have practical implications. First, the steep increase of risk makes it relatively easy to delineate a borderline where risk of the development of NIDDM starts to become unacceptable. Second, SHBG determinations and measurements of WHR are fairly easily performed on a population screening basis. Third, when such women are found they could be given advice or treatment to prevent the development of NIDDM.

References

1. Achard C, Thiers J. Le virilism pilaire et son association à l'insufficience glycolytique (diabète à femmes de barbe). Bull Acad Natl Med (Paris) 1921;86:51–55.
2. Stein IF, Leventhal ML. Amenorrhea associated with bilateral polycystic ovaries. Am J Obstet Gynecol 1935;29:181–187.
3. Chang RJ, Nakamura RM, Judd HL, Kaplan SA. Insulin resistance in nonobese patients with polycystic ovarian disease. Clin Endocrinol 1983;57:356–363.
4. Jialal I, Naiker P, Reddi K, Moddley J, Joubert M. Evidence for insulin resistance in nonobese patients with polycystic ovarian disease. Clin Endocrinol Met 1987;64:1 066–1 069.
5. Rebuffe'-Scrive M, Cullberg G, Lundberg PA, Lindstedt G, Björntorp P. Anthropometric variables and metabolism in polycystic ovarian disease. Horm Metab Res 1989; in press.
6. Burghen GA, Givens JR, Kitabchi AE. Correlation of hyperandrogenism with hyperinsulinism in polycystic ovarian disease. J Clin Endocrinol Med 1980;50:113.
7. Shoupe D, Kumar D, Lobo RA. Insulin resistance in polycystic ovary syndrome. Am J Obstet Gynecol 1983;147:588.
8. Evans PJ, Hoffman RG, Kalkhoff RK, Kissebah AH. Relationship of androgenic activity to body fat topography, fat cell morphology and metabolic aberrations in menopausal women. J Clin Endocrinol Metab 1983;57:304–310.
9. Kissebah AH, Evans DJ, Peiris A, Wilson CR. Endocrine characteristics of regional obesities: role of sex steroids. In: Vague J, et al., eds. Metabolic complications of human obesities. Amsterdam: Excerpta Medica, 1985;115–130.
10. Shoupe D, Lobo RA. The influence of androgens on insulin resistance. Fertil Steril 1984;41:385–388.
11. Landon JC, Wynn V, Samols E. The effect of anabolic steroids on blood sugar and plasma insulin levels in man. Metabolism 1963;12:924–930.
12. Beck P. Contraceptive steroids. Modification of carbohydrate and lipid metabolism. Metabolism 1973;22:841–855.
13. Cohen JC, Hickman R. Insulin resistance and diminished glucose tolerance in power lifters ingesting anabolic steroids. J Clin Endocrinol Metab 1987;64:960–964.
14. Billiar RB, Richardson D, Schwartz R, Posner B, Little B. Effect of chronically elevated androgen and estrogen on the glucose tolerance test and insulin response in female rhesus monkeys. Am J Obstet Gynecol 1987;157:1 297–1 302.
15. Barbieri RL, Ryan KJ. Hyperandrogenism, insulin resistance, and acanthosis nigricans syndrome: a common endocrinopathy with distinct pathophysiologic features. Am J Obstet Gynecol 1983;147:90–101.
16. Barbieri RJ, Makris A, Ryan KJ. Insulin stimulates androgen accumulation in incubations of human ovarian stroma and theca. Obstet Gynecol 1984;64:73.
17. Cara JF, Rosenfield RL. Potentiation of LH-induced stimulation of androgen synthesis in rat theca-

interstitial (TI) cells by insulin-like growth factor-I (IGF-I) and insulin (Abstract). In: Proceedings of Sixty-ninth Annual Meeting of The Endocrine Society, Indianapolis, Indiana, June 10–12, 1987:44.

18. Geffner ME, Kaplan SA, Bersch N, Golde DW, Landaw EW, Chang RJ. Persistence of insulin resistance in polycystic ovarian disease after inhibition of ovarian steroid secretion. Fertil Steril 1986;45: 327–333.

19. Madsbad S, Gluud C, Bennett P, Krarup T. Rapid changes in plasma androgens during insulin withdrawal in male Type I (insulin-dependent) diabetics. J Endocrinol Invest 1986;9:21–24.

20. Poretsky L, Kalin MF. The gonadotropic function of insulin. Endocrinol Rev 1987;8:132–139.

21. Adashi EY, Hsueh AJW, Yen SSC. Insulin enhancement of luteinizing hormone and follicle-stimulating hormone release by cultured pituitary cells. Endocrinology 1981;108:1 441–1 451.

22. Nestler JE, Clove JN, Strauss JF III et al. The effects of hyperinsulinemia on serum testosterone, progesterone, dehydroepiandrosterone sulfate, and cortisol levels in normal women and in women with hyperandrogenism, insulin resistance, and acanthosis nigricans. J Clin Endocrinol Metab 1987; 64:180–184.

23. Dunaif A, Mandeli J, Fluhr H, Dobrjansky A. The impact of obesity and chronic hyperinsulinemia on gonadotropin release and gonadol steroid secretion in the polycystic ovary syndrome. Clin Endocrinol Metab 1988;66;I:131–139.

24. Alper MM, Garner PR. Elevated serum dehydroepiandrosterone sulfate levels in patients with insulin resistance, hirsutism, and acanthosis nigricans. Fertil Steril 1987;47:255–258.

25. Schriock ED, Buffington CK, Hubert GD, et al. Clin Endocrinol Metab 1988;66:1 329–1 331.

26. Lundgren H, Bengtsson C, Blohme G, Lapidus L. Adiposity and adipose tissue distribution in relation to incidence of diabetes in women: results from a prospective population study in Gothenburg, Sweden. Int J Obesity 1989; in press.

27. Stern MP, Haffner SM, Katz MS, Dunn JF. The relationship of sex hormones to hyperinsulinemia and hyperglycemia. Metabolism 1988;37:683–688.

28. Seidell JC, Cigolini M, Deurenberg P, Oosterlee A, Doornbos C. Fat distribution, androgens and metabolism in non-obese women. Am J Clin Nutr 1989; in press.

29. Peiris AN, Meuller RA, Struve MF, Smith GA, Kissebah AH. Relationships of androgenic activity to splanchnic insulin metabolism and peripheral glucose utilization in premenopausal women. J Clin Endocrinol Metab 1987;64:162–169.

30. Reference deleted.

31. Krotkiewski M, Björntorp P. Muscle tissue in obesity with different distribution of adipose tissue, effects of physical training. Int J Obesity 1986;10:331–341.

32. Hom FG, Goodner CJ. Insulin dose-response characteristics among individual muscle and adipose tissues measured in the rat in vivo with [³H]2-deoxyglucose. Diabetes 1984;33:153–159.

33. James DE, Jenkins AB, Kraegen EW. Heterogenity of insulin action in individual muscles in vivo: euglycemic clamp studies in rats. Am J Physiol 1985;248:E567–E574.

34. Lillioja S, Young AA, Culter CL, et al. Skeletal muscle capillary density and fiber type are possible determinants of in vivo insulin resistance in man. J Clin Invest 1987;80:415–425.

35. Lithell M, Lindegärde F, Hellsing K, et al. Body weight skeletal muscle morphology and enzyme activities in relation to fasting serum insulin concentration and glucose tolerance in 48-year-old men. Diabetes 1981;30:19–25.

36. Lindgärde F, Erickson KF, Lithell H, Saltin B. Coupling between dietary changes, reduced body weight, muscle fiber size and improved glucose tolerance in middle-aged men with impaired glucose tolerance. Acta Med Scand 1982;212:99–106.

37. Komi PV, Viitasalo HT, Havn M, Thorstensson A, Sjödin B, Karlsson J. Skeletal muscle fibers and muscle enzyme activities in monozygous and dizygous twins of both sexes. Acta Physiol Scand 1977; 100:385–392.

38. Danneskjold-Samsoe B, Grimby G. The influence of prednisolone on the muscle enzymes in patients with rheumatoid arthritis. Clin Sci 1986;71:693–701.

39. Rebuffé-Scrive M, Krotkiewski M, Elfverson J, Björntorp P. Muscle and adipose tissue morphology and metabolism in Cushing's syndrome. J Clin Endocrinol Metab 67:6:1 122–1 128.

40. Krotkiewski M, Kral J, Karlsson J. Effects of castration and testosterone substitution on body composition and muscle metabolism in rats. Acta Physiol Scand 1980;109:233–237.

41. Suzuki S, Yamamuro T. Long-term effects of estrogen on rat skeletal muscle. Exp Neurol 1985;87: 291–299.

42. Holmäng A, Björntorp P. Effects of testosterone on insulin sensitivity and muscle morphology of female rats. Int J Obesity 1989;13(Suppl 1):65.

43. Björntorp P. Obesity and diabetes. In: Alberti KGMM, Krall P, eds. The Diabetes Annual, Vol. 4. Amsterdam: Elsevier, 1988;615–622.

44. Lapidus L, Bengtsson C, Larsson B, Pennert K, Rybo E, Sjöström L. Distribution of adipose tissue and risk of cardiovascular disease and death: a 12 year follow-up of participants in the population study of women in Gothenburg, Sweden. Br Med J 1984;289:1 257–1 261.

© 1989 Elsevier Science Publishers B.V. (Biomedical Division)
Frontiers of diabetes research: current trends in non-insulin-dependent diabetes mellitus
K.G.M.M. Alberti and R. Mazze, editors

CHAPTER 5

Epidemiology of complications of NIDDM

EVELINE ESCHWEGE[1], ANNIE LACROUX[1], LAURE PAPOZ[1],
ANNICK FONTBONNE[1] and DOMINIQUE COSTAGLIOLA[2]

[1]*INSERM, Unité 21, 16 avenue Paul Vaillant-Couturier, 94807 Villejuif Cedex, and*
[2]*INSERM, Unité 263, Université Paris VII, 2 Place Jussieu, 75251 Paris Cedex 05, France*

Introduction

Non-insulin-dependent diabetes mellitus (NIDDM) is the most common of the two types of diabetes, since it concerns 80 to 85% of those with diabetes. Often remaining undiagnosed, the severity of NIDDM relates to its complications. For different reasons, the epidemiology of NIDDM complications is not easy to document.

1. Maturity-onset diabetes often remains asymptomatic for a long period; its diagnostic criteria suffer from a lack of precision: 25 to 63% of NIDDM subjects are diagnosed following a routine test [1]; in 1 to 14% of cases, this diagnosis is made after complications have occurred.
2. Most of the published studies deal with both types of diabetes, and even if NIDDM patients are the most numerous, it is often not easy to distinguish them from the whole sample.
3. NIDDM complications are frequently asymptomatic at onset for the patient, and are not systematically investigated. Their diagnosis does not (or cannot) rely on perfectly standardized methods. Furthermore, differences exist in requirements for measures of the disease in epidemiological studies and in clinical medicine.

For each complication considered, retinopathy, nephropathy, neuropathy and macrovascular diseases, the methods of assessment, the prevalence and incidence data*, and the associated risk factors will be considered.

$$*\text{Prevalence (\%)} = \frac{\text{No. existing diabetic complication cases at a point in time}}{\text{No. individuals in the population at risk at same point in time}} \times 100$$

Incidence (per 1 000 person-years) ($^0/_{00}$/yr) =

$$\frac{\text{No. new diabetic complication cases diagnosed in study period}}{\text{Person-years of observation of subjects at risk during study period}} \times 1\,000$$

Ophthalmological complications

These are considered as the most disabling complications, since they may lead to total loss of vision. In the United States, approximately 8% of those who are legally blind are reported to have diabetes as the cause [2]. Cataracts, glaucoma and corneal diseases are associated with diabetes, but retinopathy, characterized by alterations in the small blood vessels in the retina, is the most studied complication.

Diagnostic criteria

Diagnosis relies on eye fundus examination carried out on each eye, according to well-defined procedures [3]. Several classifications, based on a morphological description of the lesions, have been proposed in order to assess severity of diabetic retinopathy. Roughly, two main categories are defined, according to whether new vessels are present or not: background retinopathy (the less severe), and proliferative retinopathy, which has a rather poor prognosis. Each one is divided into levels of severity, the number of which varies according to the author [4]. However, preproliferative retinopathy should be given special attention because it may induce macular oedema, almost as severe as proliferative retinopathy.

TABLE 1

Retinopathy: prevalence data in NIDDM patients

	NIDDM patients (n)	Age at examination (years)	Prevalence rates (%)	
			Any retinopathy	Proliferative retinopathy
Pima Indians (1976) [6]	765	> 15	18%	1.1%
Framingham Eye Study (1988) [7]	209 (175)[a]	52–85	20%	2%
Falster Island (DK) (1980) [8]	367	35–92	47%	Not given
Rochester, MN (1986) [9]	1 004 (875)[a]	30–80	3%	Not given
Wisconsin ESDR (1984) [5]	1 370 (696)[a]	30–87	54% (39%)[a]	8.5% (3%)[a]
Poole Area (UK) (1982) [10]	474	30–95	23%	8.3%
Hopi-Navajo Indians (1983) [11]	137 (87)[a]	20–99	36%	4%

[a] Non-insulin-treated.

Prevalence

According to different population-based studies of NIDDM patients recruited on criteria unrelated to retinopathy, prevalence varies from 3 to 54% (Table 1) [5–11] for any retinopathy, and from 1.1% to 8.5% for proliferative retinopathy. Prevalence of blindness was around 2% for NIDDM [2].

Incidence

Very few population-based data are available on the incidence and progression of retinopathy. Incidence of background retinopathy varied from $15.6^0/_{00}$/yr to $65^0/_{00}$/yr and that of proliferative from 0.8 to $3.6^0/_{00}$/yr (Table 2) [9,12–14]. There are very few studies on the incidence of legal blindness except for the UDGP newly diagnosed diabetics, aged 20–79 yrs, in whom the five-year incidence of blindness was 3.8% or less in each treatment group [12].

Associated and/or risk factors of retinopathy

Incidence as well as prevalence rate has to be related to associated or risk factors of diabetic retinopathy (Table 3) [5,6,8,9,12,13]. Firstly, of the three possible risk factors, age at eye examination, age at diagnosis and duration of diabetes, only duration of diabetes is important, the other factors playing only an indirect part. The longer the duration of diabetes, the more often retinopathy is observed. Secondly, regarding

TABLE 2

Incidence of retinopathy in NIDDM patients

	NIDDM patients (n)	Age at examin. (years)	Duration of follow-up (years)	Patients with retinopathy (n)	Type of retinopathy	Incidence rate ($^0/_{00}$/yr)
Rochester (1986) [9]	1 031	30–80	25	170	Any	15.6
				14	Prolif.	0.8-1.4
Pima Indians (1980) [14]	196	> 25	6	a	Backgr.	33–65
Radcliffe Infirmary, Oxford (1984) [13]	150	> 66	7	55	Backgr.	52
UGDP[a] (1982) [12]	619	20–77	12.5	137	Mild	23–25
				20	Pre-prolif.- + prolif.	0.8–3.6

[a] Oral hypoglycemic agents excluded.

TABLE 3
Retinopathy, associated (or risk) factors in NIDDM patients

	Pima [6]	Wisconsin [5]	Rochester [9]	Radcliffe [13]	Falster (DK) [8]	UGDP [12]
Age at diagnosis	No	Yes[b]	Yes	a	a	a
Age at eye examination	No	No	No	No	a	a
Duration of diabetes	Yes	Yes	Yes	Yes	Yes	Yes
Blood glucose control (BG level or HbA$_1$)	Yes	Yes	Yes	Yes	Yes	No
Insulin use	Not relevant	Yes	No	No	a	No
Blood pressure	Yes	Yes	No	a	a	a
BMI	Yes, negatively	Yes[b], negatively	Yes, positively	a	a	a
Smoking	a	No	No	a	a	a
Sex	No	No	No	No	a	a

[a] Not given.

[b] Only related to severity of retinopathy.

blood glucose control, there is little doubt that retinopathy tends to be more prevalent and more severe in groups of patients who have more severe and/or less well controlled diabetes [13]. However, the UGDP results [12] did not suggest any reduction in the incidence of retinopathy in the best blood-glucose controlled group. Finally, other factors considered to be related to diabetic retinopathy, such as insulin use, body mass index, smoking habits, sex, and blood pressure, have, up to now, no consistent data to support any definite conclusion.

Renal complications

The kidneys of diabetic patients undergo many functional and morphological changes before the clinical appearance of diabetic nephropathy, which is marked by the development of constant proteinuria. In NIDDM patients, proteinuria occurs early after clinical diagnosis of diabetes but does not generally herald progressive renal insufficiency. A classification system following five stages of renal involvement [15] which was defined for IDDM patients does not completely fit NIDDM subjects, considering especially cardiovascular disease which may give rise to microalbuminuria. However, four levels can be defined according to albumin excretion rate: (1) less than 30 μg/min, (2) between 30 and 200 μg/min, (3) persistently greater than 200 μg/min (persistent proteinuria – overt diabetic nephropathy) and (4) end-stage renal fail-

TABLE 4
Prevalence of renal complications

	NIDDM patients (n)	Age at 1st exam. (years)	Criteria for proteinuria (μg/ml)	Prevalence rate (%)	Prevalence at DM diagnosis (%)
Pima Indians (1974) [16]	404	15–75	> 30	22.4	b
Navajo Indians (1983) [11]	137	20–99	> 30	31	b
Wisconsin (1984) [17]	1 294	30–80	> 30	15.1	12.2
Rochester, MN (1988) [18]	1 031	30–80	> 40	8.2	8.2
Mogensen (1979) [19]	791	30–100	> 30	24	b
Aarhus, DK (1987) [20]	503 (162)[a]	50–75	> 16 > 200	30 5	6.5
Geneva (1982) [21]	510 (165)[a]	42–92	> 150 mg/24 h	48	16
Fredericia, DK (1986) [22]	211	60–74	> 30	26	16

[a] Non-insulin-treated.
[b] Not given.

ure (renal insufficiency). Urine collection procedures, urinary albumin concentrations and serum creatinine measurements are well standardized.

Prevalence

Most of the studies to date were derived from clinic populations and suffer from selection and ascertainment bias. Furthermore, NIDDM and IDDM were often mixed. Prevalence of renal complications, defined as proteinuria higher than 30 μg/ml, varied from 8.2% to 31% in population-based studies [11,16–18], the highest values being observed for a US Indian population (Table 4), and from 24 to 48% in clinic populations [19–22]. At diagnosis of diabetes, microalbuminuria was present in 6 to 16% of subjects [15].

Incidence

Incidence data are scarce, since most of the clinic population studies were aimed at analysing the role of microalbuminuria as a risk factor for death, rather than investigating its characteristics and conditions of occurrence. The annual incidence rate varied from 15.3⁰/₀₀/yr to 25⁰/₀₀/yr in two population-based studies (Table 5) [8,12,14,23]; the highest rate has been observed in Pima Indians [23]. These rates have to be compared to those observed in the UGDP [12]: for patients not treated with oral hypoglycemic agents, after a 12.5-year follow-up, the cumulative incidence of

TABLE 5
Incidence of renal complications in NIDDM patients

	NIDDM patients (n)	Age (years)	Duration of follow-up (years)	Criteria for proteinuria (μg/ml)	Incidence rate (⁰/₀₀/yr)
Rochester (1988) [8]	1 031	30–80	25	> 40	15.3
Pima Indians					
(1980) [14]	196	> 25	6	> 30	6.6–30
(1988) [23]	–	–	20	> 30	25
UGDP (1982) [12]	619ᵃ	20–77	12.5	+ +twice	6.3– 9.4
				> 100	1.7– 4.8

ᵃOral hypoglycemic agents excluded.

urine protein 2+ or more at two consecutive quarterly follow-up examinations varied from 7.9 to 11.8%; the corresponding rate for urine protein > 1 g/l varied from 2.1 to 5.8%. In NIDDM patients, end-stage renal failure was infrequent and a $0.26^0/_{00}$/yr incidence rate was observed [17]. Renal complications in NIDDM patients were moderately severe: cause of death in a 10-year follow-up as reported by Mogensen et al. [15] in 416 NIDDM patients was uremia for only 2.3%. In addition, as recently reported by Danish and English workers [20,22,24], proteinuria in NIDDM was a strong predictor of total and cardiovascular mortality and morbidity, and was independent of the other usual risk factors.

Associated and risk factors

Few studies are available on the incidence of proteinuria risk factors; the development of persistent proteinuria appears to be more strongly associated with aging than with the duration of diabetes. Presence of retinopathy was also found to be predictive of microalbuminuria in most studies. Male gender, higher blood glucose levels and higher blood pressure are controversial as risk factors [16,18–21]. Afro-Caribbean or Asian NIDDM patients could be more exposed to advanced or end-stage renal failure than European subjects [25]. Such studies are, however, rare and their analyses too limited, except for the Rochester Study [18], so that no definite conclusions are possible. Microalbuminuria in NIDDM patients should be investigated in specific studies.

Neuropathy in NIDDM

Disturbances of the peripheral nervous system in diabetes are so common as to be considered together with retinopathy and nephropathy as one of the major later complications. Unfortunately diabetic neuropathy encompasses a variety of clinical pictures, and the lack of consistency in the basic definition together with the poor quality of epidemiological data make the results of the few studies done to date difficult to compare. The measurement of diabetic neuropathy goes from objective complaints (pain, weakness, chronic diarrhea, neurotropic ulcers, orthostatic hypotension, sexual impotence in men), through ankle jerk and malleolar vibratory perception, to apparently more objective and reproducible electrophysiological studies of nerve conduction velocity in motor and sensory perception thresholds, or to cardiovascular autonomic function tests as summarized by Ewing [28]. Among many classifications, that proposed by Canal and Pozza [26], derived from Brown and Asbury [27], is the most satisfactory. However, because of the range of definitions and measurements, diabetic neuropathy has rarely been the object of epidemiological research and there are very few available data for all diabetics and even fewer for NIDDM patients.

Prevalence and incidence

According to Melton [29] the prevalence of neuropathy in diabetes varies from 10% to 52% for objective signs, 35% to 62% for general signs or subjective complaints, and up to 100% for abnormalities of motor conduction velocity. In the Rochester population-based study, the prevalence [30] of neuropathy in 995 NIDDM patients aged 30–80 years was 10%, 3/4 of them suffering from distal neuropathy and 1/10 from carpal tunnel syndrome (Table 6) [11,30].

In the same cohort of NIDDM patients, who were followed for 25 years and were free of neuropathy at first diagnosis, the actuarially estimated cumulative incidence of distal polyneuropathy was 4% at 5 years and it rose to 15% at 20 years. After 20

TABLE 6
Prevalence of neuropathy in NIDDM patients

	NIDDM patients (n)	Age at examination (years)	Patients with neuropathy (n)	Prevalence rate (%)
Rochester (1978) [30]	995	30–80	108	10 (72 distal polyneurop., 12 carpal tunnel, 6 mononeuropathy, 10 others)
Hopi and Navajo Indians (1983) [11]	137 (87)[a]	20–99	16	12

[a] Non-insulin-treated.

years of follow-up, the cumulative incidence of carpal tunnel syndrome was 1.3%, of mononeuropathy 0.6%, of autonomic neuropathy 0.3% and of all other neuropathies 1.1% [30].

Associated or risk factors

In diabetic patients as well as in non-diabetics, ageing is the factor most commonly associated with neuropathy. Duration of diabetes, independently of age, was also demonstrated as a risk factor for all types of neuropathy: prevalence of abnormal parasympathetic or sympathetic cardiovascular tests as well as carpal tunnel syndrome increased from 0 to 20–30% between one and ten years of diabetes duration [26]. Hyperglycemia is another possible major risk factor in the pathogenesis of neuropathy. There are, however, no consistent epidemiological data to sustain a definitive conclusion, particularly in NIDDM patients [31]. There is a need for clear definitions and standardized measurements to analyse the frequency and natural history of diabetic neuropathy.

Macrovascular complications in NIDDM

The term 'macrovascular' disease is used to describe diseases of the coronary, cerebral and peripheral circulation, in contrast to 'microvascular' disease, which is the general term used to describe retinopathy, nephropathy and neuropathy complications specific to diabetes mellitus. Accompanying disorders of macrovascular diseases are based on atherosclerosis. Diabetic patients, on average, have quantitatively more atherosclerosis than non-diabetic patients, but it is not qualitatively different. In addition, atherosclerotic coronary heart disease, the most common of the macroangiopathies, is considered as the main cause of death among NIDDM patients [32].

Assessment of data on large-vessel diseases in NIDDM is difficult for several reasons, such as lack of sensitivity and specificity of diagnostic criteria of vascular diseases, survivorship bias of prevalence studies for cardio- and cerebrovascular diseases; furthermore, very few population-based studies are available where NIDDM patients have been examined separately. Diagnosis of large-vessel diseases relies either on clinical or ECG data, or on death certificates for heart disease (HD); on clinical data or death certificates for stroke; on clinical data only for peripheral vascular disease.

1. Heart disease (HD)

Prevalence
The prevalence of vascular heart disease (coronary heart disease or congestive heart

failure) in population-based studies [32,33] varied, according to clinical examination, from 2 to 20.9% in males and 1.6 to 15.7% in females depending on age at the time of diagnosis of DM. The ratio of diabetics to non-diabetics was always greater in young people than in older ones: HD appears earlier in diabetics than in normoglycemic patients. Prevalence of abnormalities on resting ECG varied from 9 to 29% [32] according to the Whitehall definition [34]. Higher prevalence rates derived from clinic populations were observed: for example up to 44% in a center-assisted educational program for the Münich area [35]; however, such data suffer from selection and ascertainment bias.

Incidence [12,36–43]
Most of the reliable heart disease incidence data are derived from large population-based studies of coronary heart disease risk factors where NIDDM patients could be examined separately. There were wide differences in age-adjusted incidence rates according to study populations: the highest incidence rates in NIDDM patients are observed in the US, 13 to $39^0/_{00}$/yr [36], closely followed by the UK, 10 to $14^0/_{00}$/yr [40], with France far behind, $4^0/_{00}$/yr [43] (Table 7).

Risk factors
Risk factors for heart disease have been analysed mainly in population-based studies including the usual (and rather small) proportion of diabetic patients, with a risk consistently 2 to 3 times higher than in non-diabetic patients. Very few studies on risk factors have been carried out in diabetic patients per se. In these studies, the following points deserve to be remembered:

(1) Prevalence and incidence of heart disease in NIDDM did not differ consistently between males and females according to the different epidemiological studies [36–40]. Thus, NIDDM female subjects had a coronary risk almost identical to that of NIDDM males, in contrast to what is observed in non-diabetic patients, where men are approximately twice as exposed as women [38].

(2) There was no independent association between heart disease and duration of diabetes [35,40–42,44].

(3) Univariate analysis showed, according to the different studies, that age, smoking habits, blood pressure, cholesterol, triglycerides and insulin levels were predictors of HD [36–38,41–43,45–47]. However, multivariate analysis revealed the major role of hypertriglyceridemia, the long-lasting marker of insulin resistance, which is also associated with relative insulin deficiency [35,43]. When determining macrovascular risk, hyperglycemia and degree of blood glucose control were not associated with heart disease: so, in NIDDM patients, a deleterious lipid profile, perhaps related to long-term insulin action/secretion defects, was more important than hyperglycemia [48,49].

TABLE 7

Incidence of coronary heart disease (CHD) mortality in NIDDM

	NIDDM patients (n)	Age at exam. (years)	Duration of follow-up (years)	CHD deaths (n)	Incidence rate (%/yr)
Framingham (1979) [36]	239 (146)[a]	30–62	20	42	M: 39.1[c]
					F : 22.2
Evans County (1980) [37]	158	Not given	4.5	7	b
					b
Rancho-Bernardo (1983) [38]	343 (338)	40–79	7	24	b
Chicago Heart (1986) [39]	Known: M: 377	35–64	9	44	12.4[c]
	F : 170	"	"	170	3.4
	Newly M: 1163	"	"	48	4.2
	diagn.: F : 708	"	"	708	1.1
Whitehall[d] (1988) [40]	Known: 121	40–64	15	21	9.9–13.9[c]
	Newly				
	diagn.: 56	"	"	17	28.0
	IGT: 999	"	"	101	6.7
Paris Prospect. Study[d] (1989) [43]	Known: 135	43–54	15	6	4.2
	Newly				
	diagn.: 158	"	"	5	2.9
	IGT: 690	"	"	20	2.7
Bedford (1982) [41]	Known: 122	< 50–70	10	26	13[c]
	IGT: 241				
Schwabing (1985) [42]	362	40–84	5	39	21.5
UGDP [12] (1982)	619[e]	20–77	12.5	46	1.3–1.4

[a] Non-insulin-treated.

[b] Not given.

[c] Age-adjusted.

[d] Men only.

[e] Oral hypoglycemic agents excluded.

(4) In recent studies [20,22,24,50], microalbuminuria was a strong predictor of total and cardiovascular mortality and morbidity. Although this association could be explained in part by an effect of elevated blood pressure on both arterial disease and albumin excretion rate, multivariate analysis showed that at least part of the urinary albumin hyperexcretion with cardiovascular disease and death was independent of associated elevated blood pressure.

2. Cerebrovascular disease (CVD)

Few epidemiological data are available on stroke in NIDDM patients: as observed for heart disease, diabetes was considered as one of the risk factors for stroke in most of the population-based studies (risk of stroke was 2 to 4 times higher in diabetics than in non-diabetics) [51]. However, stroke occurs at an older age than heart disease; besides, the number of cases in the different studies was too small to extract reliable information for NIDDM.

Prevalence of CVD in population-based studies, according to clinical examination, varied from roughly 5 to 13% depending on age [51].

The incidence rate (Table 8) based on stroke as a cause of death varied between $4.3^0/_{00}$/yr to $10.1^0/_{00}$/yr (age-adjusted rate) in the US [52–55], $0.75^0/_{00}$/yr in the Whitehall Study [56], and $1.0^0/_{00}$/yr in the Paris Prospective Study (unpublished data).

Associated risk factors: both sexes are equally affected [53–55]. There is considerable evidence that hypertension is a major risk factor for cerebral infarction [57]; consequently, the relationship between diabetes and stroke might be due to an increased prevalence of hypertension among diabetic individuals. However, in the Framingham population [54], as in the Rancho-Bernardo [52] or the Honolulu Study [55], the impact of diabetes on the occurrence of cerebral infarction was substantial and independent of other risk factors. In the Rochester population [53], poor control and long duration of diabetes appeared as risk factors for stroke, but blood pressure was not considered in the analysis.

TABLE 8
Incidence of cerebrovascular mortality in NIDDM

	NIDDM patients (n)	Age at examin. (years)	Duration of follow-up (years)	Deaths (n)	Incidence rate ($^0/_{00}$/yr)
Whitehall [56]	121	40–64	10	3	0.75[a]
Paris Prospect. Study (unpublished)	293	43–54	15	4	1.0
Rancho-Bernardo [52]	320	50–79	12	b	M: 4.3[a]
					F: 6.1
Rochester[a] [53]	1 010	− 30–80 +	2.5	113	10.1
Framingham [54]	239	30–62	20	b	M: 4.7[a]
					F: 6.2
Honolulu [55]	690	45–69	12	43	5.1

[a] Age-adjusted.
[b] Not given.

82

3. Peripheral vascular disease (PVD)

With regard to heart disease and cardiovascular complications, the epidemiology of peripheral vascular disease suffers from the lack of DM population-based studies and of the mixture, in the few general population studies, of NIDDM and IDDM patients [58]. In addition, the diagnostic criteria are multiple (pulse deficit, intermittent claudication, gangrene or amputation), not well standardized, and can only rely on clinical examination.

Prevalence of PVD

In the Rochester population-based study [59] the prevalence of absent peripheral pulses was around 10.5%. At the time of diagnosis of diabetes, 8% of the population had absent pulses. This percentage is similar to the 10.3% observed at baseline in the recently diabetes-diagnosed UGDP [60] patients. Among them 4.6% also had intermittent claudication (Table 9).

Incidence of PVD

Using peripheral pulse deficit as the diagnostic criterion the incidence of peripheral vascular disease varied between 16.9 and $27^o/_{oo}$ person/yr [59–61]. Incidence of intermittent claudication varied between 8.4 and $29^o/_{oo}$/yr, the highest rates being observed in the UGDP male and female subjects [60,61] (Table 10). Data regarding gangrene are too scarce to allow a correct estimation of either prevalence or incidence. However, in the Rochester Study [59], the crude incidence of new episodes of gangrene

TABLE 9

Prevalence of peripheral vascular disease among NIDDM patients

	NIDDM patients (n)	Age (years)	Measurement	PVD (n)	Prevalence rate (%)
Rochester [59]	724	30–80	Pulse deficit	76	10.5
			Gangrene	10	a
UGDP [60]	619[b]	20–77	Pulse deficit	63	10.3
			Intermittent claudic.	28	4.6
			Gangrene	0	0
Hopi-Navajo [11]	137	20–99	Pulse deficit		
			Amputation	18	13.0
			Intermittent claudic.		

[a] Not given.

[b] Oral hypoglycemic agents excluded.

TABLE 10
Incidence of peripheral vascular disease among NIDDM patients

	NIDDM patients (n)	Age (years)	Follow-up duration (years)	Criterion	PVD (n)	Incidence rate (⁰/₀₀/yr)
Rochester [59]	1 073	30–80	25	Pulse deficit	159	M: 26.2[a]
						F: 16.9
				Gangrene	37	b
Framingham [61]	239	30–62	16	Intermittent claudic.	b	M: 12.6[a]
						F: 8.4
UGDP [60]	619[c]	20–77	14	Pulse deficit	b	M: 27
						F: 27
				Intermittent claudic.	b	M: 29
						F: 19
				Amputations	19	b

[a] Age-adjusted.
[b] Not given.
[c] Oral hypoglycemic agents excluded.

among the 145 diabetics who were gangrene-free at the first diagnosis of pulse deficit was 29.6⁰/₀₀/yr for men and 37.1 for women.

Associated risk factors of PVD

Age was the most important risk factor: incidence of absent pulses varied from 0 before 39 years to more than 25 after 80 years [59]. With regard to heart disease, NIDDM male and female subjects had a similar risk of PVD, in contrast to non-diabetic subjects where men are more at risk than women [59–61]. Acting independently of age, duration of diabetes and levels of blood glucose were risk factors of peripheral vascular disease: incidence rates roughly doubled after 10 years of diabetes in comparison with less than 10 years [59]. In the Framingham Study [61] as well as in the UGDP [60], elevated blood glucose level was also predictive of peripheral vascular disease, but all these observations have to be confirmed in other studies, where the role of peripheral neuropathy is also considered.

Macrovascular diseases are undoubtedly associated with NIDDM. They are more severe and occur at an earlier age in NIDDM than in non-diabetics; women as well as men are concerned, unlike non-diabetic subjects where men are more at risk than women. However, they are inconsistently related to characteristics of diabetes, duration of disease, and blood glucose level. So, as suggested by Jarrett [48,49] and supported by observations of different population-based studies [12,40,42–44,62],

84

NIDDM and macrovascular diseases may only be associated diseases and not causally related, and NIDDM may occur more frequently in individuals predisposed to develop vascular diseases.

Conclusions

Epidemiology of complications of NIDDM is even more confused than that of IDDM, because most of the complications of NIDDM are age-related and non-specific and because the date of onset of NIDDM is often uncertain, so that asymptomatic hyperglycemia may have been present for years. The most reliable and unbiased data are incidence rates provided by population-based studies in NIDDM patients who initially had no complications and who were followed for at least 5 to 10 years. Retinopathy is the most specific, the most frequent and the most directly diabetes-related complication. Proteinuria, half as common, may occur early after the clinical diagnosis of diabetes but does not generally herald progressive renal insufficiency. It has to be related to age-associated cardiovascular disease but high blood pressure and hyperinsulinemia have also to be accounted for. Moreover, the indisputable role of diabetes per se in the progression of nephropathy is difficult to isolate from ageing.

Very little is known about neuropathy due to lack of well-defined diagnosis. In addition, ageing is a real confounding factor. Macrovascular complications have to be considered more as associated diseases than as specific complications, even if the most frequent, coronary heart disease, is the primary cause of death for NIDDM patients. The incidence rates were 2 to 3 times higher in NIDDM patients than in non-diabetics for coronary heart disease, 3 to 4 times higher for stroke, and 4 to 6 times higher for peripheral vascular disease. Several hypotheses have been advanced to explain the importance of the role of macrovascular disease in diabetics, including a greater frequency of hypertension, proteinuria, lipid abnormalities and hyperinsulinemia. These factors are particularly operative in generally overweight NIDDM patients. Moreover, the absence of association between risk of vascular disease and characteristics of diabetes (duration [40–48], blood glucose control [12,44]) supports the hypothesis that macrovascular disease and NIDDM are associated disorders [63–65], possibly linked genetically [48,49].

References

1. Costagliola D, Chwalow AJ, Simon D, Eschwège E. Some key factors in the clinical diagnosis of non-insulin dependent diabetes: a multinational comparison. Diabète Métab 1989;15:51–52.
2. Klein R, Klein BEK. Vision disorders in diabetes. In Diabetes in America. Diabetes Data Compiled

1984. Chapter XIII. NIH Publication 85-1468. US Department of Health and Human Services, 1984; 1–36.

3. Bennett PH. Recommendations on the standardization of methods and reporting of tests for diabetes and its microvascular complications in epidemiologic studies. Diabetes Care 1979;2:98–104.

4. Davis MD. Diabetic retinopathy: a clinical overview. Diabetes Metab Rev 1988;4:291–322.

5. Klein R, Klein BEK, Moss SE, Davis MD, DeMets DL. The Wisconsin epidemiologic study of diabetic retinopathy. III. Prevalence and risk of diabetic retinopathy when age at diagnosis is 30 or more years. Arch Ophthalmol 1984;102:527–532.

6. Dorf A, Ballintine EJ, Bennett PH, Miller M. Retinopathy in Pima Indians. Relationships to glucose level, duration of diabetes, age at diagnosis of diabetes and age at examination in a population with a high prevalence of diabetes mellitus. Diabetes 1976;25:554–560.

7. Hiller R, Sperduto RD, Podgor MJ, Ferris FL, Wilson PWF. Diabetic retinopathy and cardiovascular disease in type II diabetics. The Framingham heart study and the Framingham eye study. Am J Epidemiol 1988;128:402–409.

8. Nielsen NV, Ditzel J. Prevalence of macro- and microvascular disease as related to glycosylated hemoglobin in type I and II diabetic subjects. An epidemiologic study in Denmark. Horm Metab Res 1985;Suppl 15:19–23.

9. Ballard DJ, Melton III LJ, Dwyer MS, Trautmann JC, O'Fallon WM, Palumbo PJ. Risk factors for diabetic retinopathy: a population-based study in Rochester, Minnesota. Diabetes Care 1986;9: 334–342.

10. Houston A. Retinopathy in the Poole area: an epidemiological enquiry. In: Eschwège E, ed. Advances in Diabetes Epidemiology, INSERM Symposium No. 22: Amsterdam: Elsevier 1982;199–206.

11. Rate RG, Knowler WC, Morse HG, Bonnell MD, McVey J, Cherzvenak CL, Smith MG, Pavanich G. Diabetes mellitus in Hopi and Navajo Indians. Prevalence of microvascular complications. Diabetes 1983;32:894–899.

12. The University Group Diabetes Program. Effect of hypoglycemic agents on vascular complications in patients with adult-onset diabetes. VIII, Evaluation of insulin therapy: final Report. Diabetes 1982;31, suppl 5:1–81.

13. Howard-Williams J, Hillson RM, Bron A, Awdry P, Mann JI, Hockaday TDR. Retinopathy is associated with higher glycaemia in maturity-onset type diabetes. Diabetologia 1984;27:198–202.

14. Pettit DJ, Knowler WC, Lisse JR, Bennett PH. Development of retinopathy and proteinuria in relation to plasma-glucose concentrations in Pima Indians. Lancet 1980;ii:1 050–1 052.

15. Mogensen CE, Schmitz A, Christensen CK. Comparative renal pathophysiology relevant to IDDM and NIDDM patients. Diabetes Metab Rev 1988;4:453–483.

16. Kamenetzky SA, Bennett PH, Dippe SE, Miller M, LeCompte PM. A clinical and histologic study of diabetic nephropathy in the Pima Indians. Diabetes 1974;23:61–68.

17. Herman WH, Teutsch SM. Kidney diseases associated with diabetes. Diabetes Data Compiled 1984. Chapter XIV. NIH Publication 85-1468. US Department of Health and Human Services, 1984;1–28.

18. Ballard DJ, Humphrey LL, Melton III LJ, Frohnert PP, Chu CP, O'Fallon WM, Palumbo PJ. Epidemiology of persistent proteinuria in type II diabetes mellitus. Diabetes 1988;37:405–412.

19. Mogensen CE. A complete screening of urinary albumin concentration in an unselected diabetic outpatient clinic population. Diabetologia 1979;16:165–171.

20. Schmitz A, Vaeth M. Microalbuminuria: a major risk factor in non-insulin-dependent diabetes. A 10-year follow-up study of 503 patients. Diabetic Med 1988;5:126–134.

21. Fabre J, Balant LP, Dayer PG, Fox HM, Vernet AT. The kidney in maturity onset diabetes mellitus: a clinical study of 510 patients. Kidney Int 1982;21:730–738.

22. Damsgaard EM, Mogensen CE. Microalbuminuria in elderly hyperglycaemic patients and controls. Diabetic Med 1986;3:430–435.

23. Knowler WC, Kunzelman CL. Population comparisons of the frequency of diabetic nephropathy. In: Morgensen CE, ed. Kidney and Hypertension in Diabetes Mellitus. Boston: Martin Nijhoff, 1988; 25–32.

24. Jarrett RJ, Viberti GC, Argyropoulos A, Hill RD, Mahmud U, Murrells TJ. Microalbuminuria predicts mortality in non-insulin-dependent diabetes. Diabetic Med 1984;1:17–19.

25. Allawi J, Rao PV, Gilbert R, Scott G, Jarrett RJ, Keen H, Viberti GC, Matter HM. Microalbuminuria in non-insulin-dependent diabetes: its prevalence in Indian compared with Europid patients. Br Med J 1988;296:462–464.

26. Canal N, Pozza G. Clinical aspects of peripheral neuropathies in diabetes. In: Andreani D, Crepaldi G, DiMario U, Pozza G, eds. Diabetic Complications: Early Diagnosis and Treatment. New York: John Wiley & Sons, 1987;155–165.

27. Brown MJ, Asbury AK. Diabetic neuropathy. Ann Neurol 1984;15:2–12.

28. Ewing DJ. Quantification of autonomic neuropathy in diabetes mellitus. In: Eschwège E, ed. Advances in Diabetes Epidemiology, INSERM Symposium No. 22. Amsterdam: Elsevier, 1982;261–268.

29. Melton III LJ, Dyck PJ. Clinical features of the diabetic neuropathies. In: Dyck PJ, Thomas PK, Asbury AK, Winegrad AI, Porte D, eds. Diabetic Neuropathy. Philadelphia: WB Saunders, 1987; 27–35.

30. Palumbo PJ, Elveback LR, Whisnant JP. Neurologic complications of diabetes mellitus: transient ischemic attack, stroke, and peripheral neuropathy. Adv Neurol 1978;19:593–601.

31. Porte D. The role of metabolic control in the onset and development of diabetic neuropathy. In: Andreani D, Crepaldi G, DiMario U, Pozza G, eds. Diabetic Complications: Early Diagnosis and Treatment. New York: John Wiley & Sons, 1987;123–131.

32. Barrett-Connor E, Orchard T. Diabetes and heart disease. Diabetes Data Compiled 1984, Chapter XVI. NIH Publication 85-1468. US Department of Health and Human Services, 1984;1–40.

33. Palumbo PJ, Elveback LR, Connolly DC. Coronary heart disease and congestive heart failure in the diabetic. In: Scott RC, ed. Clinical Cardiology and Diabetes. Vol. 1. Mount Kisco, New York: Futura 1981;13–27.

34. Fuller JH, Shipley MJ, Rose G, Jarrett RJ, Keen H. Coronary heart disease risk and impaired glucose tolerance: The Whitehall Study. Lancet 1980;i:1373–1376.

35. Standl E, Stiegler H, Janka HU, Mehnert H. Risk profile of macrovascular disease in diabetes mellitus. Diabète Métab 1988;14:505–511.

36. Kannel WB, McGee DL. Diabetes and cardiovascular risk factors: The Framingham study. Circulation 1979;1:8–13.

37. Heyden S, Heiss G, Bartel AG, Hames CG. Sex differences in coronary mortality among diabetics in Evans County, Georgia. J Chron Dis 1980;33:265–273.

38. Barrett-Connor E, Wingard DL. Sex differential in ischemic heart disease mortality in diabetics: a prospective population-based study. Am J Epidemiol 1983;118:489–495.

39. Pan WH, Cedres LB, Liu K, Dyer A, Schoenberger JA, Shekelle RB, Stamler R, Smith D, Colette P, Stamler J. Relationship of clinical diabetes and asymptomatic hyperglycemia to risk of coronary heart disease mortality in men and women. Am J Epidemiol 1986;123:504–516.

40. Jarrett RJ, Shipley MJ. Type 2 (non-insulin-dependent) Diabetes Mellitus and Cardiovascular Disease – putative association via common antecedents; further evidence from the Whitehall study. Diabetologia 1988;31:737–740.

41. Jarrett RJ, McCartney P, Keen H. The Bedford Survey: ten year mortality rates in newly diagnosed diabetics, borderline diabetics and normoglycaemic controls and risk indices for coronary heart disease in borderline diabetics. Diabetologia 1982;22:79–84.

42. Janka HU. Five year incidence of major macrovascular complications in diabetes mellitus. Horm Metab Res 1985;suppl series,15:15–19.

43. Fontbonne A, Eschwège E, Cambien F, Richard JL, Ducimetière P, Thibult N, Warnet JM, Claude JR, Rosselin GE. Patients with impaired glucose tolerance or diabetes in the Paris prospective study: hypertriglyceridaemia is a risk factor of coronary heart disease mortality. Diabetologia: in press.

44. Panzram G. Mortality and survival in type 2 (non-insulin-dependent) diabetes mellitus. Diabetologia 1987;30:123–131.

45. Kannel WB, McGee DL. Diabetes and glucose tolerance as risk factors for cardiovascular disease. Diabetes Care 1979;2:120–126.

46. Jarrett RJ, Shipley MJ. Mortality and associated risk factors in diabetes. Acta Endocrinol 1985; 110,suppl 272:21–26.

47. Kawate R, Yamakido M, Nishimoto Y, Bennett PH, Hamman RF, Knowler WC. Diabetes mellitus and its vascular complications in Japanese migrants on the island of Hawaii. Diabetes Care 1979;2: 161–170.

48. Jarrett RJ. Type 2 (non-insulin-dependent) diabetes mellitus and coronary heart – chicken, egg or neither? Diabetologia 1984;26:99–102.

49. Jarrett RJ. Is insulin atherogenic? Diabetologia 1988;31:71–75.

50. Viberti GC, Keen H. The patterns of proteinuria in diabetes mellitus. Diabetes 1984;33:686–692.

51. Kuller LH, Dorman JS, Wolf PA. Cerebrovascular disease and diabetes. Diabetes Data Compiled 1984. Chapter XVII. NIH Publication 85-1468. US Department of Health and Human Services, 1984;1–18.

52. Barrett-Connor E, Khaw KT. Diabetes mellitus: an independent risk factor for stroke? Am J Epidemiol 1988;128:116–123.

53. Roehmoldt ME, Palumbo PJ, Whisnant JP, Elveback LR. Transient ischemic attack and stroke in a community-based diabetic cohort. Mayo Clin Proc 1983;58:56–58.

54. Wolf PA, Kannel WB, Verter J. Current status of stroke risk factors. In: Barnett HJM, ed. Neurologic Clinics. Philadelphia: WB Saunders, 1983;317–343.

55. Abbott RD, Donahue RP, MacMahon SW, Reed DM, Yano K. Diabetes and the risk of stroke. The Honolulu heart programme. JAMA 1987;257:949–952.

56. Fuller JH, Shipley MJ, Rose G, Jarrett RJ, Keen H. Mortality from coronary heart disease and stroke in relation to degree of glycaemia: the Whitehall study. Br Med J 1983;287:867–870.

57. Kuller LH. Epidemiology of stroke. Adv Neurol 1978;19:281–311.

58. Palumbo PJ, Melton LJ. Peripheral vascular disease and diabetes. Diabetes Data Compiled 1984. Chapter XV. NIH Publication 85-1468. US Department of Health and Human Services, 1984;1–17.

59. Melton III LJ, Macken KM, Palumbo PL, Elveback LR. Incidence and prevalence of clinical peripheral vascular disease in a population-based cohort of diabetic patients. Diabetes Care 1980;3:650–654.

60. Kreines K, Johnson E, Albrink M, Knatterud GL, Levin ME, Lewitan A, Newberry W, Rose FA. The course of peripheral vascular disease in non-insulin-dependent diabetes. Diabetes Care 1985;8: 235–243.

61. Kannel WB, McGee DL. Diabetes and cardiovascular disease. The Framingham study. JAMA 1979;241:2035–2038.

62. Pyörälä K, Savolainen E, Kaukola S, Haapakoski J. Plasma insulin as coronary heart disease risk factor: relationship to other risk factors and predictive value during 9 1/2 year follow-up of the Helsinki policemen study population. Acta Med Scand 1985 (suppl);701:38–52.

63. Horan MJ. Diabetes and hypertension. Diabetes Data Compiled 1984. Chapter XVII. NIH Publication 85-1468, US Department of Health and Human Services, 1984;1–22.

64. Modan M, Halkin H, Almog S, Lusky A, Eshkol A, Shefi M, Shitrit A, Fuchs Z. Hyperinsulinemia: a link between hypertension, obesity and glucose tolerance. J Clin Invest 1985;75:809–817.

65. Reaven GM. Role of insulin resistance in human disease. Diabetes 1988;37:1595–1607.

CHAPTER 6

Risk factors for vascular complications of NIDDM

PETER H. BENNETT, ROBERT G. NELSON, DAVID J. PETTITT and
WILLIAM C. KNOWLER

*National Institute of Diabetes and Digestive and Kidney Diseases, Phoenix Epidemiology and Clinical
Research Branch, 1550 East Indian School Road, Phoenix, AZ 85014, U.S.A.*

Introduction

Non-insulin-dependent diabetes (NIDDM) is associated with the development of a variety of vascular complications which are responsible for most of the morbidity and the excess mortality associated with diabetes. The clinical manifestations of these complications are seen particularly in the eye (background and proliferative retinopathy), the kidney (diabetic nephropathy and end-stage renal disease), peripheral blood vessels (intermittent claudication, gangrene and amputation) and the heart (coronary heart disease). Often several of these complications are present simultaneously in the same patient, suggesting that they have similar causes and represent a systemic vascular disease. Some of these complications are not specific as they occur in non-diabetics. In NIDDM, some complications, such as coronary heart disease, affect the arteries and appear to represent a more severe or extensive degree of atherosclerosis than is seen in nondiabetic subjects. Other complications, such as background and proliferative retinopathy, which may result in visual loss, and intercapillary glomerular sclerosis, which gives rise to diabetic nephropathy and end-stage renal disease, affect capillaries and arterioles in particular and are found almost exclusively in those with diabetes.

There is a voluminous literature that attempts to relate complications to the duration and severity of diabetes, yet despite many investigations it is still uncertain whether or not the severity of hyperglycemia and lack of glycemic control are the major determinants and to what extent other factors play an important role. It is also recognized that some diabetics do not develop clinically severe vascular disease and live a normal lifespan in spite of diabetes of prolonged duration. Furthermore the relative frequencies of heart disease and renal disease, the complications that contribute most to excess mortality in NIDDM, vary considerably among diabetics in different parts of the world [1].

Mortality

Mortality rates among those with NIDDM substantially exceed rates among nondiabetics. Fig. 1 shows the age-adjusted death rates among U.S. whites aged 40–77 years at baseline, obtained in a nine-year follow-up study of the First National Health and Nutrition Examination Survey (NHANES I) [2]. The data are representative of persons of European origin in the United States and the findings are similar to other less representative studies of mortality and NIDDM. Among both men and women the age-adjusted death rate is twice as high in diabetics as nondiabetics. Compared with the nondiabetic population of similar age, the relative risk of death from cardiovascular disease among the diabetics is 2.6 in men and 2.4 in women. Even after adjusting for age, cigarette smoking, systolic blood pressure, serum cholesterol and body mass index the excess risk for cardiovascular disease mortality among the diabetics remains almost unchanged (2.6 for men and 2.2 for women), yet the majority of the excess cardiovascular disease mortality is attributable to ischemic heart disease. In contrast, among persons with diabetes from populations of non-European origin such as the Japanese, Chinese in Hong Kong, and the Pima Indians of Arizona, the proportion of deaths attributable to renal disease exceeds that due to ischemic heart disease [1]. In Japan, in fact, the death rate from ischemic heart disease among diabetics is only slightly higher than in the general population [3].

The fact that the classical risk factors for coronary heart disease (smoking, hyper-

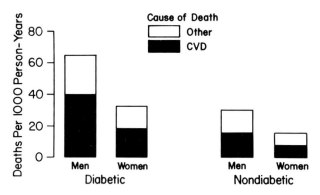

Fig. 1. Age-adjusted death rates in U.S. whites, aged 40–77 years at baseline, over a nine-year follow-up period according to self-reported diagnosis of diabetes at baseline. Adapted from Kleinman et al. [2].

tension and hypercholesterolemia) account for only a minor proportion of the excess coronary artery disease in subjects of European origin suggests that diabetes per se or hyperglycemia is perhaps the major determinant of the excess of coronary heart disease attributed to diabetes. On the other hand, diabetes does not appear to result in an equivalent increase in deaths attributable to coronary heart disease in non-European populations. Moreover, Jarrett has pointed out that if diabetes itself were the important factor one would expect to see an increase in the incidence of coronary heart disease with increasing duration of diabetes after age is taken into account, and this does not appear to be the case [4]. Furthermore, from the University Group Diabetes Project (UGDP) study [5], there is no evidence that the lower blood glucose levels in patients with NIDDM randomized to treatment with variable doses of insulin resulted in any reduction in the death rates attributable to cardiovascular causes compared with subjects treated with diet or a fixed insulin dose whose blood glucose levels were consistently higher over the 12.5-year follow-up period. Thus, risk factors – other than hyperglycemia and the classical risk factors for atherosclerosis – also appear to be important.

Risk factors

There have been two significant difficulties in documenting and understanding the risk factors for vascular complications in NIDDM. First, the onset of the disease is often insidious, and unless an entire population is examined systematically at regular intervals it is difficult to know when the disease began. Second, as many of the serious complications are associated with premature death, cross-sectional studies of risk factors and complications, which only permit examination of survivors, may seriously underestimate and distort conclusions about the relative importance of risk factors, particularly in older subjects or those with long duration of diabetes. Among the Pima Indians we have had the opportunity to study a cohort with NIDDM longitudinally. We have administered glucose tolerance tests to the entire population at regular intervals to ascertain the onset of NIDDM, and have defined presence or absence of various risk factors in persons with diabetes (as well as in those without) on a periodic basis and ascertained the presence or absence of complications at these same examinations. Consequently we are in the process of constructing a more complete account of the factors that precede the development of complications and their natural history [6–10].

The relationships of a number of risk factors to the development of many of the more serious vascular complications of NIDDM are summarized in Table 1. Several factors influence the development of many different types of complication. For example, duration of diabetes is related to the development of each of the complications

TABLE 1

Risk factors (and relative risks[a]) for vascular complications of NIDDM in Pima Indians (adapted from Refs. 6–10)

Risk factor	Proteinuria	Proliferative retinopathy	Amputation	End-stage renal disease
2-h glucose conc.	**	(1.3)	**	NR
Insulin Rx	***	3.5	NR	NR
Proteinuria	NA	2.5	2.2	****
Hypertension	***	2.2	(1.4)	3.8
Absent achilles tendon reflex	NR	4.4	1.2	NR
Medial arterial calcification	2.4	NR	4.8	NR
Renal insufficiency	NA	4.8	NR	****

( ), not significant.
**, $p < 0.01$.
***, $p < 0.001$.
****, present in all cases.
NR, not reported.
NA, not applicable.
[a] Incidence rate ratios, adjusted for age, sex and duration of diabetes.

listed. On the other hand, although the two-hour post-load plasma glucose level is not a significant risk factor for the development of proliferative retinopathy or fatal coronary heart disease, it is significantly associated with the development of protein-uria and the occurrence of amputation. Those receiving treatment with insulin have a higher incidence of each of the complications wherever this has been examined. Proteinuria is a risk factor, not only for the development of end-stage renal disease as would be expected, but also for the development of proliferative retinopathy, am-putation and fatal coronary heart disease. Hypertension is strongly related to the de-velopment of proteinuria, end-stage renal disease and proliferative retinopathy, but perhaps surprisingly was not significantly associated with the development of fatal coronary heart disease or with the need for amputation. On the other hand, medial arterial calcification is strongly related to the development of coronary heart disease and amputation, and was also a predictor of increased overall mortality [7].

From these studies it is apparent that subjects who develop these serious complica-tions of NIDDM share a variety of risk factors. The duration of diabetes is common to all, and those who receive treatment with insulin are at higher risk than those treat-ed otherwise. Moreover, factors other than the duration or severity of hyperglycemia, such as proteinuria and hypertension, influence the appearance of most of these com-plications. The occurrence of these two features increases the risk of developing serious complications even after accounting for increases that can be attributed to the duration and degree of glycemia or the type of treatment.

In view of the degree of interrelationships among the risk factors themselves, as well as among the complications, the time sequence in which abnormalities develop or can be detected is critical to developing an understanding of the pathogenesis of the complications and to defining subgroups of the diabetic population who are at particular risk of developing some or all of them. To do so, detailed longitudinal investigations of subjects with NIDDM are needed from the time of onset of their diabetes until one or more of these serious complications develop.

Proteinuria

Besides predicting the development of end-stage renal disease, proteinuria is an important predictor for development of proliferative retinopathy, amputation and fatal coronary heart disease. Furthermore, among the Pima Indians virtually all the excess mortality attributable to diabetes occurs among those with proteinuria [11]. In addition, both Jarrett et al. and Mogensen have shown that albumin excretion above the normal range predicts increased mortality [12,13] but, in contrast to the Pimas, where most of the increased deaths are due to uremia, in the European populations the majority of the excess mortality is attributable to heart disease.

As shown in Fig. 2, the age-adjusted death rates among Pima Indians aged 45 and over are similar in diabetics without proteinuria and in the nondiabetic population. On the other hand, the mortality rate among diabetics with proteinuria is 3.5 times

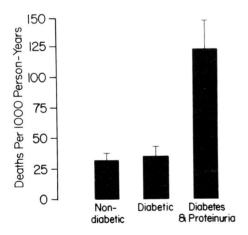

Fig. 2. Age-sex-adjusted death rates (and 95% confidence intervals) in nondiabetic Pima Indians aged ≥ 45 years, and in diabetics without and with proteinuria. From Nelson et al. [11].

as high as in those without. Furthermore, in diabetics with proteinuria diabetes duration is no longer significantly associated with increasing mortality, suggesting that the proteinuria, rather than duration of diabetes, is the more critical factor that determines the risk of death. Similar relationships have been described for mortality and for the incidence of coronary heart disease in insulin-dependent diabetes (IDDM) [14,15]. Among the Pima diabetics with proteinuria, the excess deaths are mainly attributable to coronary heart disease and diabetic renal disease, with death rates from the latter exceeding those from coronary heart disease by a ratio of about 2 to 1.

Thus proteinuria is a risk factor for the development of end-stage renal disease, coronary heart disease, proliferative retinopathy and amputation and is a predictor of all the excess mortality attributable to diabetes. The serious complications of NIDDM and the excess mortality in NIDDM among the Pima Indians can, therefore, be attributed to the development of proteinuria. These findings indicate that proteinuria is a marker of increased risk for various vascular complications, and possibly that the determinants of proteinuria per se may be the same as those responsible for the complications that ultimately lead to death. Consequently, the development of proteinuria appears to represent a key step or be a key indicator of processes that lead to excess mortality in NIDDM as well as for the development of many of the other serious but non-fatal complications such as proliferative retinopathy and amputation.

Risk factors for proteinuria
Among the Pima the incidence of proteinuria increases progressively with increasing duration of diabetes so that the cumulative incidence reaches 50% after 20 years of the disease [9]. The rate of development of proteinuria is not related to sex or age of onset of diabetes but is a function of the duration and severity of diabetes as assessed either by the post-load plasma glucose levels at the time of diagnosis or the selection of insulin as the required form of treatment, and blood pressure (Fig. 3). In each diabetes duration category, subjects who are treated with insulin and those with the highest post-load plasma glucose levels at diagnosis have the highest incidence of proteinuria. The incidence of proteinuria is significantly related to systolic and diastolic blood pressure after controlling for age, sex and duration of diabetes – a relationship which persists even after stratification by the simultaneous two-hour plasma glucose concentration.

The cumulative incidence of proteinuria with increasing diabetes duration in Pima Indians is at least as great as in cohorts of insulin-dependent diabetics followed at the Steno Memorial Hospital or the Joslin Clinic [9]. The incidence of proteinuria, therefore, appears to be as high in NIDDM as in IDDM when subjects of similar duration are compared. Furthermore, among the Pima the incidence of proteinuria in those with up to 15 years duration of diabetes is similar to that reported in

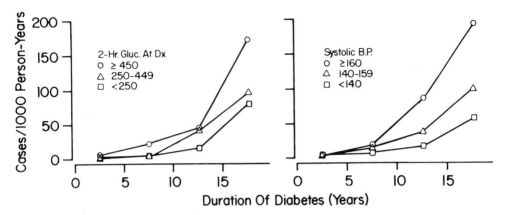

Fig. 3. Incidence of proteinuria in Pima Indians with NIDDM according to two-hour post-load plasma glucose level (mg/dl) at time of diagnosis of NIDDM and systolic blood pressure (mmHg). From Pettitt and Bennett [9].

NIDDM in the predominantly Caucasian population of Rochester, MN, in spite of the considerably higher average age of onset of NIDDM in the Rochester population [16].

Blood pressure

Higher blood pressures and higher sodium-lithium counter-transport activity have been reported in insulin-dependent diabetics who developed nephropathy when compared with individuals with diabetes of similar duration who did not have nephropathy [17,18]. These findings suggest that blood pressure elevation may have a pathogenetic role in nephropathy in IDDM. Blood pressure is associated with proteinuria in NIDDM [19,20], and the incidence of clinical proteinuria is related to blood pressure among the Pima (vide supra). Less severe degrees of proteinuria, as reflected by lower but abnormal albumin excretion, are also related to the level of glycemia and blood pressure [21]. Furthermore, higher blood pressure even before the onset of diabetes predicts the occurrence of excessive albumin excretion after the development of NIDDM [22].

Higher blood pressure, therefore, is a risk factor not only for the occurrence of elevated albumin excretion early in the course of NIDDM, but also for the progression of more severe proteinuria to end-stage renal disease. In a similar way, blood pressure elevation is also associated with a greater incidence of background retinopathy within the first few years of diabetes [23], and is an important risk factor for the development of proliferative retinopathy among those who already have background retinopathy [10].

The genesis of complications

Knowledge of the sequence of events is critical to understanding causation. In the sequence of events that leads to the development of the more severe complications of diabetes, the development of proteinuria (and background retinopathy) signals an enhanced risk of development of end-stage renal disease, coronary heart disease and proliferative retinopathy as well as an increased risk for amputation. A possible schema for the development of vascular complications is shown in Fig. 4. In NIDDM increased albumin excretion and proteinuria may appear relatively soon after the onset of diabetes. Thus, in NIDDM, the development of proteinuria appears to represent an early indicator of the likelihood of serious vascular disease.

Elevated blood pressure predicts the development of proteinuria as well as being a risk factor for the development of more severe background and proliferative retinopathy, renal insufficiency and end-stage renal disease. The observation that prediabetic blood pressure predicts abnormal albumin excretion after the development of diabetes suggests that there may be interaction between the presence of higher blood pressure and diabetes which produces a vasculopathy that is progressive. Alternatively, higher blood pressure in the prediabetic state may perhaps represent an underlying vasculopathy that, once diabetes develops, becomes progressive and accelerated,

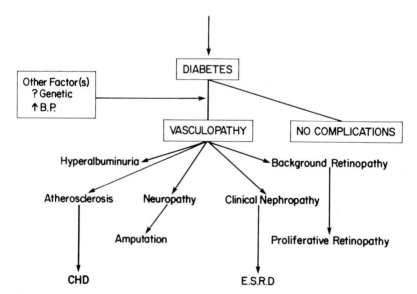

Fig. 4. Schema for development of vascular complications. Evidence of vasculopathy may be recognized soon after the development of NIDDM or may develop later. The recognition of vasculopathy signals an increased likelihood of the development of many of the more serious vascular complications of NIDDM.

leading to severe complications more rapidly and more frequently than would otherwise be the case. A further possibility is that the susceptibility to vascular disease is the result of inherited characteristics which are first clearly recognizable when proteinuria develops.

The concept that vascular complications of diabetes may have a component of susceptibility which is separate from the susceptibility to diabetes itself was first suggested by studies of insulin-dependent diabetes. Higher blood pressures in the parents of those with IDDM who subsequently developed nephropathy than among those who did not [17,18] suggest the possibility of an inherent susceptibility to vascular complications. Among the Pima Indians, because of the high frequency of NIDDM and its relatively early age of onset, it has been possible to examine the risk of developing proteinuria and renal insufficiency in offspring with NIDDM according to whether or not their parents with NIDDM developed similar complications [24]. We have recently shown that the likelihood of offspring having proteinuria is related to proteinuria among the diabetic parents. When both parents have diabetes and proteinuria the risk is higher than when only one diabetic parent is so affected. When one parent is affected the risk for the offspring is about twice that which pertains when neither parent is affected. Furthermore, if a parent with diabetes develops renal insufficiency, the risk of the diabetic offspring developing renal insufficiency is enhanced many-fold. Thus, there is a familial component to susceptibility to the development of vascular disease, which seems likely to be inherited, and which is determined independently of the susceptibility to NIDDM itself.

Conclusions

Vascular complications are responsible for most of the excessive morbidity and mortality associated with NIDDM. Yet, despite many years duration, some subjects with diabetes escape the serious vascular complications while others develop progressive systemic vascular disease which produces proliferative retinopathy, coronary heart disease and/or end-stage renal disease and other complications that result in morbidity and premature mortality. From the Pima Indian experience it appears that in NIDDM the development of proteinuria signals that a subject is at high risk of developing serious vascular complications. The mechanisms underlying the appearance of proteinuria are obscure, but their elucidation might lead to understanding why not all subjects with NIDDM develop the serious vascular complications of the disease. If so, innovative strategies to prevent their occurrence or delay their progression in the subgroup at higher risk might be possible.

Future investigations are needed to determine why certain individuals with proteinuria develop particular types and combinations of complications. It seems likely that other factors (e.g. age of onset of diabetes; specific genetic determinants, such as genes that relate to lipoprotein metabolism; and environmental factors) will determine who develops which combination of these possible outcomes. On the other hand, the risk factors for the development of proteinuria, possibly the earliest clearly recognizable indication of the propensity to develop these complications, include the severity of the diabetes and blood pressure. The fact that proteinuria and renal insufficiency in diabetic parents predicts the risk of developing renal disease in diabetic offspring also strongly suggests that there are determinants of susceptibility to vascular disease which are inherited separately from that of NIDDM itself.

These features suggest the possibility that even among those with NIDDM who are susceptible to the development of vascular disease, its rate of progression and course can perhaps be modified by interventions which lower blood pressure or modify the degree of glycemia. The observational data suggest that the potential for preventing or delaying the progression of complications by lowering blood pressure may be at least as great as that which might be attained by intensive glycemic control. An ability to identify diabetics who are susceptible to vascular disease, and those who are not, will have important therapeutic implications and could lead to more intensive and better directed intervention to delay the onset or progression of the vascular complications. While much remains to be learned about the determinants of vascular disease in NIDDM, recent developments suggest that additional knowledge may lead to radical changes in the management of NIDDM in the future.

References

1. Head J, Fuller J, WHO Multinational Study Group. International variations in mortality among diabetic patients: the WHO multinational study of vascular disease in diabetics (1989) (submitted for publication).
2. Kleinman JC, Donahue RP, Harris MI, Finucane FF, Madans JH, Brock DB. Mortality among diabetics in a national sample. Am J Epidemiol 1988;128:389–401.
3. Sasaki A, Komado K, Horiuchi N. A changing pattern of causes of death in Japanese diabetics. Observations over fifteen years. J Chron Dis 1978;31:433–444.
4. Jarret RJ. Type 2 (non-insulin-dependent) diabetes mellitus and coronary heart disease – chicken, egg or neither? Diabetologia 1984;26:99–102.
5. University Group Diabetes Program. Effects of hypoglycemic agents on vascular complications in patients with adult-onset diabetes. VIII. Evaluation of insulin therapy: final report. Diabetes 1982;31 (Suppl 5):1–81.
6. Nelson RG, Gohdes DM, Everhart JE, Hartner JA, Zwemer FL, Pettitt DJ, Knowler WC. Lower-extremity amputations in NIDDM. 12-yr follow-up study in Pima Indians. Diabetes Care 1988;11:8–16.
7. Everhart JE, Pettitt DJ, Knowler WC, Rose RA, Bennett PH. Medial arterial calcification and its association with mortality and complications of diabetes. Diabetologia 1988;31:16–23.

8. Nelson RG, Newman JM, Knowler WC, Sievers ML, Kunzelman CL, Pettitt DJ, Moffett CD, Teutsch SM, Bennett PH. Incidence of end-stage renal disease in Type 2 (non-insulin-dependent) diabetes mellitus in Pima Indians. Diabetologia 1988;31:730–736.
9. Pettitt DJ, Bennett PH. Incidence of proteinuria in type 2 diabetes mellitus in the Pima Indians. Kidney Int 1989;35:681–687.
10. Nelson RG, Wolfe JA, Horton MB, Pettitt DJ, Bennett PH, Knowler WC. Proliferative retinopathy in NIDDM: incidence and risk factor in Pima Indians. Diabetes 1989;36:435–440.
11. Nelson RG, Pettitt DJ, Carraher MJ, Baird HR, Knowler WC. Effect of proteinuria on mortality in NIDDM. Diabetes 1988;37:1 499–1 504.
12. Jarret RJ, Viberti GC, Argyropoulos A, Hill RD, Mahmud V, Murrells TJ. Microalbuminuria predicts mortality in non-insulin-dependent diabetes. Diabetic Med 1984;1:17–19.
13. Mogensen CE. Microalbuminuria predicts clinical proteinuria and early mortality in maturity-onset diabetes. N Engl J Med 1984;310:356–360.
14. Borch-Johnsen K, Kragh-Andersen P, Deckert T. The effect of proteinuria on relative mortality in type 1 (insulin-dependent) diabetes mellitus. Diabetologia 1985;28:590–596.
15. Jensen T, Borch-Johnsen K, Kofoed-Enevoldsen A, Deckert T. Coronary heart disease in young type 1 (insulin-dependent) diabetic patients with and without diabetic nephropathy: incidence and risk factors. Diabetologia 1987;30:144–148.
16. Ballard DJ, Humphrey LL, Melton J, Frohnert PP, Chu C-P, O'Fallon WM, Palumbo PJ. Epidemiology of persistent proteinuria in type II diabetes mellitus. Diabetes 1988;37:405–412.
17. Viberti GC, Keen H, Wiseman MJ. Raised arterial pressure in parents of proteinuric insulin dependent diabetics. Br Med J 1987;295:515–517.
18. Krolewski AS, Canessa M, Warram JH, Laffel LMB, Christlieb AR, Knowler WC, Rand LI. Predisposition to hypertension and susceptibility to renal disease in insulin-dependent diabetes mellitus. N Engl J Med 1988;318:140–145.
19. Kamenetzky SA, Bennett PH, Dippe SE, Miller M, LeCompte PM. A clinical and histologic study of diabetic nephropathy in the Pima Indians. Diabetes 1974;23:61–68.
20. Klein R, Klein BEK, Moss S, DeMets DL. Proteinuria in diabetes. Arch Intern Med 1988;148:181–186.
21. Nelson RG, Kunzelman CL, Pettitt DJ, Saad MF, Bennett PH, Knowler WC. Albuminuria in non-insulin-dependent diabetes in Pima Indians. (submitted for publication)
22. Knowler WC, Bennet PH, Nelson RG, Saad MF, Pettitt DJ. Blood pressure before the onset of diabetes predicts albuminuria in type 2 (non-insulin-dependent) diabetes. Diabetologia 1988;37:509A.
23. Knowler WC, Bennett PH, Ballintine EJ. Increased incidence of retinopathy in diabetics with elevated blood pressure. N Engl J Med 1980;302:645–650.
24. Pettitt DJ, Saad MF, Bennett PH, Nelson RG, Knowler WC. Familial predisposition to renal disease in two generations of Pima Indians with non-insulin-dependent diabetes mellitus. (submitted for publication)

CHAPTER 7

Primary prevention of non-insulin-dependent diabetes mellitus: a dream or reality?

JAAKKO TUOMILEHTO

Department of Epidemiology, National Public Health Institute, Mannerheimintie 166, 00280 Helsinki, Finland

Introduction

Non-insulin-dependent diabetes mellitus (NIDDM) is a condition with chronic hyperglycemia, not fully understood, but it is associated with severe long-term complications, and with large human and economic burdens and costs. Epidemiologic data from various parts of the world suggest that NIDDM affects 3–10% of adults in most European populations, that it is increasing in most populations and that in some American Indians, Asian Indians and Pacific Islanders it has already reached epidemic proportions [1]. Diabetes seriously affects the quality of life because of its complications, and the life of diabetic patients is clearly shortened. These facts make the questions of preventing NIDDM important.

In 1921 Joslin [2] was already calling for attempts 'to devote time not alone to treatment (of diabetes) but, still more, to prevention'. He was especially suggesting interventions against obesity. It is astonishing that, despite all the resources used in diabetes research, the hypothesis of weight control in the prevention of NIDDM has not been scientifically tested in proper population-based studies. The list of serious attempts at primary prevention of diabetes is not long [3]. Uncertainty still exists as to whether the data available are sufficient to make prevention of NIDDM attainable, but very little can be learned about prevention of NIDDM without making the attempt.

Prevention strategies

Primary prevention has been defined as any measure designed to reduce the incidence of a certain disease in a population by reducing the risk of its onset. In other words this means that the risk attributable to certain factors in a disease is modified by influencing the levels of these factors. Non-insulin-dependent diabetes mellitus (NIDDM) is clearly a multifactorial and heterogeneous disorder. Therefore, preventive measures for NIDDM, to be fully effective in a population, must be based on modification of several potential risk factors simultaneously. With regard to the search for risk factors for NIDDM this will also mean that estimates of attributable risks for various factors are needed, but they are usually derived from univariate analyses of epidemiological data and, therefore, they must be interpreted with caution.

Assuming that NIDDM is preventable, there are two components of the implementation of primary prevention:

(1) a population strategy, for altering the life-style and those environmental determinants which are the underlying causes of NIDDM;
(2) a high-risk strategy, for screening for individuals at special high risk for NIDDM and bringing preventive care to them.

However, the critical questions concerning the prevention of NIDDM are: what should we try to prevent, if we hope to prevent NIDDM? The majority of subjects with NIDDM will develop coronary heart disease (CHD) or other types of cardiovascular disease (CVD). Are these the main issues in the prevention of NIDDM? Or is the main issue the prevention of symptomatic hyperglycemia? Or should we aim the preventive efforts to avoid a heterogeneous multimetabolic syndrome which may include hyperglycemia, hyperinsulinemia, hypertension, hyperlipidemia and obesity? There is no doubt that hyperglycemia is a deleterious condition which is toxic to β-cells [4], but it can be argued that it would be wrong to take a totally glycemic view of NIDDM and to ignore the other components of this syndrome [5,6].

As little can be done to change genetic susceptibility, which is important in the development of NIDDM, the principal challenge, although not the only one in diabetes prevention, will be the modification of environmental factors identified as being associated with the risk of NIDDM in particular populations. Hence, the central element in the planning of any NIDDM prevention activity is the characterization of the chief behavioural and environmental determinants of NIDDM. Another important issue is to understand the mechanisms of their action in the target population or in genetically susceptible individuals. Epidemiological studies have provided new insights into putative determinants of NIDDM, but data are still limited. In particular, there are only a few prospective studies in this field. Moreover, many such studies have been performed in unusual populations with a high prevalence of NIDDM, and these results may not be fully representative of other populations owing to the hetero-geneity of NIDDM.

Putative risk factors of NIDDM can be reviewed, paying particular attention to their potential role in the primary prevention of NIDDM. For this it is essential to determine the 'population attributable risk'. Using a univariate approach the relative importance of different individual risk factors can be determined by calculating from the incidence of the exposed (I_e) and nonexposed (I_o) populations and the total population (I_p). Thus, the population attributable risk is:

$$\frac{I_p - I_o}{I_p} = \frac{P_e\,(\mathrm{RR}-1)}{1 + P_e\,(\mathrm{RR}-1)};$$

where P_e = prevalence of the factor in the population; RR = risk ratio I_e/I_o.

The population attributable risk provides a rough estimate of the proportion of the disease that could be eliminated by eliminating the risk factor. The only way to obtain these essential risk estimates is to carry out population-based surveys using standard methods, and, if possible, to follow the survey cohorts longitudinally.

Determinants of NIDDM

1. Genetic susceptibility and the prevention of NIDDM

The risk of NIDDM is determined by genetic factors, social conditions, behavioural patterns and chance. The evidence for an important genetic contribution to the etiology of NIDDM comes from several sources. NIDDM has a strong familial aggregation, and it has been estimated that almost 40% of the siblings of NIDDM patients can expect to develop diabetes assuming a maximum life expectancy of 80 years [7]. Twin studies have shown that there is about 90% concordance for NIDDM in monozygotic twins [8]. Striking differences in NIDDM prevalence between ethnic groups, sometimes even living in the same environment, also speak for a genetic connection [9–12].

It can be argued that environmental factors unmask this susceptibility in genetically predisposed individuals, but specific genetic markers or determinants still remain to be identified. Several markers independent of blood glucose concentration which have been proposed have failed to provide further understanding of this problem [13,14]. This may actually mean that there is no single specific genotype which carries the susceptibility to NIDDM, but that environmental exposures may result in NIDDM in many different genotypes. If this is true, it will have great influence in the choice of strategies for primary prevention of NIDDM, because it implies that it may not be feasible to identify genetically susceptible individuals for potential intervention.

2. Obesity

A strong, graded and consistent association has been demonstrated between obesity and NIDDM. As many as 80% of the NIDDM patients are obese at the time of onset of the disease. The incidence of NIDDM increases exponentially with an increasing degree of obesity. The obese children of diabetic parent(s) have a much higher risk of developing NIDDM than obese persons with non-diabetic parents [15]. Thus, the genetic susceptibility and obesity seem to act synergistically. It is clear that there is heterogeneity in the occurrence of obesity and its impact on insulin resistance and glucose intolerance between populations.

Complications of obesity are shown to be more increased in android (excess fat in upper part of the body) than in gynoid (excess fat in gluteal-femoral parts of the body) obesity [16–18]. The findings from several studies have suggested that this association is more pronounced in women than in men. There is some evidence that subjects with predominantly upper-body fat distribution are more insulin-resistant than equally heavy subjects with predominantly lower-body fat [19].

TABLE 1

The proportion of obese subjects among diabetic subjects in men and women aged 20–59 in 12 populations with high risk of diabetes

Population	Number of diabetic subjects		Proportion of diabetic subjects with high BMI			
	Men	Women	BMI ≥ 27		BMI ≥ 29	
			Men (%)	Women (%)	Men (%)	Women (%)
Cook Islands	20	35	65.0	80.0	50.0	74.3
Niue	22	39	54.5	69.2	40.9	51.3
New Caledonia- Noumea	43	53	83.7	84.9	72.1	79.2
Fiji-Melanesian	13	29	53.8	79.3	30.8	55.2
Fiji-Asian Indian	65	78	21.5	56.4	9.2	37.2
Fiji-Lakeba	11	11	72.7	72.7	36.4	72.7
New Caledonia-Loyalty	9	18	66.7	66.7	33.3	55.6
Western Samoa	25	36	76.0	80.6	68.0	69.4
Tuvalu	3	13	100.0	92.3	100.0	92.3
Nauru	73	78	80.8	96.2	71.2	87.2
Kiribati	79	72	69.6	69.4	50.6	56.9
Nauru -82	140	168	92.9	92.3	84.3	88.1
Malta	40	62	57.5	80.6	42.5	67.7
Total	543	692	70.9	80.6	57.8	70.4

Among the Pacific Island populations [20] and in Malta, for instance, the vast majority of the diabetic subjects were obese at the time of the survey. As a whole 70.9% of diabetic men and 80.6% of diabetic women had a body mass index (BMI) $\geq$ 27.0 kg/m^2, and 57.8% of men and 70.4% of women a BMI $\geq$ 29.0 kg/m^2 (Table 1). In a longitudinal study of Finnish men aged 40–59 years [21], the baseline BMI was a significant predictor of developing diabetes during the subsequent 25-year follow-up. The baseline BMI was a stronger predictor than the change in BMI during the follow-up (Table 2). The effect of BMI on the risk of diabetes was clear in the younger age group, aged 40–49 years at baseline, and slightly less among the 50–54-year-olds. However, the population attributable risk of high BMI at baseline was only about 10%. About 20% of diabetes of these men could have been prevented by keeping the BMI below 27 kg/m^2. Therefore, other factors besides obesity must be evaluated for their potential in primary prevention of NIDDM.

TABLE 2
Risk of diabetes by body mass index in middle-aged Finnish men

Initial body-mass index level (kg/m^2)	Diabetes at 25-year follow-up					
	40–49 yrs		50–59 yrs		Total	
	n	%	n	%	n	%
BMI < 27.0 at baseline	227	18.5	102	32.5	349	22.8
BMI at 15 years						
< 27.0	146	17.1	71	31.0	237	19.0
$\geq$ 27.0	81	21.0	31	35.5	112	25.0
BMI $\geq$ 27.0 at baseline	35	34.3	22	50.0	57	40.4
Total	262	20.6	124	35.5	386	25.4
Population attributable risk for BMI < 27.0 at baseline	11.4%		8.5%		10.2%	
Population preventable fraction for BMI < 27.0 both at baseline and at 15 years	21.4%		16.9%		18.9%	

Only those subjects are included whose fasting time before the oral glucose tolerance test was more than 3 hours and who were examined during the morning hours.

3. Physical inactivity

Regular physical activity improves glucose tolerance in patients with NIDDM through increasing insulin sensitivity [22]. In non-diabetic people the positive effect of physical training on glucose tolerance seems to be only small. It has also been suggested that physical activity could partially prevent the deterioration of glucose tolerance with ageing [23]. At present, epidemiological data on the role of physical activity in the etiology of NIDDM or in the worsening of glucose tolerance are still scarce, but show promise. A lower prevalence of diabetes was found in female former college athletes as compared to non-athletes using a retrospective questionnaire method, with a relative risk of 2.24 [24]. Results from cross-sectional studies suggest that physical inactivity is an independent risk factor of NIDDM [25–27]. In Malta, the age-standardized two-year risk of NIDDM was consistently and inversely related to the level of physical activity (Table 3). The risk of NIDDM was especially high in subjects with a positive family history for NIDDM and who were physically inactive.

TABLE 3

Risk of diabetes in Maltese people by physical activity and family history of diabetes during a two-year follow-up in Malta

Diabetes at follow-up	Baseline situation				
	High or moderate physical activity		Low physical acitivty		Total
	Family history negative (n)	Family history positive (n)	Family history negative (n)	Family history positive (n)	(n)
No	68	17	65	9	159
Yes	12	5	15	5	37
Total	80	22	80	14	196
Incidence of diabetes	15.0%	18.8%	22.7%	35.7%	18.9%
Risk ratio	1.00	1.25	1.51	2.38	
Population attributable risk for:					
Low physical activity			11.7%		
Family history of diabetes and low physical activity together			8.9%		

However, the population attributable risk for physical inactivity was only 11.7% and for the joint effect of family history and inactivity only 9%.

4. Dietary fats

There is good evidence that saturated fatty acids and diets high in saturated fats raise serum cholesterol levels [28]. Diets high in saturated fats also have a blood-pressure-elevating effect [29] and they are associated with insulin resistance, a fore-runner of NIDDM [30]. Himsworth, who first suggested insulin resistance over 50 years ago [31], also suggested that it may have something to do with a diet rich in saturated fats. Surprisingly few data exist about the effects of dietary fats on the development of NIDDM as compared to the studies of effects on serum lipids. Moreover, most of the existing data are from short-term studies. It was suggested that the lower prevalence of diabetes among vegetarian Seventh-Day Adventists in California was related to the reduced fat intake [32]. Recently, much research has been devoted to determining the metabolic effects of different groups of dietary fatty acids. However, only a few studies have examined the intake or composition in serum of fatty acids. Faas et al. [33] reported that diabetic subjects had higher palmitic acid (saturated) and lower linoleic acid (polyunsaturated) concentrations than non-diabetic control subjects. Diets rich in polyunsaturated or monounsaturated fatty acids seem to augment insulin secretion significantly more than a diet comprised primarily of saturated fatty acids [34,35]. The mechanism is unknown, but this ability of unsaturated fatty acids to enhance insulin secretion may in part explain geographic and ethnic differences in the risk of NIDDM.

Hyperinsulinemia and insulin resistance

It is well known that a large proportion of patients with NIDDM also have hypertension, and it has been suggested that hyperinsulinemia is a link between hypertension and glucose intolerance [40,41]. Hypertensive patients seem to exhibit insulin resistance [42] and they also show an inverse correlation between HDL cholesterol concentration and hyperinsulinemia [40].

Reaven and his coworkers, who have further elaborated the hypothesis proposed by Himsworth [31], have even suggested that this 'syndrome X' with multiple metabolic abnormalities leading to cardiovascular disease is really a consequence of insulin resistance [5,36]. This has important implications for the approach to the prevention of NIDDM. Moreover, if we are also aiming at preventing major complications associated with NIDDM, it is indeed necessary to apply a relatively broad approach to tackle multiple metabolic abnormalities, such as hypertension, hypercholesterolemia, obesity, hyperinsulinemia, etc. In most populations in the world this would imply the application of the population strategy for the prevention of non-communicable diseases, which has also been recently proposed by others [43–45].

Obese individuals often produce excessive quantities of insulin after glucose challenge, but insulin seems to be ineffective as glucose tolerance is relatively impaired even in the face of massive hyperinsulinemia. Data from several studies have suggested that these populations at high risk for NIDDM have more hyperinsulinemia than can be accounted for by their adiposity alone [37,38].

In normal-weight individuals, impaired glucose tolerance is a feature of either impaired insulin secretion or insulin resistance. In the obese subjects with IGT, however, insulin resistance is consistently present whereas impaired secretion is not found. However, in people with IGT, low plasma insulin levels after glucose load seem to predict a worsening to NIDDM [39].

Impaired glucose tolerance (IGT) and prevention of NIDDM

It is well documented that people with IGT may worsen to overt diabetes [37,39,46–49]. IGT may be a critical stage in the development of NIDDM, because it is detectable and treatment may prevent or delay its progression. It might be con-

TABLE 4

The risk of diabetes mellitus in people with normal and impaired (IGT) glucose tolerance during a 6-year follow-up in Nauru and during a 2-year follow-up in Malta

Diabetes at follow-up	Glucose tolerance at baseline				
	Nauru			Malta	
	Normal (n)	IGT (n)	Total (n)	Normal (n)	IGT (n)
No	201	38	239	117	40
Yes	14	13	27	18	14
Total	215	51	266	135	54
Incidence of diabetes	6.5	25.5	11.3	13.3%	25.9%
Risk ratio for IGT		3.92		1.95	
Population attributable risk for IGT during the follow-up		42.5%		8.9%	

sidered as the first recognizable stage in the process from genetic susceptibility to NIDDM, and therefore it could be important with regard to the prevention of NIDDM. IGT is, however, a heterogeneous category which contains not only individuals who are indeed either in transition or already at an early stage of NIDDM, but also people whose casual 2-hour blood glucose values are high by random testing only [64]. Recent results from the Finnish study show that in a repeated glucose tolerance test 3 out of 4 subjects with IGT at the first measurement will no longer fulfill the criteria for IGT (Table 4).

IGT is a significant problem in terms of number of people affected. The prevalence of IGT increases with age up to about 65 years, where it may exceed 20% in some populations [21,50,51]. The duration of the IGT phase varies markedly. Some people may stay in this category for a long period, whereas others may develop overt diabetes without this intermediate stage being diagnosed at all. The present criteria for IGT are arbitrary and under debate [52] and the association between the 'baseline' blood glucose level and the subsequent risk of NIDDM is probably linear or exponential without any clear threshold.

The rate of progression from IGT to diabetes is about 2 to 3% per year in studies carried out in the UK and USA (Table 5). In the populations where the occurrence of diabetes was not very high about half of those with IGT seemed to return to normal in a ten-year follow-up [39,46,53–55]. It is likely in populations which have a higher prevalence of diabetes that a greater proportion of those with IGT will develop diabetes [56–58], as shown in Pima Indians [59] and Nauruans [49].

It is noteworthy that a large number of individuals with IGT may not develop NIDDM even in high-risk populations. In Nauru, IGT was associated with a four-fold risk of diabetes over 6 years (Table 6). At baseline about 20% had IGT, and the population attributable risk for developing diabetes was 42.5%, suggesting that

TABLE 5

Value of a casual screening for oral glucose tolerance test in the diagnosis of IGT (Tuomilehto et al., unpublished)

		Standardized, repeated test					
		IGT		Not IGT		Total	
		n	%	n	%	n	%
Screening test	IGT	65	22.8	220	77.2	285	100
	Not IGT	22	5.4	388	94.6	410	100
Total		87	12.5	608	87.5	695	100

screening for IGT could be useful. In Malta, the risk of diabetes among subjects with IGT was less, two-fold. In the Maltese study population over 35 years of age the prevalence of IGT was about 10%, and the population attributable risk for developing diabetes was 8.9%. This indicates that in Malta screening for IGT would detect only a small proportion of new cases of NIDDM that could potentially be prevented, and screening for IGT would probably not be an efficient method of identifying high-risk individuals for preventive measures.

Comment

Until the present time, only a few studies have attempted to test measures for primary prevention of diabetes despite the fact that extensive research into the etiology and natural history of diabetes mellitus has increased our knowledge about different types of diabetes. Too little is known and too few controlled long-term studies have attempted to provide data about preventing the worsening to diabetes in subjects who are considered to be at high risk for NIDDM. Thus, the data base for the potential for primary prevention is still to a great extent indirect. Preventive trials and also community-based prevention programs are needed, especially in the populations where the prevalence of diabetes is known to be high or has clearly increased during recent decades.

TABLE 6
Incidence of diabetes in persons with IGT in different studies

Study	Reference	Treatment	Subjects	Follow-up (years)	Incidence of diabetes/year (%)
Whitehall, UK	53	Yes/No*	204	5	2.6
Malmöhus, Sweden	54	No	59	10	2.9
''		Yes	147	10	1.2
''		No	22	10	3.2
''		Yes	25	10	2.0
Bedford, UK	55	Yes/No*	241	10	1.5
Nauru	56	No	51	6	4.2
Tokyo, Japan	39	No	288	9	1.9
Israel	57	No	83	3	3.7
Pima Indians, USA	58	No	697	5	5.4
'' ''	58	No	411	10	4.8

* In these clinical trials those subjects treated or not treated with hypoglycemic drugs were pooled, as this treatment variable had no significant effect on the outcome.

When choosing the prevention strategy, the most appropriate intervention should try to restore biological normality, i.e. the normal distribution of the outcome parameter. In most situations, such a result can be best achieved by modification of risk factors in the population as a whole, i.e. by the population approach. It can, however, be argued that in NIDDM the whole population distribution of blood glucose does not have to be shifted to the higher levels as is the case with blood pressure distribution with increasing prevalence of hypertension, but it is rather the upper tail of the blood glucose distribution which becomes more pronounced. Thus, if we were able to identify those individuals who are going to be affected the high-risk approach might prove particularly useful. However, according to present knowledge such high-risk individuals may be those who are obese, physically inactive or with a family history of NIDDM. In many populations they are so numerous that they would include more than half of the adult population, and thus it would be unrealistic to assume that the prevention of NIDDM could be solved by the high-risk approach, which is based on individual counselling and treatment.

The focus on glycemic control has resulted in a lack of attention to the other major risk factors of CVD such as high blood pressure, smoking and dyslipidemia, which together with hyperglycemia and hyperinsulinemia determine the fate of people with NIDDM and IGT. There are two possibilities of influencing the natural history of the disease. The first is to identify a risk category (obesity, IGT, etc.) and to start intervention procedures at that relatively late stage (Fig. 1, Alternative A). The main objective of this kind of prevention will be to increase the triggering level of the underlying disease (e.g. symptomatic NIDDM) by specific treatment. Even though it may be possible to postpone the symptomatic stage of the disease, the effect on life-expectancy and severe complications is not always significant. This may explain some of the disappointing findings from studies in diabetes [60] and the fact that some treatments of hypertension have had only a slight effect on the risk of myocardial infarction [61]. The second alternative for prevention is an early, less specific intervention which would slow the progression of the pathophysiological process (e.g. metabolic abnormalities related to diet). Such an intervention may not affect the triggering level of the disease, but would change the natural course of the disease (Fig. 1, Alternative B). This approach has been successfully used in the prevention of CHD, both in clinical trials [62] and in community-based programmes [63]. There may be a positive interaction between the two alternatives for prevention presented here. Thus, in reality one should not attempt to consider either one of them exclusively, but both of them jointly.

In conclusion, the dream of primary prevention of NIDDM, which has existed for a long time [2], may only become reality with systematic research efforts. However, there are good grounds for believing that we know enough about the determinants and natural history of NIDDM to actually attempt the prevention of NIDDM.

Preventing or delaying end-points: Alternative A

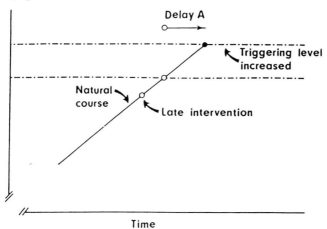

Preventing or delaying end-points: Alternative B

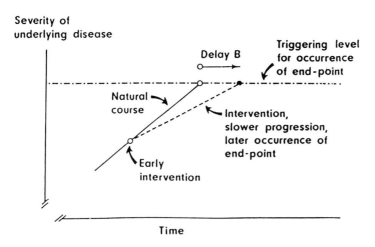

Fig. 1. Two different ways of preventing disease end-points (e.g. NIDDM). Alternative A describes the mode of prevention based on the increase in the triggering level of an end-point (symptomatic hyperglycemia/diabetic complications), and Alternative B the effect of an early intervention which would result in a slower progression of the underlying pathogenetic process.

While controlled unifactorial and multifactorial trials may be an important step on the way towards preventing NIDDM, population-based programs to address the issue of multiple metabolic disorders, including glucose intolerance, will very likely be the real solution. Through the healthier lifestyles of individuals and health promotion in the community the prevalence and the rate of complications of NIDDM may be reduced, keeping in mind that the eradication of NIDDM is clearly utopian.

References

1. Zimmet P. Type 2 (non-insulin-dependent) diabetes – an epidemiological overview. Diabetologia 1982;22:399–411.
2. Joslin EP. The prevention of diabetes mellitus. JAMA 1921;76:79–84.
3. Tuomilehto J, Wolf E. Primary prevention of diabetes mellitus. Diabetes Care 1987;10:238–248.
4. Reahy LJ, Bonner-Weir GC. Minimal chronic hyperglycemia is a critical determinant of impaired insulin secretion after an incomplete pancreatectomy. J Clin Invest 1988;81:1407–1414.
5. Reaven GM. Role of insulin resistance in human disease. Diabetes 1988;37:1595–1607.
6. Editorial. Type 2 diabetes or NIDDM: looking for a better name. Lancet 1989;i:589–591.
7. Köbberling J, Tillil H. Empirical risk figures for first-degree relatives of non-insulin-dependent diabetes. In: Köbberling J, Tattersall R, eds. The genetics of diabetes mellitus. London: Academic Press, 1982:201–210.
8. Barnett AH, Eff C, Leslie RDG, Pyke DA. Diabetes in identical twins – a study of 200 pairs. Diabetologia 1981;20:87–93.
9. West KM. Epidemiology of diabetes and its vascular lesions. New York: Elsevier, 1978.
10. King H, Zimmet P, Bennett P, Taylor R, Raper LR. Glucose tolerance and ancestral genetic admixture in six semi-traditional Pacific populations. Genetic Epidemiol 1984;1:315–328.
11. Zimmet P. Epidemiology of diabetes mellitus. In: Ellenberg M, Rifkin H (eds). Diabetes mellitus – theory and clinical practice, 3rd edn. New York: Med Exam Pub Co Inc, 1983;451–468.
12. Ekoe J-M. Recent trends in prevalence of diabetes mellitus syndrome in the world. Diabetes Res Clin Pract 1986;1:249–264.
13. Rotwein PS, Chirgwin J, Province M, et al. Polymorphism in the 5'-flanking region of the human insulin gene: a genetic marker for non-insulin dependent diabetes. N Engl J Med 1983;308:65–71.
14. O'Rahilly S, Wainscoat JS, Turner RC. Type 2 (non-insulin dependent) diabetes mellitus. New genetics for old nightmares. Diabetologia 1988;31:407–414.
15. Knowler WC, Pettit DJ, Savage PJ, Bennett PH. Diabetes in Pima Indians: contributions of obesity and parental diabetes. Am J Epidemiol 1981;113:114–156.
16. Vague J. The degree of masculine differentiation of obesities: a factor determining predisposition to diabetes, arteriosclerosis, gout and uric calculus disease. Am J Clin Nutr 1956;4:20–34.
17. Larsson B, Svärdsudd K, Welin L, et al. Abdominal adipose tissue distribution, obesity, and risk of cardiovascular disease and death: 13 year follow up of participants in the study of men born in 1913. Br Med J 1984;288:1401–1404.
18. Stern MP, Haffner SM. Body fat distribution and hyperinsulinemia as risk factors for diabetes and cardiovascular disease. Arteriosclerosis 1986;6:123–130.
19. Krotkiewski M, Björntorp P, Sjöström L, Smith U. Impact of obesity on metabolism in men and women: importance of regional adipose tissue distribution. J Clin Invest 1983;72:1150–1162.
20. Zimmet P, Taylor R, King H. Diabetes in the Pacific: an epidemiological perspective. In: Eschwège E, ed. Advances in diabetes epidemiology, INSERM Symposium No. 22. New York: Elsevier, 1982.

21. Tuomilehto J, Nissinen A, Kivelä S-L, et al. Prevalence of diabetes mellitus in elderly men aged 65 to 84 years in eastern and western Finland. Diabetologia 1986;29:611–615.

22. Kemmer FW, Berger M. Exercise and diabetes mellitus: physical activity as a part of daily life and its role in the treatment of diabetic patients. Int J Sports Med 1983;4:77–88.

23. Seals DR, Hagberg JM, Allen WK, et al. Glucose tolerance in young and older athletes and sedentary men. J Appl Physiol 1984;56:1 521–1 535.

24. Frisch RE, Wyshak G, Albright TE, Albright NL, Schiff I. Lower prevalence of diabetes in female former college athletes compared with nonathletes. Diabetes 1986;35:1 101–1 105.

25. Taylor R, Ram P, Zimmet P, Raper LR, Ringrose H. Physical activity and prevalence of diabetes in Melanesian and Indian men in Fiji. Diabetologia 1984;27:578–582.

26. Cederholm J, Wibell L. Glucose tolerance and physical activity in a health survey of middle-aged subjects. Acta Med Scand 1985;217:373–378.

27. Berntorp K, Lindgärde F. Impaired physical fitness and insulin secretion in normoglycaemic subjects with familial aggregation of type 2 diabetes mellitus. Diabetes Res 1985;2:151–156.

28. Keys A, Anderson JT, Grande F. Serum cholesterol response to changes in the diet. Metabolism 1965;14:747–787.

29. Puska P, Iacono JM. Blood pressure and dietary fat. In: Bulpitt CJ, ed. Handbook of hypertension, Vol. 6: Epidemiology of hypertension. Amsterdam: Elsevier 1985;230–248.

30. Ferrannini E, Barret EJ, Bevilacqua S, DeFronzo RA. Effect of fatty acids on glucose production and utilisation in man. J Clin Invest 1983;72:1 737–1 747.

31. Himsworth HP. Diet and incidence of diabetes mellitus. Clin Sci 1935;2:117–148.

32. Philips RL, Lemon FR, Beeson WL, Kuzma JW. Coronary heart disease mortality among Seventh-day Adventists with differing dietary habits: a preliminary report. Am J Clin Nutr 1978;31:S191–S198.

33. Faas Fh, Dang AQ, Norman J, Carter WJ. Red blood cell and plasma fatty acid composition in diabetes mellitus. Metabolism 1988;37:711–713.

34. Lardinois CK, Starich GH, Mazzaferri EL, DeLett A. Polyunsaturated fatty acids augment insulin secretion. J Am Coll Nutr 1987;6:507–515.

35. Eck M, Wynn JO, Carter WJ, et al. Fatty acid desaturation in experimental diabetes mellitus. Diabetes 1979;28:479–485.

36. Golay A, Swislocki ALM, Chen YD-I, Reaven GM. Relationship between plasma free fatty acid concentration, endogenous glucose production and fasting hyperglycemia in normal and non-insulin dependent diabetic individuals. Metabolism 1987;36:692–696.

37. Bennett PH, Knowler WC, Pettitt DJ, Carraher MJ, Vasquez B. Longitudinal studies of the development of diabetes in the Pima Indians. In: Eschwège E, ed. Advances in diabetes epidemiology. Amsterdam: Elsevier, 1982;65–74.

38. King H, Zimmet P, Pargeter K, Raper LR, Collins V. Ethnic differences in susceptibility to noninsulin-dependent diabetes: a comparative study of two urbanized Micronesian populations. Diabetes 1984;33:409–415.

39. Kadowaki T, Miyake Y, Hagura R, et al. Risk factors for worsening to diabetes in subjects with impaired glucose tolerance. Diabetologia 1984;26:44–49.

40. Fuh MM-T, Shieh S-M, Wu D-A, Chen Y-DI, Reaven GM. Abnormalities of carbohydrate and lipid metabolism in patients with hypertension. Arch Int Med 1987;147:1 035–1 038.

41. Modan M, Halkin H, Almog S, et al. Hyperinsulinemia. A link between hypertension, obesity and glucose intolerance. J Clin Invest 1985;75:809–817.

42. Ferranini E, Buzzigoli G, Bonadona R, et al. Insulin resistance in essential hypertension. N Engl J Med 1987;317:350–358.

43. Grabauskas V, Tuomilehto J. Integration of diabetes control with other non-communicable diseases.

In: Tuomilehto J, Zimmet P, King H, Pressley M, eds. Diabetes mellitus, primary health care prevention and control. Singapore: International Diabetes Federation, International Press, 1982;51–60.

44. Glasunov IS, Grabauskas V, Holland WW, Epstein FH. An integrated programme for the prevention and control of noncommunicable diseases. A Kaunas report. J Chron Dis 1983;36:419–426.

45. Epstein FH, Holland W. Prevention of chronic diseases in the community – one-disease versus multiple-disease strategies. Int J Epidemiol 1983;12:135–137.

46. Crombie DL, Pike LA, Malins JM, FitzGerald MG, Goodwin RP, Thompson J. Ten-year follow-up report on Birmingham Diabetes Survey of 1961. Br Med J 1976;2:35–37.

47. Hawthorne VM, Cowie CC. Some thoughts on early detection and intervention in diabetes mellitus. J Chronic Dis 1984;37:667–669.

48. O'Sullivan JB, Mahan CM. Blood sugar levels, glycosuria and body weight related to development of diabetes mellitus. JAMA 1965;194:117–122.

49. Sicree R, Zimmett P, King H, Coventry J. Plasma insulin response among Nauruans: prediction of deterioration in glucose tolerance over 6 years. Diabetes 1987;36:179–186.

50. Zimmet P, Taylor R, Ram P, et al. Prevalence of diabetes and impaired glucose tolerance in the biracial (Melanesian and Indian) population of Fiji: a rural-urban comparison. Am J Epidemiol 1983;118:673–688.

51. Harris MI, Hadden WC, Knowler WC, Bennett PH. Prevalence of diabetes and impaired glucose tolerance and plasma glucose levels in U.S. population aged 20–74 yr. Diabetes 1987;36:523–534.

52. Jarrett RJ. Do we need IGT? Diabetic Med 1987;4:544–545.

53. Jarrett RJ, Keen H, Fuller JH, McCartney P. Worsening to diabetes in men with impaired glucose tolerance ('borderline diabetes'). Diabetologia 1979;16:25–30.

54. Sartor G, Schersten B, Carlstrom S, Melander A, Norden A, Persson G. Ten-year follow-up of subjects with impaired glucose tolerance: prevention of diabetes by tolbutamide and diet regulation. Diabetes 1980;29:41–49.

55. Keen H, Jarret RJ, McCartney P. Ten year follow-up of the Bedford survey (1962–1972): glucose tolerance and diabetes. Diabetologia 1982;22:73–78.

56. King H, Zimmet P, Raper LR, Balkau B. The natural history of impaired glucose tolerance in the Micronesian population of Nauru: a six year follow-up study. Diabetologia 1984;26:39–43.

57. Modan M, Karasik A, Halkin H, et al. Effect of past and concurrent body mass index on prevalence of glucose intolerance and type 2 (non-insulin-dependent) diabetes and on insulin response: the Israel study of glucose intolerance, obesity and hypertension. Diabetologia 1986;29:82–89.

58. Knowler WC, Pettitt DJ, Everhart JR, Slaine KS, Bennett PH, Mott D. Rate of deterioration of impaired glucose tolerance to diabetes and the effects of age, obesity, and serum insulin (abstract). Diabetologia 1986;29:558a.

59. Knowler WC, Bennett BH, Hamman RF, Miller M. Diabetes incidence and prevalence in Pima Indians: a 19-fold greater incidence than in Rochester, Minnesota. Am J Epidemiol 1978;108:497–504.

60. University Group Diabetes Program. Mortality results. Diabetes 1970;19(Suppl 2).

61. Macmahon SW, Cutler JA, Furberg CD, Payne GH. The effects of drug treatment for hypertension on morbidity and mortality from cardiovascular disease: a review of randomised controlled trials. Prog Cardiovasc Dis 1986;24(suppl 1):99–118.

62. Hjerman I, Velve Byre K, Holme I, Leren P. Effect of diet and smoking intervention on the incidence of coronary heart disease. Report from the Oslo study group of a randomized trial in healthy men. Lancet 1981;ii:1303–1310.

63. Puska P, Nissinen A, Salonen JT, et al. The community-based strategy to prevent coronary heart disease: conclusions from the ten years of the North Karelia project. Annu Rev Public Health 1985;6:147–193.

Screening for non-insulin-dependent diabetes mellitus

Frontiers of diabetes research: current trends in non-insulin-dependent diabetes mellitus
K.G.M.M. Alberti and R. Mazze, editors

CHAPTER 8

Screening for undiagnosed non-insulin-dependent diabetes

MAUREEN I. HARRIS

National Diabetes Data Group and World Health Organization Collaborating Center for Diabetes, National Institute of Diabetes and Digestive and Kidney Diseases, National Institutes of Health, Westwood Building, Room 620, Bethesda, MD 20892, U.S.A.

Introduction

Over the past decade, the scope of non-insulin-dependent diabetes (NIDDM) in the United States and its extensive impact on the American people have become more fully appreciated [1]. NIDDM is a highly prevalent disorder whose morbidity and mortality are excessive, and any efforts to control or prevent its impact would be welcome. One method to be considered for such control and prevention is to detect NIDDM in its early stages in order to institute appropriate treatment, including pharmacological therapy and behavioral and lifestyle changes. This report presents a discussion of factors in favor of such screening.

In the past, screening for NIDDM has been controversial because of five issues:

1. Lack of a consensus on definitions of diabetes and diagnostic criteria for the various types of the disease;

2. Lack of accurate information about prevalence of NIDDM, both diagnosed and undiagnosed, in the population;

3. Lack of appreciation for the morbidity that persons with undiagnosed NIDDM incur before their diagnosis;

4. Lack of understanding regarding the identity, magnitude and effect of risk factors for complications of NIDDM;

5. Lack of methods to modify risk factors or to intervene effectively in the pathogenesis of NIDDM.

These five factors are indeed formidable deterrents to screening for NIDDM. However, in the past decade, significant advances have been made so that each of these controversies has been diminished or eliminated entirely, and a position can now be taken to endorse screening for NIDDM. The following data support this position.

Definitions of diabetes and diagnostic criteria for the various types of the disease

Significant research in England and the United States during the 1960s and 1970s was directed toward this topic [2–6]. These studies involved long-term observations on adults who had been administered oral glucose tolerance tests, and the findings were that the renal and retinal complications of diabetes were almost exclusively confined to individuals whose 2-h glucose values were ≥ 200 mg/dl (11.1 mmol/l). Based on these results, the National Diabetes Data Group (NDDG) of the National Institutes of Health and the World Health Organization (WHO) promulgated recommendations for definition of NIDDM and diagnostic criteria which are now widely accepted [7–9]. These are shown in Table 1.

TABLE 1

Definition and diagnostic criteria for NIDDM recommended by the National Diabetes Data Group [7] and the World Health Organization [8,9]

Definition:
   Hyperglycemia meeting diagnostic criteria shown below
   Insulin levels may be decreased, increased, or normal
   Often characterized by hyperinsulinemia and insulin resistance
   Patients are not ketosis-prone under basal conditions
   Patients may require insulin for control of symptoms or fasting hyperglycemia
   Onset is generally after age 40, but may occur at any age
   Most patients are obese
   Includes patients with onset of diabetes in youth or young adulthood from families in which dominant
      inheritance of NIDDM appears to occur

Diagnostic criteria:
   (A) Classical symptoms of diabetes together with abnormal plasma glucose values
or (B) Fasting plasma glucose ≥ 140 mg/dl*
or (C) Plasma glucose ≥ 200 mg/dl at 2 h after 75 g oral glucose challenge**

* 97% of those with fasting plasma glucose ≥ 140 mg/dl in the 1976–80 U.S. National Health and Nutrition Examination Survey also have plasma glucose ≥ 200 mg/dl at 2 h after a 75 g oral glucose challenge (criterion C).
** The National Diabetes Data Group criteria stipulate that the plasma glucose value at 0.5, 1 or 1.5 h after 75 g oral glucose should also be ≥ 200 mg/dl; however, in practice, 95% of persons meeting the 2-h criteria also have midtest values ≥ 200 mg/dl. Only 25% of persons with 2-h values ≥ 200 mg/dl have fasting plasma glucose ≥ 140 mg/dl.

It is unlikely that criterion A would be encountered in a screening situation, since the severe symptoms characteristic of diabetes would already have led to a diagnosis. This seems to be the primary route by which most persons with NIDDM are identified, that is, they are already quite symptomatic. Criterion B is inadequate in a screening situation, since only 25% of persons with undiagnosed NIDDM have fasting plasma glucose $\geq$ 140 mg/dl (7.8 mmol/l) [10]. Consequently, criterion C is the most desirable to use for screening. In sum, the first controversy appears to have been eliminated, since a consensus now exists on definitions and diagnostic criteria for NIDDM that has its basis in sound scientific research.

Accurate information about prevalence of NIDDM, both diagnosed and undiagnosed, in the population

Since the NDDG/WHO recommendations on diagnostic criteria, there has been an explosion of new studies worldwide using the 75 g oral glucose challenge. The findings show that significant proportions of adults meet criteria for NIDDM but have not yet been diagnosed. They also indicate that undiagnosed NIDDM is widespread, affecting not only urban industrialized nations but also rural underdeveloped countries. In the United States, 3.4% of adults aged 20–74 years have been diagnosed as having diabetes and 3.4% meet oral glucose tolerance test criteria for diabetes but have not been diagnosed [11] (Table 2). Hence there are as many cases that have not been diagnosed as cases that have, and undiagnosed diabetes represents 50% of all

TABLE 2

Relative prevalence of diagnosed and undiagnosed NIDDM in U.S. populations aged 20–74 years

Population	Percent with diagnosed diabetes	Percent with undiagnosed diabetes	Undiagnosed as percent of total diabetes
Total U.S.			
Both sexes	3.4	3.4	50
Male	2.9	3.0	51
Female	3.8	3.9	50
White	3.2	3.2	51
Black	5.3	4.8	47
Mexican American	5.4	4.1	43

Data are derived from the U.S. National Health and Nutrition Examination Survey (1976–80) [11] and the Hispanic Health and Nutrition Examination Survey (1982–84) [12]. Diagnosed diabetes is defined as having a medical history of diabetes diagnosed by a physician. Undiagnosed diabetes is defined using criteria B and C from Table 1 for persons with no medical history of diabetes.

diabetes. When these rates are applied to the current population, there are over 5 million adults in the United States who have diabetes but do not know it. For Blacks and Mexican Americans, higher rates of NIDDM are found, but essentially half of diabetes is undiagnosed in these populations also (Table 2).

Prevalence of NIDDM is even greater than indicated in Table 2 when specific age groups are considered. As shown in Fig. 1, the rate is low at the youngest ages, and about 5% have undiagnosed diabetes at age 45–54 years. Among older ages, however, as many as 10% of persons have undiagnosed diabetes. Certain other high-risk populations can be identified when family history of diabetes and obesity, in addition to

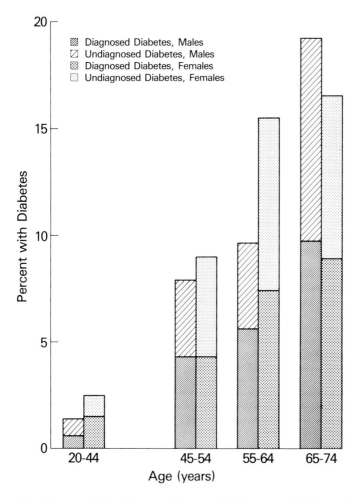

Fig. 1. Percent of the U.S. population aged 20–74 years with diagnosed and undiagnosed diabetes, NHANES II, 1976–80 (Ref. 11).

age, are considered in screening for NIDDM. The recommended screening test would involve administering a 75 g oral glucose challenge, taking a 2-h blood sample, and measuring glucose concentration, with 200 mg/dl being the cutoff to define diabetes. In Table 3, all persons aged 20–74 years serve as the reference population, constituting 100% of the group. If screening were conducted in this age group, 3.4% would be found to have undiagnosed NIDDM, and this would detect 100% of all undiagnosed diabetics aged 20–74 years. If screening were restricted to persons aged 40–74 years, only 53% of the population would have to be screened. The yield of positive screenees would rise to 6.3%, an 85% increase over a rate of 3.4%. Few diabetics would be missed, since 93% of persons with undiagnosed NIDDM are aged 40–74 years. Family history of diabetes appears to be an inadequate screening factor. If screening is conducted in those aged 20–74 years who report having a family history of diabetes, 24% of the population would have to be tested and the positive screenee rate would be 5.7%, but only 37% of persons with undiagnosed NIDDM would be detected. Thus 63% of persons would not be detected, and this does not appear to be a desirable situation.

TABLE 3
Screening for undiagnosed NIDDM in U.S. populations

Screened group	Percent of all persons aged 20–74 yr	Percent with undiagnosed NIDDM	Percent of all undiagnosed NIDDM aged 20–74 yr
All races			
Age 20–74	100	3.4	100
Age 40–74	53	6.3	93
Age 20–74 and family history of diabetes	24	5.7	37
Age 20–74 and PDW $\geq$ 120%	34	6.7	64
Age 40–74 and PDW $\geq$ 120%	22	10.0	61
Age 40–74 and PDW $\geq$ 140%	8	16.2	37
Age 40–74 and PDW $\geq$ 140% and family history of diabetes	3	28.5	20
Black			
Age 20–74	100	5.0	100
Age 40–74	52	9.7	96
Mexican American			
Age 20–74	100	4.4	100
Age 40–74	36	10.0	82

PDW (percent desirable weight) $\geq$ 120% is equivalent to BMI $\geq$ 27 for men and $\geq$ 25 for women [7].
Data are derived from the U.S. National Health and Nutrition Examination Survey (1976–80) and the Hispanic Health and Nutrition Examination Survey (1982–84) [11,12].

Yields of positive screenees can be increased even more, but a greater proportion of missed cases will occur. Compared with testing persons aged 20–74 years, if obesity is added as a criterion (i.e., only persons who are both aged 20–74 years and 20% over ideal body weight are screened) 34% of the population would have to be tested, 6.7% would be found positive for diabetes, and 64% of diabetics would be discovered. If age 40–74 years and 120% of ideal body weight were simultaneously used as screening criteria, only one-fifth of the population would be tested, one in 10 would be found to have undiagnosed diabetes, and 61% of NIDDM would be discovered. Raising the obesity level to 140% of ideal body weight for persons aged 40–74 years eliminates 92% of the population from the group needing to be screened. Sixteen percent of screenees would be found to have diabetes, but only 37% of diabetics would be captured. Finally, if family history were added to this combination of screening criteria, only 3% of adults would have to be screened, 28.5% of these would be diabetic, but only 20% of cases would be detected.

Blacks and Mexican Americans have rates of NIDDM that are greater than those in the general population [11,12]. For Blacks, the rate of undiagnosed diabetes at age 20–74 years is 5% (Table 3). If screening were restricted to persons aged 40 years and older, only 52% of Blacks would have to be screened, the rate of positive screenees would rise to 9.7%, and 96% of all Blacks with undiagnosed diabetes would be detected. For Mexican Americans, the underlying rate is 4.4%. If persons aged 40 years and older were screened, only 36% of persons would be screened, 10% would be found to have undiagnosed diabetes, and this would capture 82% of all cases.

Which of these groups would be the best group to screen? This is a decision to be made by those organizing the screening, but there are certainly sufficient data to document any position one wishes to take. In sum, the second controversy appears to have been eliminated, for there are now very good data on prevalence of undiagnosed NIDDM in the population.

Where should screening take place? An appropriate location is offices of physicians providing primary medical care. Data from the U.S. National Ambulatory Medical Care Survey indicate that over 600 million visits are made to office-based physicians in the United States each year. Of these, 268 million are to primary-care physicians, sites that would be ideal for diabetes screening. An additional location is the offices of obstetricians and gynecologists, which many women use as their only source of primary medical care; 57 million visits were made to these physicians during 1985. Literally millions of blood glucose measurements are conducted annually. In 1985, there were 24 million such tests conducted during visits to office-based physicians in which the patient did not have a medical history of diabetes. Thus, there is ample opportunity to screen for diabetes during the regular primary medical care provided by U.S. physicians.

Morbidity incurred by persons with undiagnosed NIDDM before diagnosis

Undiagnosed diabetes is not, by any means, a benign condition. Indeed, significant morbidity is often present at diagnosis. Table 4 presents data on the prevalence of retinopathy at diagnosis of NIDDM and shows that up to 29% of newly diagnosed patients present with this complication. Jarrett [20] has developed an estimate of the minimum duration of NIDDM necessary before retinopathy, which is probably the earliest developing complication of NIDDM, becomes evident. He followed 240 men with IGT in the Whitehall study, and screened them for NIDDM during 10 years. He found that retinopathy began developing 5 years after onset of diabetes. It has been estimated by others that diabetes remains undiagnosed for approximately 10 years in an unscreened population. If this is true, and if there is no retinopathy during the first 5 years after onset of diabetes, then in the second 5 years retinopathy is developing during a time when diabetes is totally untreated. Undoubtedly, other morbidity is also occurring during the period after onset and before diagnosis, since a number of studies have shown that a significant percentage of patients have micro- and macrovascular complications at the time of diagnosis, as illustrated in Table 4. We may be very remiss in not detecting persons with undiagnosed diabetes in order to institute appropriate therapy.

Identity, magnitude and effect of risk factors for complications of NIDDM

Most people familiar with diabetes agree that hyperglycemia is a necessary, although

TABLE 4
Prevalence of retinopathy at diagnosis of NIDDM

	Percent with retinopathy	Reference
Patients at the University of Wales College of Medicine, Cardiff	29.0	13
Patients in the U.K. NIDDM Prospective Diabetes Study	23.8	14
Non-Hispanic Whites in Colorado	16.7	15
Non-Hispanic Whites in Texas	14.2	16
Mexican Americans in Colorado	18.8	15
Mexican Americans in Texas	15.7	16
Patients at the Birmingham General Hospital Clinic, U.K. (age 30+)	8.0	17
Chinese in Jiaxianqiao area	6.8	18
Micronesians in Nauru	5.9	19

126

perhaps not sufficient, condition leading to development of the complications of diabetes. Fig. 2 illustrates therapies currently used to control blood glucose levels in persons with NIDDM in the United States. Approximately 26% are treated with insulin, 35% with oral agents, 14% with diet alone, and the remaining 25% with none of these therapies. In practice, however, most people with NIDDM are receiving no pharmacological or dietary treatment for the disease. When people with undiagnosed diabetes are taken into account, only 13% of those with NIDDM are taking insulin, only 18% are using oral agents, 7% are using a diet alone, and the remaining 62% are receiving no therapy. This latter group includes those who have not been diagnosed, representing 50% of all persons with NIDDM, who are receiving no medical treatment *in any form* for their diabetes.

Numerous studies have suggested that development of microvascular complications in NIDDM is directly correlated with the degree of glycemia, and many people believe that strict control of blood glucose will reduce the frequency of these complications. Virtually all diabetologists now endorse the goal of improved glycemic control when this can be attained by the nonpharmacological interventions of dietary and lifestyle modification, which convey little risk to the patient. Many also endorse use of oral antidiabetic therapy and insulin in patients whose blood glucose levels cannot be maintained at an appropriate level with dietary therapy alone. Indeed, as

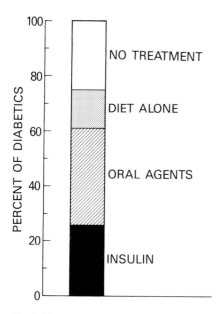

Fig. 2. Therapy for blood glucose control in patients with diagnosed diabetes aged 20–74 yrs, NHANES II, 1976–80 (Ref. 1).

shown in Fig. 2, 60% of patients with established NIDDM are being treated pharmacologically. However, blood glucose levels in patients with NIDDM are far from satisfactory. Table 5 presents data on blood glucose control in persons with NIDDM
from recently published studies. Values in the nondiabetic U.S. population are shown
in the first line and for those with NIDDM in the remaining lines. It is obvious that
values for persons with established diabetes, who have fasting glucose ranging from
164 to 224 mg/dl, elevated 2-h or postprandial glucose and glycosylated hemoglobin

TABLE 5

Plasma glucose values of adults without diabetes and with NIDDM

	Mean plasma glucose (mg/dl)		Glycosylated hemoglobin	Reference
	Fasting	Nonfasting		
Without diabetes				
Representative sample of nondiabetic adults, U.S.	91	97*	ca. 5–7%	11,21
Patients with established diabetes				
Hospital outpatient department, Boston	199		8.5%	22
Hospital outpatient clinic, Indiana	217	332**	10.7%	23
Hospital outpatient clinic, Missouri	224			24
Community patients, Michigan	30% > 180		9.5%	25
Community patients, Wisconsin			9.6%	21
Navajo Indians, Arizona		245**		26
WHO Multinational Study (age 35+)				27
Using insulin	221			
Not using insulin	164			
Primary health care centers, Stockholm, Sweden			9.4%	28
Representative sample of patients, Western Australia		180**	10.7%	29
Known diabetic patients, Nauru		352		19
Newly diagnosed patients, U.K.	205			30
Undiagnosed NIDDM detected during screening				
Population sample, U.S.	132	262*		11
Population sample, Israel			7.8%	31
Population sample, Nauru		289*		19

* 2 h after 75 g oral glucose.
** Postprandial or random glucose.

well above the normal range, are significantly higher than those of nondiabetics. The last section of Table 5 shows plasma glucose concentrations for persons with undiagnosed NIDDM detected in surveys of three populations. Although their values are lower than those of established diabetics, they are still significantly higher than those of nondiabetics. It is just such subjects, with milder cases of NIDDM, in which the most success in controlling blood glucose might be achieved with nonpharmacological interventions. Therefore, it is possible that greater effectiveness in controlling blood glucose levels might result if screening for undiagnosed diabetes were to occur, so that persons would be detected in the early stages of glucose intolerance and brought under medical care sooner than they currently are.

Many studies have shown that, in addition to glucose, there are two key risk factors for retinopathy. One is duration of diabetes since diagnosis, and evidence has been discussed above for believing that NIDDM often remains untreated for 10 years, during the latter 5 years of which retinopathy is evident. Duration may be a proxy for sustained exposure to elevated blood glucose levels. Hence the effect of duration might be reduced by effective blood glucose control. Duration has been found to be a risk factor in many studies of Caucasians in the United States [16,32,33] and England [17,34] and among Japanese [35], Chinese [18], Micronesians in Nauru [36], Hispanics in Texas [16], Pima Indians [37], Oklahoma Indians [38] and in the WHO Multinational Study [39,40]. The second variable is systolic blood pressure, which is amenable to dietary and pharmacological treatment. Blood pressure has been shown to be a risk factor for retinopathy in many studies of NIDDM. The same two variables, duration of diabetes and systolic blood pressure, have also been documented to be risk factors for proteinuria in a number of populations. They may also be important in the development of neuropathy.

A number of variables are considered to be risk factors for macrovascular disease, which is about twice as frequent in NIDDM as in nondiabetic subjects. These factors include blood pressure, cholesterol, obesity, cigarette smoking, low HDL levels and triglycerides. All of these variables can be modified, and intervention for these risk factors is certainly warranted in persons with diabetes, even if methods for blood glucose control are less than fully successful.

Methods to modify risk factors or to intervene effectively in the pathogenesis of NIDDM

The argument has been put forward that 'little can be done for diabetes, so why should we screen for the disease?' However, much has occurred to make this argument antiquated. Certainly, intervention in risk factors for micro- and macrovascular disease discussed above is possible and is desirable. Some developments in the past

10–15 years that have improved the outlook for 'what we can do for diabetes' are shown in Table 6. This is a formidable list indeed, and its indicates that there is a great deal available for treatment of people with NIDDM, either pharmacologically or with lifestyle and behavioral changes.

Taken together, the data presented above constitute a strong argument that previous deterrents to screening have, to a large extent, been overcome. Should the decision be made to devote resources to screening for undiagnosed diabetes, with concomitant medical treatment, pharmacological therapy and patient education to induce behavioral and lifestyle changes, there exists a sound basis for this decision.

TABLE 6
Advances in treatment and prevention of diabetes and its complications

Purified insulins
Synthesis and manufacture of commercial human insulin
New insulin-delivery devices
Second-generation oral agents
Increased emphasis on tight regulation of blood glucose
New devices and techniques to measure blood glucose
Self-monitoring of blood glucose
Measurement of glycosylated hemoglobin as an indicator of long-term blood glucose control
More eclectic health-care team for management of diabetes
Development of patient education and patient support groups
National certification of qualified diabetes health education programs
Third-party payment for diabetes patient education
Use of therapeutic shoes in diabetic patients
Laser photocoagulation for treatment of retinopathy
Focal laser treatment for diabetic macular edema
Early vitrectomy for diabetic vitreous hemorrhage
Methods for measurement of microalbuminuria
Improved renal dialysis methods
Larger proportion of diabetic patients accepted for renal replacement therapy
Pancreas transplantation
New medications for treatment of elevated blood pressure
National High Blood Pressure Education Program
New medications for treatment of hypercholesterolemia
National Cholesterol Education Program
U.S. Surgeon General's Report on Smoking and Health and the National Smoking Education Program
Intense public pressure against smoking
Clinical trials in progress of aldose reductase inhibitors, ACE-inhibitors, and nonenzymatic glycosylation inhibitors

130

References

1. Harris MI, Hamman RF (eds.). Diabetes in America. DHHS Publication Number NIH 85-1468. Washington DC: U.S. Government Printing Office, August 1985.
2. Birmingham Diabetes Survey Working Party. Ten-year follow-up report on the Birmingham Diabetes Survey of 1961. Br Med J 1976;2:35–37.
3. Jarrett RJ, AlSayeah H. Impaired glucose tolerance – defining those at risk of diabetes complications. Diabetologia 1978;15:243–247.
4. Jarrett RJ, Keen H, Fuller JH, et al. Worsening of diabetes in men with impaired glucose tolerance. Diabetologia 1979;16:25–30.
5. O'Sullivan JB, Mahan CM. Prospective study of 352 young patients with chemical diabetes. N Engl J Med 1968;278:1 038–1 041.
6. Bennett PH, Rushforth NB, Miller M, LeCompte PM. Epidemiologic studies of diabetes in the Pima Indians. Recent Prog Horm Res 1976;32:333–371.
7. National Diabetes Data Group. Classification and diagnosis of diabetes mellitus and other categories of glucose intolerance. Diabetes 1979;28:1 039–1 056.
8. World Health Organization. Report of the Expert Committee on Diabetes. WHO Technical Report Series, No. 646, Geneva, 1980.
9. World Health Organization. Diabetes mellitus – Report of a WHO study group. WHO Technical Report Series, No. 727, Geneva, Switzerland, 1985.
10. Harris MI, Hadden WC, Knowler WC, Bennett PH. International criteria for the diagnosis of diabetes and impaired glucose tolerance. Diabetes Care 1985;8:562–567.
11. Harris MI, Hadden WC, Knowler WC, Bennett PH. Prevalence of diabetes and impaired glucose tolerance and plasma glucose levels in U.S. population aged 20–74 yr. Diabetes 1987;36:523–534.
12. Harris MI. Diabetes in Hispanics, Whites, and Blacks in the U.S. population: epidemiologic correlates. Diabetes Care, submitted for publication.
13. Dolben J, Owens DR, Young S, Vora J, Atiea J, Dean J, Luzio S. Retinopathy at presentation in Type 2 (non-insulin-dependent) diabetic patients. Diabetic Med 1988;5(suppl 2):20.
14. Aldington SJ, Kohner EM, Nugent A. Retinopathy at entry in the United Kingdom prospective diabetes study (UKPDS) of maturity onset diabetes. Diabetic Med 1987;4:355.
15. Hamman RF, Mayer EJ, Moo-Young G, Hildebrandt W. Prevalence of retinopathy among Anglos and Hispanics with noninsulin-dependent diabetes mellitus (NIDDM): the San Luis Valley diabetes study. Diabetes 1988;37 (suppl 1):113A.
16. Haffner SM, Fong D, Stern MP, Pugh JA, Hazuda HP, Patterson JK, Van Heuven WAJ, Klein R. Diabetic retinopathy in Mexican Americans and non-Hispanic whites. Diabetes 1988;37:878–884.
17. Soler NG, Fitzgerald MG, Malins JM, Summers ROC. Retinopathy at diagnosis of diabetes, with special reference to patients under 40 years of age. Br Med J 1969;3:567–569.
18. Lin DQ. The primary and specialized health care for diabetics. WHO Bull 1985;6:11–14.
19. Zimmet P, King H, Taylor R, et al. The high prevalence of diabetes mellitus, impaired glucose tolerance and diabetic retinopathy in Nauru – the 1962 survey. Diabetes Res 1984;1:13–18.
20. Jarrett RJ. Duration of non-insulin-dependent diabetes and development of retinopathy: analysis of possible risk factors. Diabetic Med 1986;3:261–263.
21. Klein R, Klein BEK, Moss SE, Shrago ES, Spennetta TL. Glycosylated hemoglobin in a population-based study of diabetes. Am J Epidemiol 1987;126:415–428.
22. Nathan DM, Singer DE, Godine JE, Harrington CH, Perlmuter LC. Retinopathy in older Type II diabetics. Association with glucose control. Diabetes 1986;35:797–801.
23. Vinicor F, Cohen SJ, Mazzuca SA, et al. Diabeds: a randomized trial of the effects of physician and/ or patient education on diabetes patient outcomes. J Chron Dis 1987;40:345–356.

24. Hopper SV, Miller JP, Birge C, Swift J. A randomized study of the impact of home health aids on diabetic control and utilization patterns. Am J Public Health 1984;74:600–602.
25. Hiss RG. Diabetes in communities. Michigan Diabetes Research and Training Center, University of Michigan Press, Ann Arbor, Michigan, 1986.
26. O'Connor PJ, Fragneto R, Coulehan J, Crabtree BF. Metabolic control in non-insulin-dependent diabetes mellitus: factors associated with patient outcomes. Diabetes Care 1987;10:697–701.
27. West KM, Ahuja MMS, Bennett PH, et al. Interrelationships of microangiopathy, plasma glucose and other risk factors in 3 583 diabetic patients: a multinational study. Diabetologia 1982;22:412–420.
28. Rosenqvist U, Carlson A, Luft R. Evaluation of comprehensive program for diabetes care at primary health-care level. Diabetes Care 1988;11:269–274.
29. Knuiman MW, Welborn TA, McCann VJ, Stanton KG, Constable IG. Prevalence of diabetic complications in relation to risk factors. Diabetes 1986;35:1 332–1 339.
30. Multi-centre study. UK prospective study of therapies of maturity-onset diabetes. I. Effect of diet, sulphonylurea, insulin or biguanide therapy on fasting plasma glucose and body weight over one year. Diabetologia 1983;24:404–411.
31. Modan M, Halkin H, Karasik A, Lusky A. Effectiveness of glucosylated hemoglobin, fasting plasma glucose, and a single post load plasma glucose level in population screening for glucose intolerance. Am J Epidemiol 1984;119:431–444.
32. Dwyer MS, Melton LJ, Ballard DJ, Palumbo PJ, Trautmann JC, Chu CP. Incidence of diabetic retinopathy and blindness: a population-based study in Rochester, Minnesota. Diabetes Care 1985;8:316–322.
33. Klein R, Klein BE, Moss SE, Davis MD, DeMets DL. The Wisconsin epidemiologic study of diabetic retinopathy. III. Prevalence and risk of diabetic retinopathy when age at diagnosis is 30 or more years. Arch Ophthalmol 1984;102:527–532.
34. Burditt AF, Caird FI, Draper GJ. The natural history of diabetic retinopathy. Q J Med 1968;37:303–317.
35. Oohashi H, Mihara T, Hirata Y. Prevalence of diabetic microangiopathy and neuropathy among Japanese diabetics in the Tokyo area: related to the WHO new diagnostic criteria. Tohoku J Exp Med 1983;141 (suppl):367–373.
36. King H, Balkau B, Zimmet P, Taylor R, Raper LR, Borger J, Heriot W. Diabetic retinopathy in Nauruans. Am J Epidemiol 1983;117:659–667.
37. Knowler WC, Bennett PH, Ballintine EJ. Increased incidence of retinopathy in diabetics with elevated blood pressure. N Engl J Med 1980;302:645–650.
38. West KM, Erdreich LJ, Stober JA. Risk factors for retinopathy and nephropathy in diabetes: a detailed study. Diabetes 1980;29:501–508.
39. Jarrett RJ, Keen H. The WHO multinational study of vascular disease in diabetes. 3. Microvascular disease. Diabetes Care 1979;2:196–201.
40. Diabetes Drafting Group. Prevalence of small vessel and large vessel disease in diabetic patients from 14 centers: the World Health Organization multinational study of vascular disease in diabetics. Diabetologia 1985;28:615–640.

CHAPTER 9

To screen or not to screen for NIDDM

DAVID M. NATHAN

Diabetes Unit and Department of Medicine, Massachusetts General Hospital, and Harvard Medical School, Boston, MA, U.S.A.

Introduction

The initial enthusiasm for widespread screening of asymptomatic populations has waned with performance of careful cost/benefit analyses and recognition of limited medical care resources. Careful guidelines for diseases appropriate for screening have emerged based on consideration of the disease incidence and severity, and availability of acceptable, relatively inexpensive screening methods and treatment modalities that are effective in the asymptomatic phase [1–6]. Thus, screening for hypertension, hyperlipidemia and breast and prostate cancers in selected populations is widely accepted as an efficient and relatively inexpensive means of decreasing long-term morbidity and mortality. Other diseases, such as non-insulin-dependent diabetes, albeit highly prevalent and associated with significant morbidity and mortality, have not withstood scrutiny as appropriate disease targets for screening. The purpose of this paper is to review data relevant to the arguments regarding screening for non-insulin-dependent diabetes (NIDDM) in the non-pregnant, asymptomatic population. Screening for gestational diabetes, currently recommended on the basis of demonstrated benefit for the neonate rather than the pregnant mother [7], will not be reviewed here.

Criteria for screening

The six criteria proposed by Frame and Carlson in their thorough review of periodic health screening [1] remain the standards to justify screening for a given disease

134

(Table 1). Further refinements to the criteria have been proposed, such as the use of rules of evidence to evaluate the quality of available data [2]. The Canadian Task Force [2], Institute of Medicine [3], American College of Physicians [4] and the American Medical Association [5] have all used such criteria in recommending specific screening measures.

Does NIDDM satisfy criteria for screening?

Morbidity/mortality
The long-term sequelae of NIDDM are certainly severe enough to merit attention. In addition to contributing as a major source of renal failure [8] and blindness [9] in adults, macrovascular disease associated with NIDDM causes myocardial infarctions [10], stroke [11], and amputations [12]. The Framingham study [13] and others [14,15] have documented the significant risk imparted by NIDDM, including relative risks of 2–3-fold for myocardial infarction and stroke and 4–5-fold for peripheral vascular disease compared with similarly aged non-diabetic populations. NIDDM is associated with a 10-year decrease in life-span.

Incidence
Increasing age and prevalence of obesity, the main risk factors for NIDDM, in the population of industrialized nations have led to a significant increase in the incidence of NIDDM, which ranges from 1 to 10 per 1 000 per year depending on age [16]. Prevalence approaches 10% in the U.S. population over 70 years of age.

TABLE 1
Criteria for screening*

1. Disease must have significant morbidity and/or mortality,

2. High enough incidence to justify the cost of screening, and

3. Asymptomatic phase during which detection and treatment significantly reduce morbidity or mortality.

4. Availability of methods to detect disease in its asymptomatic phase.

5. Availability of acceptable therapy.

6. Treatment of disease during asymptomatic phase must yield a result superior to that obtained by delaying treatment until symptoms appear.

* Adapted from Frame and Carlson [1].

Asymptomatic phase during which treatment is effective
Although the clinical symptoms of diabetes owing to osmotic diuresis, weight loss and dehydration lead to diagnosis of NIDDM in a large number of patients, a similar number of NIDDM patients are diagnosed solely on the basis of blood glucose testing. The National Health and Nutrition Examination Survey II (NHANES II) has estimated that 3% of the U.S. population may have asymptomatic NIDDM [17].

However, whether treatment during the asymptomatic or clinical phase benefits patients with regard to long-term complications has not been demonstrated. The largest clinical trial of treatment of NIDDM, the University Group Diabetes Program (UGDP), could not document any effect of hypoglycemic treatment on long-term outcome [18]. Thus, there are no data to support detection and treatment of asymptomatic patients, if the criterion is demonstrated ability to reduce morbidity and/or mortality.

Detection method
Previous screening studies [19–24] have used a variety of different screening methods, including tests of glycosuria and fasting and post-glucose load blood glucose levels (Table 2). While it is widely acknowledged that post-glucose-load glycemia must be tested in order to detect sensitively the presence of abnormal glucose tolerance, the specific cut-offs to diagnose diabetes versus impaired glucose tolerance versus normal have been debated strenuously (Table 3). Moreover, although a non-physiological stimulus such as the 75-g glucose tolerance test is recognized as necessary to detect NIDDM, highly variable results remain a problem [25]. Finally, although the guidelines adopted by WHO [26] and NDDG [27] are in general agreement, they are not identical [28].

Availability of acceptable therapy
Several hypoglycemic therapies are available and are effective, at least in the short

TABLE 2
Selected studies of screening for NIDDM

Study	*n*	Method
Oxford, USA (1946)	3 516	Glycosuria, 50 g carb. meal
Bergen, NOR (1956)	5 930	Glycosuria or 100 g GTT
Birmingham, UK (1962)	18 532	Glycosuria, 50 g GTT
Bedford, UK (1962)	25 700	Glycosuria, 50 g GTT
Ibstock, UK (1964)	4 379	Glycosuria, 50 g GTT
Cleveland, USA (1963–69)	600 000	75 g GTT
Whitehall, UK (1967–69)	18 403	50 g GTT
NHANES, USA (1976–80)	3 714	75 g GTT

136

TABLE 3
Diagnostic criteria used in screening studies

Study	Diagnostic criteria
Oxford	Venous post-pran. > 170 mg/100 dl
Bergen	Cap. FBG > 120, 2 H > 180 mg/100 dl
Birmingham	Cap. FBG > 130 mg/100 dl
Ibstock	Cap. BG 1 H > 160, 2 H > 120 mg/100 dl
Bedford	Cap. BG 2 H > 120 mg/100 dl
Cleveland	Cap. BG 2 H > 139 mg/100 dl
Whitehall	Cap. BG 2 H > 200 mg/100 dl
NHANES	FPG > 140, 2 H > 200 mg/100 dl

Cap., capillary; FBG, fasting blood glucose; FPG, fasting plasma glucose.

term, at lowering blood glucose levels [29,30]. As noted, the ability of these therapies to reduce long-term complications is unproved.

Demonstration of superior outcome with therapy in asymptomatic phase compared with waiting for symptoms to develop
Hypoglycemic therapy has not been demonstrated to decrease morbidity or mortality in the asymptomatic phase. In fact, the UGDP recruited newly diagnosed (< 1 yr) asymptomatic subjects and therefore represented an intervention study in the asymptomatic phase of NIDDM.

Other arguments for and against screening

In addition to the unproved prospect of decreasing long-term vascular complications, three other putative benefits of detection and treatment of NIDDM in the asymptomatic period have been advanced:
(1) Proponents of screening have suggested that early detection of NIDDM would lead to increased medical care and improved health status. The Cleveland Screening program [31] demonstrated that subjects identified as having NIDDM had more physician contact within two months of diagnosis compared with subjects who screened negative.
(2) Another proposed benefit of diagnosing NIDDM is the added motivation to lose weight in obese patients. The Cleveland program [31] demonstrated significant weight loss (2.88% decrease in average weight) at 3 years in subjects screened positive compared with subjects who screened negative (−0.17% wt loss). The difference in weight loss, however, did not persist at 5 years [24].

(3) The last argument in favor of screening involves the detection of impaired glucose tolerance (IGT) rather than NIDDM. Since IGT is a major risk factor for the development of NIDDM (Fig. 1), investigators have argued that detection and treatment of IGT might decrease the development of NIDDM. Of the three studies to examine this hypothesis, the Bedford [32] and Whitehall [33] studies have not demonstrated a salutary effect of diet with tolbutamide or phenformin, respectively, on the evolution of IGT to NIDDM. The Malmo Study [34] suggested a beneficial effect of tolbutamide, but relied on post-randomization stratification in order to demonstrate any effect of treatment. Further studies are warranted.

The arguments against screening, in addition to the failure to demonstrate a beneficial effect of early detection and treatment, include the adverse social and economic stigma and the negative self-image imparted by the diagnosis (labelling). Although there are few data available on these putative adverse effects, job discrimination and difficulty in purchasing insurance accompany the diagnosis of NIDDM. In addition, the Cleveland Screening Program documented a significantly worse self-image in positive screened subjects compared with negative subjects when examined up to 3 years after diagnosis.

Results of previous screening studies

Although many screening trials are available for examination [19–24], only a few of them have pursued long-term follow-up to determine the impact of identifying a per-

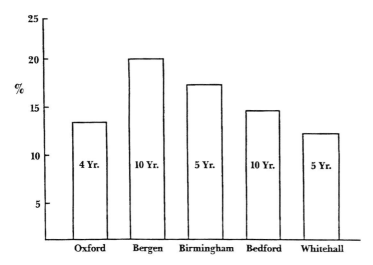

Fig. 1. Progression of IGT to NIDDM in long-term studies. Duration of follow-up noted.

138

son as having diabetes. However, several interesting observations have been made. First, the use of different glucose challenges in different populations has led to estimates of prevalence of from less than 1% to 5% (Fig. 2). Second, the progression of impaired glucose tolerance to diabetes, over a 5–10-year course, is between 14 and 21% (Fig. 1). Third, as noted, diet therapy with or without sulfonylureas or phenformin has not been demonstrated to reduce the progression of IGT to NIDDM. Finally, no obvious health benefit has accrued from the identification of persons as having NIDDM, although their self-perception of health is decreased compared with persons who screen negative.

Conclusion

The failure to demonstrate any benefit of detection and treatment of NIDDM during its asymptomatic phase militates against screening asymptomatic, non-pregnant populations.

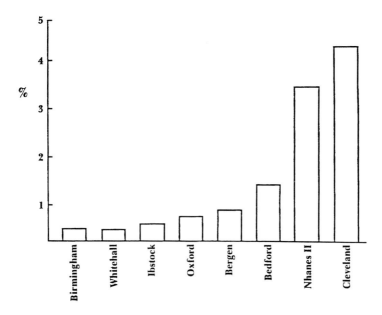

Fig. 2. Prevalence of previously undiagnosed diabetes in screening studies.

References

1. Frame SP, Carlson SJ. A critical review of periodic health screening using specific screening criteria. J Fam Pract 1975;2:123–129.
2. Canadian Task Force Report. The periodic health examination. CMA J 1979;121:1 193–1 254.
3. Fielding JE. Preventive services for the well population, in healthy people – The Surgeon General's Report on Health Promotion and Disease Prevention – Background Papers, US Dept of Health, Education, and Welfare publication (PHS) 79-55071A. Government Printing Office, 1979;277–304.
4. ACP Medical Practice Committee. Periodic health examination: a guide for designing individualized preventive health care in the asymptomatic patient. Ann Int Med 1981;95:729–732.
5. AMA Council on Scientific Affairs. Medical evaluations of healthy persons. JAMA 1983;249:1 626–1 633.
6. Oboler SK, LaForce FM. The periodic physical examination in asymptomatic adults. Ann Intern Med 1989;110:214–226.
7. American Diabetes Association. Gestational Diabetes Mellitus. Diabetes Care 1986;9:430–431.
8. Klein R, Klein BEK. Vision disorders in diabetes. In: NIH Publication No. 85-1468, August, 1985; Diabetes in America. XIII:1–36.
9. Herman WH, Teutsch SM. Kidney diseases associated with Diabetes. In: NIH Publication No. 85-1468, August, 1985; Diabetes in America. XIV:1–31.
10. Barrett-Connor E, Orchard T. Diabetes and Heart Disease. In: NIH Publication No. 85-1468, August 1985; Diabetes in America. XVI:1–41.
11. Kuller LH, Dorman JS, Wolf PA. Cerebrovascular disease and diabetes. In: NIH Publication No. 85-1468, August 1985; Diabetes in America. XVIII:1–18.
12. Palumbo PJ, Melton LJ, III. Peripheral vascular disease. In: NIH Publication No. 85-1468, August 1985; Diabetes in America. XV:1–21.
13. Kannel WB, McGee DL. Diabetes and cardiovascular disease. JAMA 1979;241:2 035–2 038.
14. Nathan DM, Singer DE, Godine JE, Perlmuter LC. Non-insulin-dependent diabetes in older patients. Am J Med 1986;837–842.
15. Singer DS, Moulton AW, Nathan DM. Diabetic myocardial infarction: interaction with other pre-infarction risk factors. Diabetes 1989;38:350–357.
16. Everhart J, Knowler WC, Bennett PH. Incidence and risk factors for non-insulin-dependent diabetes. In: NIH Publication No. 85-1468, August 1985; Diabetes in America. IV:1–35.
17. Harris MI, Hadden WC, Knowler WC, Bennett PH. Prevalence of diabetes and impaired glucose tolerance and plasma glucose levels in the U.S. population aged 20–74 years. Diabetes 1987;36:523–534.
18. University Group Diabetes Program. A study of the effects of hypoglycemic agents on vascular complications in patients with adult-onset diabetes. II. Mortality results. Diabetes 1970;19(Suppl 2):785–830.
19. Wilkerson HLC, Krall LP. Diabetes in a New England town. JAMA 1953;152:1 322–1 329.
20. Brown PE. Early diabetes: A five-year follow-up of diabetes in an English community. Lancet 1964;ii:246–248.
21. Crombie DL, Pike LA, Pinsent RJFH, Fitzgerald MG, Malins JM, Wall M. Five-year follow-up on the Birmingham diabetes survey of 1962. Br Med J 1970;3:301–305.
22. Aspevik E, Jorde R, Raeder S. The diabetes survey in Bergen, Norway, 1956. Acta Med Scand 1974;196:161–169.
23. Reid DD, Brett GZ, Hamilton PJS, Jarrett RJ, Keen H, Rose G. Cardiorespiratory disease and diabetes among middle-aged male civil servants. Lancet 1974;i:469–473.

24. Genuth SM, Houser HB, Carter JR, Merkatz IR, Price JW, Schumacher OP, Wieland RG. Observations on the value of mass indiscriminate screening for diabetes mellitus based on a five-year follow-up. Diabetes 1978;27:377–383.

25. Ganda OP, Day JL, Soeldner JS, Connon JJ, Gleason RE. Reproducibility and comparative analysis of repeated intravenous and oral glucose tolerance tests. Diabetes 1978;27:715–725.

26. Expert Committee on Diabetes Mellitus, World Health Organization; 1980; WHO Technical Report Series 646.

27. National Diabetes Data Group. Classification and diagnosis of diabetes mellitus and other categories of glucose intolerance. Diabetes 1979;1 039–1 057.

28. Massari V, Eschwège E, Valleron AJ. Imprecision of new criteria for the oral glucose tolerance test. Diabetologia 1983;24:100–106.

29. Stanik S, Marcus R. Insulin secretion improves following dietary control of plasma glucose in severely hyperglycemic obese patients. Metabolism 1980;29:346–350.

30. Nathan DM, Roussell A, Godine JG. Glyburide or insulin for metabolic control in non-insulin-dependent diabetes mellitus. Ann Intern Med 1988;108:334–340.

31. Houser HB, Mackay W, Verma N, Genuth S. A three-year controlled follow-up study of persons identified in a mass screening program for diabetes. Diabetes 1977;26:619–627.

32. Keen H, Jarrett RJ, McCartney P. A ten-year follow-up of the Bedford survey (1962–1972): Glucose tolerance and diabetes. Diabetologia 1982;22:73–78.

33. Jarrett RJ, Keen H, Fuller JH, McCartney M. Worsening to diabetes in men with impaired glucose tolerance ('Borderline Diabetes'). Diabetologia 1979;16:25–30.

34. Sartor G, Schersten B, Carlstrom S, Melander A, Norden A, Persson G. Ten-year follow-up of subjects with impaired glucose tolerance. Diabetes 1980;29:41–49.

© 1989 Elsevier Science Publishers B.V. (Biomedical Division)
Frontiers of diabetes research: current trends in non-insulin-dependent diabetes mellitus
K.G.M.M. Alberti and R. Mazze, editors

CHAPTER 10

Glycated hemoglobin: is it a useful screening test for diabetes mellitus?

DAVID E. GOLDSTEIN, RANDI R. LITTLE, JACK D. ENGLAND, HSAIO-MEI WIEDMEYER and EDITH McKENZIE

University of Missouri Health Sciences Center, Departments of Child Health, Medicine, and Pathology, One Hospital Drive, Columbia, MO 65212, U.S.A.

Introduction

Glycated hemoglobin is formed in erythrocytes as the product of a slow, continuous reaction between glucose and hemoglobin. Determination of glycated hemoglobin (GHB) is now widely used in clinical practice to monitor long-term glycemia in persons with diabetes mellitus. Studies indicate that GHB is a reliable index of average blood glucose during the preceding 2–3 months [1–5].

The potential use of GHB for diagnosis of diabetes was suggested more than a decade ago [6–8]. The appeal of the test is that it might provide a more 'true life' measure of a person's glycemic status than an oral glucose tolerance test. In addition, the GHB test requires only a single, small sample of blood collected at any time of the day, without regard to timing of prior food ingestion, recent illness or other factors that are known to affect the oral glucose tolerance test (OGTT) [9]. Many investigators have, in fact, explored the possibility of using GHB for diagnosis and/or screening for diabetes [6–8,10–38]. Results have often been conflicting and difficult to compare because of marked differences in characteristics of patient populations studied, testing procedures and criteria for diagnosis. Regardless of these methodological difficulties, taken together the studies suggest that GHB is not a reliable substitute for the OGTT – the 'gold standard' – for diagnosis of diabetes.

Thus, in 1982 Orchard and colleagues [17] reported on a comparison of the OGTT and GHB for the diagnosis of diabetes. They studied 400 first-degree relatives of patients with insulin-dependent diabetes. All those tested were thought to be free from diabetes. They found that GHB was elevated in only 37% of those found to be diabetic by OGTT. Only 25% of those with either diabetes or impaired glucose tolerance

(IGT) had an abnormal GHB value. The authors found that GHB showed a low sensitivity for diagnosis but a very high specificity (96%); the predictive value of a positive test was only 17.6%, while the predictive value of a negative test was 99%. The authors concluded that "GHB is not a valuable screening instrument for diabetes and impaired glucose tolerance, as currently diagnosed using an OGTT." The authors did speculate that perhaps persons who fit the criteria for non-insulin-dependent diabetes mellitus (NIDDM) based on OGTT, but who have a normal GHB, are not truly diabetic and thus are not at risk for diabetic complications.

In a recent literature review of data on tests of glycemia and diabetes, Singer and associates [38] also concluded that GHB is highly specific as a diagnostic tool but shows only 'modest sensitivity' compared to the OGTT. They calculated that if 50% of diabetics and 3% of non-diabetics had an abnormal GHB result, use of GHB for diagnosis would decrease the need for OGTT by more than 50% (they did not discuss how to deal with the 3% false positives). The authors suggested that since data in the literature show that GHB values below the normal mean are rarely seen in untreated diabetes, screening for diabetes should begin with a GHB test; if the result is below the normal mean value, no further testing is indicated. The authors also suggested that all diagnoses based on elevated GHB results should be confirmed with an OGTT. They 'hedged' a bit on their recommendations, cautioning that assays of GHB vary widely in their precision and that assays have not yet been standardized.

Improvements in diagnostic criteria for diabetes

In the past decade, enormous strides have been made in improving diagnostic criteria for diabetes. In 1979–80 two groups, the National Diabetes Data Group (NDDG) [39] and the World Health Organization (WHO) [40], developed similar criteria for the diagnosis of diabetes. In both systems, the diagnosis requires a fasting plasma glucose value greater than 140 mg/dl (7.8 mmol/l) or a 2-h post 75 g oral glucose load value equal to or greater than 200 mg/dl (11.1 mmol/l). The NDDG criteria for diagnosis of diabetes based on the OGTT are a bit more complicated than those of the WHO, requiring a fasting plasma glucose value of less than 115 mg/dl (6.4 mmol/l) to classify the test as normal; the WHO criteria require only that the level is less than 140 mg/dl. In addition, the NDDG recommends measurement of plasma glucose at 0.5 h, 1 h and 1.5 h after the challenge, while the WHO recommends only two values, fasting and 2-h. For both groups, the category of impaired glucose tolerance (IGT) requires a fasting plasma glucose of less than 140 mg/dl and a 2-h value between 140 and 199 mg/dl (NDDG also requires a mid-test value equal to or greater than 200 mg/dl).

In practical terms, both systems agree closely in classification of OGTTs, with approximately 99% concordance. The main difference is in prevalence of IGT, which is considerably higher using the WHO criteria. To reconcile these differences, in 1985 the NDDG recommended that the WHO system should be used because of its simpler classification scheme [41]. They further recommended that for large-scale field research or screening purposes, a 2-h post-glucose load determination should be used to decide whether a subject has diabetes, IGT or normal glucose tolerance.

Prevalence of diabetes and impaired glucose tolerance in the U.S. population

In order to consider whether GHB might be a more reliable screening test for diabetes than studies have suggested, it is first necessary to examine prevalence data for diabetes based on the OGTT. Data from the Second National Health and Nutrition Examination Survey (NHANES II) conducted by the National Center for Health Statistics (NCHS) during 1976–80 provide perhaps the best estimate of the prevalence of diabetes in the U.S. population aged 20–74 years [42]. Oral glucose tolerance testing was performed on 3 772 people with no history of diabetes. Based on WHO criteria, 3.4% were found to be diabetic, with an age-related increase in prevalence (e.g. 20–44 yr = 0.9%; 65–74 yr = 9.4%). The prevalence of prior diabetes by medical history was nearly identical to the number of previously undiagnosed cases that were discovered, with the total prevalence of diabetes 6.8% in the age range 20–74 years (age 20–44 yr = 2.0%; 45–54 yr = 8.5%; 55–64 = 13.4%; 65–74 = 18.7%). For previously undiagnosed cases, about 75% were diagnosed solely on the basis of the 2-h glucose value; the fasting plasma glucose was elevated in only about 25% of cases.

The prevalence of IGT was 11.2% overall in the age range 20–74 years (age 20–44 = 11.2%; 65–74 yr = 22.8%). The total prevalence of glucose intolerance in the U.S., including people previously diagnosed as diabetic, newly diagnosed cases and IGT, was 18% (about 42% in the age group 65–74 years). Previously diagnosed diabetes contributed to about 30% of the total glucose intolerance, while previously undiagnosed diabetes contributed 28%, and IGT accounted for 42%. Parental history of diabetes or obesity was associated with an approximate two-fold increase in all categories of glucose intolerance; both risk factors increased prevalence nearly four-fold.

Is there a diabetes epidemic?

Assuming that the NHANES II prevalence data are correct, there is, literally, a diabetes epidemic. Yet it has been strongly recommended by many experts in the field that routine screening for diabetes should not be performed except in very special

144

circumstances, such as pregnancy [38,43]. In an attempt to understand why the experts might recommend against routine screening for diabetes, it is necessary first to discuss the general question of screening for disease.

As outlined by Charup in 1981 [44], the basic premises underlying routine screening are as follows:

(1) asymptomatic adults can harbor organic disease,
(2) a periodic health examination (to include medical history, physical examination, and laboratory tests) can detect disease at an early stage,
(3) the discovery of disease can lead to its arrest, reversal or cure, and thereby reduces morbidity and mortality.

While the first two premises have been well substantiated, the third has not, with the exception of diabetes during pregnancy. There are widely differing views among diabetologists as to whether treatment to achieve specific blood glucose goals has any benefit over treatment, which has relief of symptoms as its only goal (the term 'symptoms' here refers both to those caused by hyperglycemia, such as polyuria and polydipsia, and those due to hypoglycemia). For those health professionals who believe that there are insufficient data to substantiate the claim that lowering blood glucose improves outcome, screening for diabetes would seem to have very little merit. If, on the other hand, one believes that treatment beyond relief of symptoms to achieve specific blood glucose goals can improve outcome, then routine screening for diabetes would seem to be strongly indicated.

The critical question of the benefits of treatment for diabetes to lower blood glucose levels is being addressed in a multi-center, large-scale, randomized trial, the Diabetes Control and Complications Trial (DCCT). This study, which began in 1983, includes 1 400 persons with insulin-dependent diabetes mellitus (type I), and will last 10 years [45]. In the DCCT, persons with IDDM, aged 13–39 years, are randomly assigned to one of two treatment groups. The first group is treated to eliminate symptoms of hyperglycemia, while the second group is treated both to eliminate symptoms, and to achieve specific blood glucose goals. No endpoint data are yet available from the DCCT, and the applicability of results to the treatment of NIDDM remains unknown.

In the light of current uncertainty about the benefits of improving glycemic control beyond relief of symptoms, it is not surprising that there is no consensus on screening for diabetes mellitus. Given the lack of data substantiating a clear-cut benefit of improving glycemic control beyond relief of symptoms, some health professionals believe it is ironic that many physicians who do not advocate screening for NIDDM advocate aggressive treatment of IDDM patients. Given the substantial risks of hypoglycemia in IDDM patients and the high cost of intensive treatment efforts, and, by contrast, the minimal risk and relatively low cost of treating NIDDM patients to achieve improved blood glucose levels, perhaps our treatment goals and methods are not entirely rational. Perhaps it is worth readdressing the question of diabetes screening as a necessary public health measure. Out of the enormous number of people diagnosed as having diabetes, is there a way of selecting for those individuals at greatest risk for developing diabetic complications? If those individuals could be identified from screening studies, then perhaps, even given uncertainty about the benefits of treatment to lower blood glucose levels beyond symptom relief, the risk/benefit ratio (probably better stated as the risk/potential benefits ratio) would greatly favor early diagnosis and treatment.

There are, in fact, numerous epidemiological data that provide information concerning levels of glycemia and risks of developing vascular complications of diabetes. The NIH has been conducting epidemiological studies of Pima Indians since 1965. This population has the highest reported prevalence of NIDDM, nearly 50% [46]. Studies in the Pima Indians have shown that the 3-year incidence of retinopathy and proteinuria in diabetic persons was associated with fasting plasma glucose levels above 140 mg/dl (7.8 mmol/l) and 2-h plasma glucose values above 200 mg/dl (11.1 mmol/l) at baseline. Beyond those levels, the higher the plasma glucose level, the greater is the risk of developing the complications [47]. Based on data such as these, if screening for diabetes were to be recommended, it would seem logical to concentrate on individuals with fasting plasma glucose levels above 140 mg/dl (7.8 mmol/l) *and* 2-h postglucose load values above 200 mg/dl (11.1 mmol/l). How could this be accomplished in a simple and cost-effective manner?

GHB revisited

In 1983, our group at the University of Missouri Health Sciences Center, Columbia, MO, began a study with colleagues from the Diabetes and Arthritis Epidemiology Section of the National Institute of Diabetes and Digestive and Kidney Disease in Phoenix, Arizona [48]. The purpose of the study was to evaluate in detail the use of GHB as a screening test for diabetes. Subjects were 381 individuals, most of whom were Pima Indians residing in the Gila River Indian community of central Arizona, who were already participating in the NIH longitudinal epidemiological studies on diabetes and obesity which began in 1965. All subjects underwent a standard OGTT according to WHO recommendations, and at the time of OGTT a blood sample was obtained from the subject for measurement of GHB. GHB was determined with a highly precise, high-performance liquid chromatographic system [49,50].

The mean age of the 381 study subjects was 46 years, with a range of 14–89 years, and the ratio of males to females was 1–1.69. We classified each of the study subjects into one of three OGTT classes, normal (N), impaired glucose tolerance (IGT) or diabetic (D), according to WHO criteria. Table 1 shows the number of subjects in

146

TABLE 1
Classification of study subjects into OGTT classes

| | OGTT classification | | |
	N	IGT	D
HbA$_{1c}$ (%) (mean $\pm$ SD)	5.43 $\pm$ 0.04	5.86 $\pm$ 0.72	8.45 $\pm$ 2.31
Abnormal* HbA$_{1c}$ (n)	14	27	112
Normal* HbA$_{1c}$ (n)	145	64	19
Total subjects (n)	159	91	131

N, normal; IGT, impaired glucose tolerance; D, diabetes mellitus.
Classification is according to WHO criteria.
Normal reference interval for HbA$_{1c}$ = 5.05 $\pm$ 0.50 (mean $\pm$ 2 SD).
*Normal HbA$_{1c}$ $\leqslant$ 6.03 (mean $\pm$ 1.96 SD); abnormal HbA$_{1c}$ > 6.03.

each OGTT class and mean HbA$_{1c}$ for each group. The mean HbA$_{1c}$ values for the three groups were significantly different. Fig. 1 shows the distribution of individual hemoglobin values for the three groups. Of the 159 subjects in the N group, 14 (8.8%) had slightly elevated HbA$_{1c}$ values, but none was more than 3 SD above the normal mean (the highest value was 6.37%). Most individuals classified as diabetic showed markedly elevated HbA$_{1c}$ values, but 19 subjects (15%) showed normal HbA$_{1c}$ values. Of the 91 subjects in the IGT group, only 27 (30%) had elevated HbA$_{1c}$ values. Fig. 2 shows the relationship between fasting and 2-h plasma glucose and HbA$_{1c}$ for subjects classified in the N, IGT and D groups. HbA$_{1c}$ was highly correlated with both fasting and 2-h plasma glucose (r = 0.91 and 0.88, respectively). For D subjects, there was a striking difference in the fasting and 2-h plasma glucose between those with normal HbA$_{1c}$ (n = 19) and those with high HbA$_{1c}$ (n = 112); in the D patients with normal HbA$_{1c}$ values, only one of 19 subjects had a fasting plasma glucose above 140 mg/dl (146 mg/dl). The mean fasting plasma glucose was almost 100 mg/dl lower in the normal HbA$_{1c}$ group. Similarly, the mean 2-h plasma glucose value was much lower in the normal HbA$_{1c}$ group, and in fact was only slightly above the OGTT cut-off for diagnosis of diabetes (mean 2-h plasma glucose value 219 mg/dl).

For those subjects with IGT, HbA$_{1c}$ was not correlated with 2-h plasma glucose. There was, however, a weak positive correlation between HbA$_{1c}$ and fasting plasma glucose (r = 0.23, p < 0.05).

In summary, we found, using a highly precise HPLC method for GHB (with a narrow normal range) in a population with a high prevalence of diabetes, that HbA$_{1c}$ was highly specific as a diagnostic test (91%). Almost all individuals with a normal OGTT had a normal HbA$_{1c}$ result; with a mean $\pm$ 3 SD cut-off, HbA$_{1c}$ would have been 100% specific. The HbA$_{1c}$ test was moderately sensitive (85%) in identifying sub-

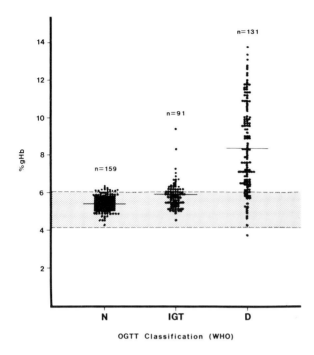

Fig. 1. GHB (specifically HbA$_{1c}$) levels in 381 subjects with normal glucose tolerance (N; $n = 159$), impaired glucose tolerance (IGT; $n = 91$), and diabetes (D; $n = 131$). Shaded area represents normal range (mean ± 1.96 SD) of HbA$_{1c}$. From Ref. 48, with permission of the American Diabetes Association, Inc.

jects with diabetes as diagnosed by OGTT, but, clearly, a normal HbA$_{1c}$ result did not exclude a diagnosis of diabetes or IGT by OGTT. However, subjects with diabetic OGTTs and normal HbA$_{1c}$ values almost always had normal fasting plasma glucose values (less than 140 mg/dl). Thus, GHB fails to identify individuals diagnosed as having diabetes if the diagnosis rests solely on the basis of the 2-h plasma glucose value. Furthermore, GHB is quite insensitive for detecting people with IGT. But, given the epidemiological studies showing that the risk of developing retinopathy and proteinuria is low if the fasting plasma glucose is less than 140 mg/dl (7.8 mmol/l), an elevated GHB should discriminate between subjects at low risk and those at high risk for developing chronic diabetic complications.

What to do until the GHB vs. complications data ship comes in?

In clinical medicine it is often necessary to make patient-care decisions which balance scientific certainty on the one hand and clinical judgment on the other hand. There

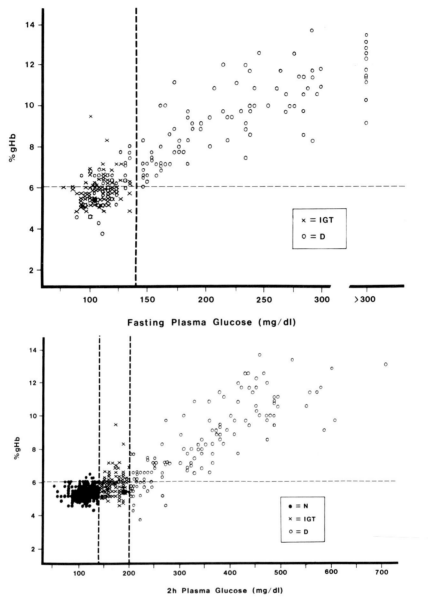

Fig. 2. Scattergrams of GHB (specifically HbA₁c) vs. fasting (upper panel) and 2-h (lower panel) plasma glucose for normal glucose tolerance (N, ●; lower panel only), impaired glucose tolerance (IGT, ×) and diabetic (D, ○) subjects. Horizontal line indicates upper limit of normal values for HbA₁c. Vertical lines indicate plasma glucose cut-offs for IGT (lower panel) and D. (Most N individuals would appear in upper panel, lower left; these points were omitted to avoid obscuring the IGT and D data points.) From Ref. 48, with permission of the American Diabetes Association, Inc.

are still quite a number of unanswered questions concerning both diabetes screening and diabetes treatment. It is not yet known for certain whether all persons diagnosed as diabetic by the OGTT (including those with normal GHB values) are at significant risk for diabetic complications. It is not yet known whether treatment of diabetes to bring blood glucose levels lower than necessary to relieve symptoms of hyperglyce-mia will delay or prevent complications. It is still not yet known whether GHB is as good as or better than a single fasting or 2-h post load plasma glucose in predicting complications of diabetes. Well-designed studies to address these and other crucial questions about diabetes are under way, but they will take time, and it is not known whether the results of the studies will provide clear-cut clinical care guidelines. In the meantime, what should be done? We believe it is time for action. It is time for the epidemiologists to put down their calculators and join forces with public health offi-cials and plan a national diabetes screening program. We recommend the following:

(1) Perform annual screening tests on all persons over 40 years of age for diabetes using GHB. Consider a test 'positive' if the result is more than 3 SD above the mean for normals.
(2) If the GHB result is 'positive', the individual should be referred for treatment. Before treatment is instituted, a fasting plasma glucose should be performed to confirm the diagnosis of diabetes.

The above recommended approach to diabetes screening would not detect many individuals who would be diagnosed as diabetic by OGTT criteria. The proposed ap-proach would, however, select for those persons at known risk for developing com-plications. It is not yet possible to determine whether such an approach would be cost-effective, since the health benefits of treatment are not clearly established. How-ever, the costs and logistics of performing large-scale GHB determinations should not present overwhelming problems. The test can be obtained by finger-prick with collection of blood into a small capillary tube or even onto filter paper with subse-quent transport to the laboratory [51]. We estimate that, for screening purposes, high-quality test results could be made available at a cost of less than $5.00 per speci-men. Standardization of GHB assays would greatly benefit a broad-based screening program [52].

Speculation

We predict that over the next few years, further progress will be made in diagnosis and treatment of diabetes mellitus. The arduous clinical trials and epidemiological studies will bear fruit and show that chronic complications of diabetes are related to the extent of hyperglycemia and that treatment to lower blood glucose levels im-proves outcome. Furthermore, we predict that GHB will be shown to identify those persons at greatest risk of developing chronic complications, and that the current diagnostic criteria for diabetes will be amended to require an elevated GHB confirmed by an elevated fasting plasma glucose or vice versa.

References

1. Jovanovic L, Peterson C. The clinical utility of glycosylated hemoglobin. Am J Med 1981;70:331–338.
2. Goldstein DE, Parker KM, England JD, et al. Clinical application of glycosylated hemoglobin measurements. Diabetes 1982;31 (Suppl. 3):70–78.
3. Gabbay KH, Sosenko JM, Banuchi GA, Mininsohn MJ, Fluckiger R. Glycosylated hemoglobins: increased glycosylation of hemoglobin A in diabetic patients. Diabetes 1979;28:337–340.
4. Gonen B, Rubenstein AH, Rochman H, Tanega SP, Horwitz DL. Haemoglobin A1: an indicator of the metabolic control of diabetic patients. Lancet 1977;ii:734–737.
5. McDonald JM, Davis JE. Glycosylated hemoglobins and diabetes mellitus. Hum Pathol 1979;10:279–289.
6. Koenig RJ, Peterson CM, Kilo C, Crami A, Williamson JR. Hemoglobin A1c as an indicator of the degree of glucose intolerance in diabetes. Diabetes 1976;25:230–232.
7. Santiago JV, Davis JE, Fisher F. Hemoglobin A1c levels in a diabetes detection program. J Clin Endocrinol Metab 1978;47:578–580.
8. Dunn PJ, Cole RA, Soeldner JS, Gleason RE. Reproducibility of HbA1 and sensitivity to various degrees of glucose intolerance. Ann Int Med 1979;91:390–396.
9. Sherwin RS. Limitations of oral glucose tolerance test in diagnosis of early diabetes. Primary Care 1977;4:255–266.
10. Dods RF, Bolmey C. Glycosylated hemoglobin assay and oral glucose tolerance test compared for detection of diabetes mellitus. Clin Chem 1979;25:764–768.
11. Ohneda A, Kobayashi T, Nihei J. Evaluation of new criteria for diagnosis of diabetes mellitus based on follow-up study of borderline diabetes. Tohoku J Exp Med 1982;137:437–444.
12. Simon D, Coignet MC, Thibult N, Senan C, Eschwege E. Comparison of glycosylated hemoglobin and fasting plasma glucose with two-hour post-load plasma glucose in the detection of diabetes mellitus. Am J Epidemiol 1985;122:589–593.
13. Dix D, Cohen P, Kingsley S, Senkbeil J, Sexton K. Glycohemoglobin and glucose tolerance tests compared as indicators of borderline diabetes. Clin Chem 1979;25:887–879.
14. Manicardi V, Bonora E, Portioli I. Comparison of glycosylated haemoglobin and OGTT in the screening of diabetes (Abstract). Diabetologia 1981;21:301.
15. Bolli G, Compagnucci P, Cartechini MG, Santeusanio F, Cirotto C, Scionti L, Brunetti P. HbA1 in subjects with abnormal glucose tolerance but normal fasting plasma glucose. Diabetes 1980;29:272–277.
16. Kesson CM, Young RE, Talwar D, Whitelaw JW, Robb DA. Glycosylated hemoglobin in the diagnosis of non-insulin-dependent diabetes mellitus. Diabetes Care 1982;5:395–398.
17. Orchard TJ, Daneman D, Becker DJ, Kuller LH, LaPorte RE, Drash AL, Wagener D. Glycosylated hemoglobin: a screening test for diabetes mellitus? Prev Med 1982;11:595–601.
18. Lester E, Frazer AD, Shepherd CA, Woodroffe FJ. Glycosylated haemoglobin as an alternative to the glucose tolerance test for the diagnosis of diabetes mellitus. Ann Clin Biochem 1985;22:74–78.
19. Modan M, Halkin H, Karasik A, Lusky A. Effectiveness of glycosylated hemoglobin, fasting plasma glucose, and a single post load plasma glucose level in population screening for glucose intolerance. Am J Epidemiol 1984;119:431–444.

20. Flock EV, Bennett PH, Savage PJ, et al. Bimodality of glycosylated hemoglobin distribution in Pima Indians: relationship to fasting hyperglycemia. Diabetes 1979;28:984–989.

21. Hall PM, Cook JGH, Sheldon J, Rutherford SM, Gould BJ. Glycosylated hemoglobins and glycosylated plasma proteins in the diagnosis of diabetes mellitus and impaired glucose tolerance. Diabetes Care 1984;7:147–150.

22. Verillo A, de Teresa A, Golia R, Nunziata V. The relationship between glycosylated hemoglobin levels and various degrees of glucose intolerance. Diabetologia 1983;24:391–393.

23. Ferrell RE, Hanis CL, Aguilar L, Tulloch B, Garcia C, Schull WJ. Glycosylated hemoglobin determination from capillary blood samples; utility in an epidemiologic survey of diabetes. Am J Epidemiol 1984;119:159–166.

24. Boucher BJ, Welch SG, Beer MS. Glycosylated hemoglobins in the diagnosis of diabetes mellitus and for the assessment of chronic hyperglycaemia. Diabetologia 1981;21:34–36.

25. Forrest RD, Jackson CA, Yudkin JS. The glycohaemoglobin assay as a screening test for diabetes mellitus: the Islington Diabetes Survey. Diabetic Med 1987;4:254–259.

26. Cederholm J, Ronquist G, Wibell L. Comparison of glycosylated hemoglobin with the oral glucose tolerance test. Diabete Metab 1984;10:224–229.

27. Jeppson JO, Jerntorp P, Sundkvist G, Englund H, Nylund V. Measurement of hemoglobin A1c by a new liquid-chromatographic assay: methodology, clinical utility, and relation to glucose tolerance evaluated. Clin Chem 1986;32:1 867–1 872.

28. Albutt EC, Nattrass M, Northam BE. Glucose tolerance test and glycosylated haemoglobin measurement for diagnosis of diabetes mellitus – an assessment of the criteria of the WHO Expert Committee on Diabetes Mellitus 1980. Ann Clin Biochem 1985;22:67–73.

29. Lev-Ran A, VanderLaan WP. Glycohemoglobins and glucose tolerance. JAMA 1979;241:912–914.

30. Goldstein DE, Soeldner S, Nathan D (for the DCCT Research Group). Feasibility of long-term, precise measurements of glycosylated hemoglobin for the Diabetes Control and Complications Trial (DCCT). Diabetes 1986;35 (Suppl1):95A.

31. Svendsen PA, Jorgensen J, Nerup J. HbA1c and the diagnosis of diabetes mellitus. Acta Med Scand 1981;210:313–316.

32. John WG, Richardson RW. Glycosylated haemoglobin levels in patients referred for oral glucose tolerance testing. Diabetic Med 1986;3:46–48.

33. Nomura Y, Nanjo K, Kawa A, et al. Reliability of HbA1c assay in the mass survey for diabetes mellitus, with special reference to the presentation and transportation of blood samples. Tohoku J Exp Med 1983;141Suppl:77–84.

34. Bitzen P-O, Schersten B. Assessment of laboratory methods for detection of unsuspected diabetes in primary health care. Scand J Prim Health Care 1986;4:85–95.

35. Becattini U, Brogioni M, Capizzano E, Biancalani L, Mersi A. Glycohemoglobin evaluation as an index of glycemic status in diabetic and prediabetic subjects. Quad Sclavo Diagn 1982;18:140–147.

36. Woo J, Swaminathan R, Cockram C, Pang CP, Mak YT, Au SY, Valance-Owen J. The prevalence of diabetes mellitus and an assessment of methods of detection among a community of elderly Chinese in Hong Kong. Diabetologia 1987;30:863–868.,

37. Starkman HS, Soeldner JS, Gleason RE. Oral glucose tolerance: relationship with hemoglobin A1c. Diabetes Res Clin Practice 1987;3:343–349.

38. Singer DE, Coley CM, Samet JH, Nathan DM. Tests of glycemia in diabetes mellitus: their use in establishing a diagnosis and in treatment. Ann Int Med 1989;110:125–137.

39. National Diabetes Data Group: Classification and diagnosis of diabetes mellitus and other categories of glucose intolerance. Diabetes 1979;28:1 039–1 057.

40. WHO Expert Committee on Diabetes Mellitus: Second Report on Diabetes Mellitus. Technical Report Series 1980;646:9–14.

152

41. Harris MI, Hadden WC, Knowler WC, Bennett PH. International criteria for the diagnosis of diabetes and impaired glucose tolerance. Diabetes Care 1985;8:562–567.
42. Harris MI, Hadden WC, Knowler WC, Bennett PH. Prevalence of diabetes and impaired glucose tolerance and plasma glucose levels in U.S. population aged 20–74 yr. Diabetes 1987;36:523–534.
43. Herron CA. Screening in diabetes mellitus: report of the Atlanta Workshop. Diabetes Care 1979;2:357–362.
44. Charup MH. The periodic health examination: genesis of a myth. Ann Int Med 1981;95:733–735.
45. The DCCT Research Group: The Diabetes Control and Complications Trial (DCCT): results of the Feasibility Phase. Diabetes Care 1987;10:1–19.
46. Knowler WC, Bennett PH, Hamman RF, Miller M. Diabetes incidence and prevalence in Pima Indians: a 19-fold greater incidence than in Rochester, Minnesota. Am J Epidemiol 1978;108:497–505.
47. Pettitt DJ, Knowler WC, Lisse JR, Bennett PH. Development of retinopathy and proteinuria in relation to plasma-glucose concentrations in Pima Indians. Lancet 1980;ii:1 050–1 052.
48. Little RR, England JE, Wiedmeyer HM, et al. Relationship of glycosylated hemoglobin to oral glucose tolerance: implications for diabetes screening. Diabetes 1988;37:60–64.
49. Clipson KL, Kandal PC, Poon M-C, Boshell BR. Hemoglobin A1c in the diagnosis of chemical diabetes mellitus. Horm Metab Res 1981;13:129–131.
50. Goldstein DE, Little RR, Wiedmeyer HM, England JD, McKenzie EM. Methods for quantifying glycosylated hemoglobins: high performance liquid chromatography and thiobarbituric acid colorimetry. In: Larner J, Pohl S, eds. Methods in diabetes research. New York: Wiley, 1986;475–504.
51. Little RR, McKenzie EM, Wiedmeyer HM, England JD, Goldstein DE. Collection of blood in filter paper for measurement of glycated hemoglobin by affinity chromatography. Clin Chem 1986;31:898.
52. Little RR, England JD, Wiedmeyer HM, et al. Interlaboratory standardization of glycosylated hemoglobin determinations. Clin Chem 1986;32:358–360.

Biochemical aspects of NIDDM

© 1989 Elsevier Science Publishers B.V. (Biomedical Division)
Frontiers of diabetes research: current trends in non-insulin-dependent diabetes mellitus
K.G.M.M. Alberti and R. Mazze, editors

CHAPTER 11

Regulation of glucose transport in diabetes

BARBARA B. KAHN[1] and SAMUEL W. CUSHMAN[2]

[1]The Charles A. Dana Research Institute and Harvard-Thorndike Laboratory of Beth Israel Hospital, Department of Medicine, Beth Israel Hospital and Harvard Medical School, Boston, MA 02215, U.S.A., and [2]Experimental Diabetes, Metabolism and Nutrition Section, Molecular, Cellular and Nutritional Endocrinology Branch, National Institute of Diabetes and Digestive and Kidney Diseases, National Institutes of Health, Bethesda, MD 20892, U.S.A.

Introduction

Glucose entry into cells is vital for mammalian survival. Impairment of glucose entry results in a catabolic state marked by hyperglycemia, dehydration and starvation, known as diabetes mellitus. The clinical observation that insulin can lower blood glucose levels and reverse the catabolic state of diabetes mellitus was made as early as 1922. However, more than 25 years passed before insights into the cellular mechanisms for this dramatically therapeutic effect of insulin emerged. In the 1950s, Levine et al. [1] proposed that insulin might stimulate the transport of glucose across the plasma membrane of target cells. Crofford and Renold [2] finally provided direct evidence for this fundamental action of insulin in 1965.

Glucose transport: general

In many mammalian cells, glucose enters by carrier-mediated facilitated diffusion, which is not regulated by insulin. By contrast, in muscle and adipose cells, where glucose transport also occurs by facilitated diffusion, it is highly regulated by insulin and other hormones. Although muscle accounts for the majority of glucose uptake in vivo, the isolated rat adipose cell has become the preferred in vitro preparation for studying the effects of insulin on glucose transport because of the relative ease of obtaining homogeneous cell suspensions [3] and the exquisite sensitivity and responsiveness of the cells to hormones.

In adipose cells from normal, lean, growing male rats, the basal rate of glucose transport is relatively low and is enhanced 20–30-fold by insulin (for a general review of hexose transport in rat adipose cells see Gliemann and Rees [4]). Maximal stimulation occurs with a near-physiological insulin concentration (6.7 nM, 1000 μU/ml) in 7–10 min. This effect is insulin-concentration-dependent and fully reversible upon removal of insulin. Kinetic experiments show that insulin stimulation results from a change in the maximum transport velocity (V_{max}) and not in the apparent affinity (K_m) of the glucose transporter for glucose. This implies that the stimulation results from an increase in the number of functional glucose transporters present in the plasma membrane of the cell or in glucose transporter intrinsic activity, i.e. glucose turnover number.

Glucose transporters

Two groups developed independent techniques to measure glucose transporter number. Wardzala et al. [5] used cytochalasin B, a potent competitive inhibitor of glucose transport, to specifically bind glucose transporters in subcellular membrane fractions prepared by differential ultracentrifugation [6,7]. Kono and colleagues [8,9] fractionated cells by sucrose density gradient centrifugation, reconstituted the fractions into artificial liposomes, and measured glucose transport activity directly. Both groups showed that in the absence of insulin (basal state), the majority of glucose transporters are in an intracellular pool associated with the low-density microsomes. With insulin stimulation, approx. 60% of the glucose transporters are lost from the low-density microsomes, concurrent with an approx. 5-fold increase in their concentration in the plasma membranes. The time course of this redistribution of glucose transporters is slightly more rapid than that for glucose transport activity but the removal of insulin with anti-insulin antiserum or collagenase fully reverses the redistribution with the same time course as the reversal of glucose transport activity [10,11].

These observations provide the basis for the translocation hypothesis of insulin action on glucose transport illustrated in Fig. 1 [6,8]; for a general review of glucose transporter translocation see Simpson and Cushman [12]. According to this model, insulin binds to its receptor in the plasma membrane (step 1), generating a signal (step 2) the nature of which is unknown. This results in the exocytic movement of membrane vesicles containing glucose transporters from an intracellular pool to the plasma membrane (step 3), where they first bind (step 4) and subsequently fuse (step 5), thus exposing glucose transporters to the extracellular medium and increasing the glucose transport rate (step 6). When insulin dissociates from its receptor because of either physiological events or experimental treatment (step 7), the process is reversed. Glucose transporters which are present in the plasma membrane are then reinternalized by an endocytic process and translocated back to the intracellular pool (step 8). Studies utilizing rat diaphragm [13,14] and cardiac muscle [15] and guinea pig [16] and human [17–19] adipose cells have indicated that this mechanism operates in other tissues and species.

Effect of anti-insulin hormones

The regulation of lipolysis in the rat adipose cell by agents such as ACTH, glucagon and β-adrenergic agonists which increase cellular cAMP concentrations through the activation of adenylate cyclase, and by agents such as adenosine, prostaglandins and nicotinic acid which decrease cellular cAMP concentrations through the inhibition of adenylate cyclase, has long been established. Similarly, the antilipolytic actions of

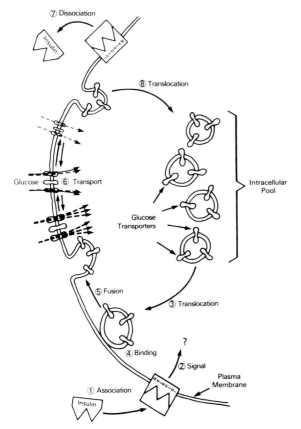

Fig. 1. Hypothetical model of the hormonal regulation of glucose transport (from Kahn and Cushman [55]).

insulin have also long been recognized although the locus of action still remains unclear. With the removal of endogenous adenosine, all of the ligands which stimulate adenylate cyclase can now be shown to inhibit insulin-stimulated glucose transport activity [20,21]. Similarly, the adenylate cyclase inhibitors such as prostaglandin E_1, nicotinic acid and N^6-phenylisopropyladenosine, a non-metabolizable adenosine analogue, prevent or reverse this inhibition. At submaximal levels, both the inhibitory actions of the lipolytic hormones/agents and the stimulatory effects of the antilipolytic hormones/agents are additive, suggesting that both actions are mediated by mechanisms distal to the interactions of the ligands with their individual receptors, perhaps at the level of the guanine nucleotide regulatory subunits of adenylate cyclase, G_s and G_i [21]. Finally, both the stimulatory action of adenosine and the inhibitory action of isoproterenol on glucose transport activity have been shown to occur through changes in the maximum transport velocity (V_{max}) [20].

However, unlike the action of insulin, this counterregulation of insulin-stimulated glucose transport activity is apparently not accompanied by corresponding changes in the number of glucose transporters in the plasma membrane [20–22]. Indeed, neither the potentiation of insulin-stimulated glucose transport activity by adenosine, nor the inhibition by isoproterenol, nor the restitution of inhibited activity by N^6-phenylisopropyladenosine is accompanied by changes in the extent of translocation of glucose transporters induced by insulin. Thus, as illustrated in Fig. 1, these ligands appear to exert their actions on the intrinsic activity of those glucose transporters present in the plasma membrane rather than through changes in the translocation process. Whether insulin itself may also have an effect on glucose transporter intrinsic activity during translocation remains to be clarified [23].

Insulin resistance

Various pathophysiological states in both rat and man are accompanied by perturbations in insulin's ability to stimulate glucose transport at the cellular level in vitro. Conditions in which a diminished glucose transport response to insulin is observed in the adipose cell, i.e. 'insulin-resistant states', include the streptozotocin-diabetic rat [24], the high-fat-fed rat [25], the aged, obese rat [26] and the fasted rat [27]. Examples in which an augmented glucose transport response to insulin is observed in the adipose cell include the chronically hyperinsulinemic rat [28–32], the chronically exercise-trained rat [33], the genetically obese Zucker fatty rat [34], the fasted/refed rat [27] and the insulin-treated streptozotocin-diabetic rat [35,36].

The streptozotocin-diabetic rat model illustrates a common mechanism for all examples of cellular insulin resistance examined to date [24]. Although the chief defect in streptozotocin diabetes is insulin deficiency, insulin resistance is also present at the cellular level. As illustrated in Fig. 2, insulin-stimulated glucose transport activity is reduced by 67% in adipose cells from diabetic rats compared with control. Glucose transporter concentration is decreased 53% in the corresponding plasma membranes in the insulin-stimulated state and 45% in the low-density microsomes in the basal state (Fig. 2). Thus, the insulin resistance appears to result from a reduced translocation of glucose transporters to the plasma membrane in response to insulin due to a depleted intracellular pool. The same mechanism is seen for the other insulin-resistant states mentioned above in spite of marked differences in nutritional status and in plasma insulin concentrations. The latter range from markedly reduced in streptozotocin diabetes to significantly elevated in obesity.

Insulin and glucose transporters

To examine the question of the role of chronic exposure to insulin in modulating cellular responsiveness to insulin, two models of chronic hyperinsulinemia have been studied: normal rats treated by injection [28,29] or infusion [30,32] of insulin, and young genetically obese Zucker fatty rats [34]. Initially, studies in normal rats treated with daily insulin injections showed that hyperinsulinemia was associated with reduced sensitivity to insulin and either no change [29] or an increase [28] in basal and maximally insulin-stimulated glucose transport activity in adipose cells. More recently, Wardzala et al. [30] showed that with constant subcutaneous insulin infusion, insulin-stimulated glucose transport activity increases 1.6–2.0-fold with no change in sensitivity to insulin.

Kahn et al. [32] investigated the mechanism for this hyperresponsiveness to insulin. In these studies, insulin-stimulated glucose transport activity was increased 55% above control. Glucose transporter concentration in the corresponding plasma mem-

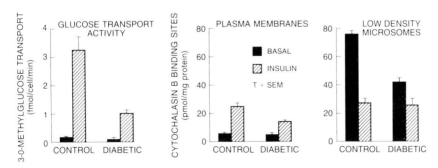

Fig. 2. Effects of streptozotocin diabetes on glucose transport activity and the subcellular distribution of glucose transporters in the isolated rat adipose cell at steady state at 37°C in the absence (basal) or presence of 6.7 nM (1000 μU/ml) insulin (from Karnieli et al. [24]).

160

branes was increased 38%. In the low-density microsomes, glucose transporter concentration was similar to control. However, the total number of glucose transporters in this fraction was increased in cells from hyperinsulinemic rats due to a 39% increase in low-density microsomal protein. Thus, the hyperresponsive insulin-stimulated glucose transport activity can be explained by a greater number of glucose transporters translocated to the plasma membrane from an enlarged intracellular pool. The additional glucose transporters appear to be the result of a generalized increase in the net synthesis of intracellular protein. A similar mechanism has been proposed to explain insulin-hyperresponsive glucose transport in adipose cells from naturally hyperinsulinemic, young, genetically obese Zucker fatty rats [34] and from physically trained rats [33].

These phenomena, however, do not clearly answer the question of the role of ambient insulin concentrations in modulating cellular responsiveness to insulin. Hyperinsulinemia in normal [32] and young Zucker fatty rats [34] appears to result in an increase in the number of glucose transporters in adipose cells and therefore in the magnitude of insulin's stimulatory effect on glucose transport. This same mechanism may be seen in the absence of hyperinsulinemia in physically trained rats [33]. Furthermore, hyperinsulinemia in aging/obese rats [26] or in adult obese Zucker fatty rats [37] is associated with an attenuated response to insulin and, in the former case, a depletion of intracellular glucose transporters.

Further complexity is introduced by studying the cellular events associated with insulin treatment of diabetic animals [35,36]. Kahn and Cushman [35] found that continuous subcutaneous insulin infusion in diabetic rats not only reversed the insulin-resistant glucose transport activity associated with diabetes but resulted in a marked, although transient, hyperresponsiveness, peaking with a 3-fold overshoot above control at 7–8 days as shown in Fig. 3, and remaining elevated for more than

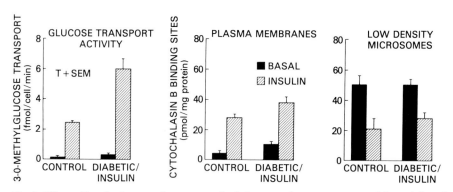

Fig. 3. Effects of insulin therapy of streptozotocin diabetes on glucose transport activity and the subcellular distribution of glucose transporters in the isolated rat adipose cell at steady state at 37°C in the absence (basal) or presence of 6.7 nM (1000 μU/ml) insulin (from Kahn and Cushman [35]).

3 weeks. Insulin therapy restored glucose transporter concentration in plasma membranes of insulin-stimulated cells from the 40%-depleted level associated with diabetes to a level approx. 35% greater than control (Fig. 3). Glucose transporter concentration in the low-density microsomes from basal cells was also restored from an approx. 45% depleted level back to normal (Fig. 3), whereas total intracellular glucose transporters were further increased owing to an approx. 2-fold increase in low-density microsomal membrane protein. Because the hyperresponsive glucose transport activity occurs through an increase in V_{max} which cannot be adequately explained by an increase in glucose transporter number, enhanced glucose transporter intrinsic activity must be invoked.

A similar reversal of cellular insulin resistance resulting in an overshoot in insulin-stimulated glucose transport activity is also seen when rats are refed after fasting [27]. These states have in common nutritional repletion after cellular starvation, which may have a unique effect on intracellular mechanisms to augment substrate entry into cells. Additionally, as noted above, acute modulation of glucose transporter intrinsic activity has been demonstrated with in vitro incubation of adipose cells with lipolytic and antilipolytic agents [20–22].

Recent data suggest that the ambient blood glucose level, independent of the insulin level, may actually regulate cellular responsiveness to insulin [38]. When diabetic rats are treated with phlorizin, which blocks renal tubular reabsorption of glucose, blood glucose is normalized, with no change in plasma insulin. This restores to normal from the depressed state associated with diabetes both in vivo glucose disposal measured by the euglycemic clamp [39] and in vitro glucose transport activity in adipose cells [38]. Studies are in progress to determine whether this is an effect on glucose transporter number, intrinsic activity, or both.

Molecular aspects of glucose transporters

With the recent cloning of the human Hep G2/rat brain glucose transporter cDNA [40,41] and gene [42], probes are now available to investigate the molecular genetic regulation of these changes in glucose transporter number and intrinsic activity. Preliminary data show a close correlation between Hep G2 glucose transporter mRNA and protein levels in adipose cells from fasted and refed rats [43], but not from diabetic rats [44], where no change in Hep G2 glucose transporter mRNA abundance is seen in spite of an approx. 65% decrease in total glucose transporter number per cell. By contrast, insulin treatment of the diabetic rat is associated with parallel increases in both total glucose transporter number (predominantly intracellular glucose transporters) and mRNA abundance. This suggests post-transcriptional regulation of glucose transporter number in diabetes, whereas at least part of the regulation with fasting, refeeding and insulin treatment of the diabetic rat is at the mRNA level.

162

Evidence is accumulating for multiple species of glucose transporters which differ at the gene and/or protein level [12,23,45] as evidenced by differences in affinity for cytochalasin B [7,12], immunoreactivity [23,45], isolectric focusing points [46] and susceptibility to neuraminidase, which desialates terminally glycosylated proteins [46]. Some of these differences appear to confer functional specificity. Thus, isoelectric focusing studies show that only one species of glucose transporter appears to be translocated to the plasma membrane in response to insulin [46]. A recent report of a monoclonal antibody which recognizes a glucose transporter exclusively in muscle and adipose cells [45] implies that the insulin-responsive glucose transporter may be immunologically distinct from a constitutive glucose transporter present in both insulin-responsive and nonresponsive tissues. Indeed, such a distinct glucose transporter has just been cloned from rat adipose cell and heart cDNA libraries [47], a rat soleus muscle library [48], a rat skeletal muscle library [49], human skeletal muscle and small intestine libraries [50] and a mouse 3T3-L1 adipocyte library [51]. In addition, genetically distinct glucose transporters have been cloned from liver [52,53] and intestinal brush border [54].

Knowledge of the sequences of these glucose transporter genes will permit studies to determine the structural features that are vital for insulin's stimulatory effect on glucose transport. Such investigations promise to enhance our understanding of the altered regulation of cellular phenomena associated with diabetes mellitus and may aid in designing more effective therapy.

Acknowledgements

The authors wish to thank their many colleagues, both former and current, for their indispensable contributions to the concepts and experimental results described here. The authors also wish to thank Elizabeth A. Guy for preparing the manuscript.

References

1. Levine R, Goldstein MS, Klein S, Huddelstun B. Action of insulin on 'permeability' of cells to free hexoses, as studied by its effect on distribution of galactose. Am J Physiol 1950;173:207–211.
2. Crofford OB, Renold AE. Glucose uptake by incubated rat epididymal adipose tissue. Rate-limiting steps and site of insulin action. J Biol Chem 1965;240:14–21.
3. Rodbell M. Metabolism of isolated fat cells. I. Effects of hormones on glucose metabolism and lipolysis. J Biol Chem 1964;239:375–380.
4. Gliemann J, Rees WD. The insulin-sensitive hexose transport system in adipocytes. Curr Top Membr Transp 1983;18:339–379.
5. Wardzala LJ, Cushman SW, Salans LB. Mechanism of insulin action on glucose transport in the isolated rat adipose cell. Enhancement of the number of functional transport systems. J Biol Chem 1978;253:8002–8005.

6. Cushman SW, Wardzala LJ. Potential mechanism of insulin action on glucose transport in the isolated rat adipose cell. Apparent translocation of intracellular transport systems to the plasma membrane. J Biol Chem 1980;255:4758–4762.

7. Simpson IA, Yver DR, Hissin PJ, Wardzala LJ, Karnieli E, Salans LB, Cushman SW. Insulin-stimulated translocation of glucose transporters in the isolated rat adipose cell: characterization of subcellular fractions. Biochim Biophys Acta 1983;763:393–407.

8. Suzuki K, Kono T. Evidence that insulin causes translocation of glucose transport activity to the plasma membrane from an intracellular storage site. Proc Natl Acad Sci USA 1980;77:2542–2545.

9. Kono T, Suzuki K, Dansey LE, Robinson FW, Blevins TL. Energy-dependent and protein synthesis-independent recycling of the insulin-sensitive glucose transport mechanism in fat cells. J Biol Chem 1981;256:6400–6407.

10. Karnieli E, Zarnowski MJ, Hissin PJ, Simpson IA, Salans LB, Cushman SW. Insulin-stimulated translocation of glucose transport systems in the isolated rat adipose cell. Time course, reversal, insulin concentration-dependency and relationship to glucose transport activity. J Biol Chem 1981;256:4772–4777.

11. Kono T, Robinson FW, Blevins TL, Ezaki O. Evidence that translocation of the glucose transport activity is the major mechanism of insulin action on glucose transport in fat cells. J Biol Chem 1982;257:10942–10947.

12. Simpson IA, Cushman SW. Hormonal regulation of mammalian glucose transport. Annu Rev Biochem 1986;55:1059–1089.

13. Wardzala LJ, Jeanrenaud B. Potential mechanism of insulin action on glucose transport in the isolated rat diaphragm. Apparent translocation of intracellular transport systems to the plasma membrane. J Biol Chem 1981;256:7090–7093.

14. Wardzala LJ, Jeanrenaud B. Identification of the D-glucose-inhibitable cytochalasin B binding site as the glucose transporter in rat diaphragm plasma and microsomal membranes. Biochim Biophys Acta 1983;730:49–56.

15. Watanobe T, Smith MM, Robinson RW, Kono T. Insulin action on glucose transport in cardiac muscle. J Biol Chem 1984;259:13117–13122.

16. Horuk R, Rodbell M, Cushman SW, Wardzala LJ. Proposed mechanism of insulin-resistant glucose transport in the isolated guinea pig adipocyte. Small intracellular pool of glucose transporters. J Biol Chem 1983;258:7425–7429.

17. Karnieli E, Chernow R, Hissin PJ, Simpson IA, Foley JE. Insulin stimulates glucose transport in isolated human adipose cells through the translocation of intracellular glucose transporters to the plasma membrane: a preliminary report. Horm Metab Res 1986;18:860–861.

18. Karnieli E, Barzilai A, Rafaeloff R, Armoni M. Distribution of glucose transporters in membrane fractions isolated from human adipose cells. Relation to cell size. J Clin Invest 1986;78:1051–1055.

19. Garvey WT, Huecksteadt TP, Matthaei S, Olefsky JM. Role of glucose transporters in the cellular insulin resistance of Type II non-insulin-dependent diabetes mellitus. J Clin Invest 1988;81:1528–1536.

20. Smith U, Kuroda M, Simpson IA. Counterregulation of insulin-stimulated glucose transport by catecholamines in the isolated rat adipose cell. J Biol Chem 1984;259:8758–8763.

21. Kuroda M, Honnor RC, Cushman SW, Londos C, Simpson IA. Regulation of insulin-stimulated glucose transport in the isolated rat adipocyte. cAMP-independent effects of lipolytic and antilipolytic agents. J Biol Chem 1987;262:245–253.

22. Joost HG, Weber TM, Cushman SW, Simpson IA. Insulin-stimulated glucose transport in rat adipose cells. Modulation of transporter intrinsic activity by isoproterenol and adenosine. J Biol Chem 1986;261:10033–10036.

23. Joost HG, Weber TM, Cushman SW. Qualitative and quantitative comparison of glucose transport activity and glucose transporter concentration in rat adipose cell plasma membranes in the basal and insulin-stimulated states. Biochem J 1987;249:155–161.

164

24. Karnieli E, Hissin PJ, Simpson IA, Salans LB, Cushman SW. A possible mechanism of insulin resistance in the rat adipose cell in streptozotocin-induced diabetes mellitus. Depletion of intracellular glucose transport systems. J Clin Invest 1981;68:811–814.

25. Hissin PJ, Karnieli E, Simpson IA, Salans LB, Cushman SW. A possible mechanism of insulin resistance in the rat adipose cell with high fat/low carbohydrate feeding. Depletion of intracellular glucose transport systems. Diabetes 1982;31:589–592.

26. Hissin PJ, Foley JE, Wardzala LJ, Karnieli E, Simpson IA, Salans LB, Cushman SW. Mechanism of insulin resistant glucose transport activity in the enlarged adipose cell of the aged, obese rat. Relative depletion of intracellular glucose transport systems. J Clin Invest 1982;70:780–790.

27. Kahn BB, Simpson IA, Cushman SW. Divergent mechanisms for the insulin resistant and hyperresponsive glucose transport in adipose cells from fasted and refed rats. Alterations in both glucose transporter number and intrinsic activity. J Clin Invest 1988;82:691–699.

28. Kobayashi M, Olefsky JM. Long-term regulation of adipocyte glucose transport capacity by circulating insulin in rats. J Clin Invest 1978;62:73–81.

29. Whittaker J, Alberti KGMM, York DA, Singh J. The effects of chronic hyperinsulinemia on insulin binding and glucose metabolism in rat adipocytes. Biochem Soc Trans 1979;7:1055–1066.

30. Wardzala LJ, Hirshman M. Pofcher E, Horton ED, Mead PM, Cushman SW, Horton ES. Regulation of glucose utilization in adipose cells and muscle following long-term experimental hyperinsulinemia in rats. J Clin Invest 1985;76:460–469.

31. Trimble ER, Weir GC, Gjinovci F, Assimacopopulos-Jeannet A, Benzi R, Renold AE. Increased insulin responsiveness in vivo consequent to induced hyperinsulinemia in the rat. Diabetes 1984;33:444–449.

32. Kahn BB, Horton ES, Cushman SW. Mechanism for enhanced glucose transport response to insulin in adipose cells from chronically hyperinsulinemic rats. Increased translocation of glucose transporters from an enlarged intracellular pool. J Clin Invest 1987;79:853–858.

33. Vinten J, Petersen LN, Sonne B, Galbo H. Effect of physical training on glucose transporters in fat cell fractions. Biochim Biophys Acta 1985;841:223–227.

34. Guerre-Millo M, Lavau M, Horne JS, Wardzala LJ. Increased number of glucose transport systems in adipocytes from young hyperinsulinemic obese Zucker rats. J Biol Chem 1985;260:2198–2201.

35. Kahn BB, Cushman SW. Mechanism for markedly hyperresponsive insulin-stimulated glucose transport activity in adipose cells from insulin-treated streptozotocin diabetic rats. Evidence for increased glucose transporter intrinsic activity. J Biol Chem 1987;262:5118–5124.

36. Karnieli E, Armoni M, Cohen P, Kanter Y, Rafaeloff R. Reversal of insulin resistance in diabetic rat adipocytes by insulin therapy. Restoration of pool of glucose transporters and enhancement of glucose transporter activity. Diabetes 1987;36:925–931.

37. Cushman SW, Zarnowski MJ, Franzusoff AJ, Salans LB. Alterations in glucose metabolism and its stimulation by insulin in isolated adipose cells during the development of genetic obesity in the Zucker fatty rat (a preliminary report). Metabolism 1978;27(Suppl 2):1930–1940.

38. Kahn BB, Cushman SW, Shulman GI, DeFronzo RA, Rosetti L. Reversal of insulin-resistant glucose transport in adipose cells from diabetic rats by normalization of plasma glucose without insulin therapy. Clin Res 1987;35:507A.

39. Rossetti L, Smith D, Shulman GI, Papachristou D, DeFronzo R. Correction of hyperglycemia with phlorizin normalizes tissue sensitivity to insulin in diabetic rats. J Clin Invest 1987;79:1501–1515.

40. Mueckler MM, Caruso C, Baldwin SA, Panico M, Blench I, Morris HR, Allard JW, Lienhard GE, Lodish HF. Sequence and structure of a human glucose transporter. Science 1985;229:941–945.

41. Birnbaum MJ, Haspel HC, Rosen OM. Cloning and characterization of cDNA encoding the rat brain glucose-transporter protein. Proc Natl Acad Sci USA 1986;83:5784–5788.

42. Fukumoto H, Seino S, Imura H, Seino Y, Bell GI. Characterization and expression of human HepG2/erythrocyte glucose-transporter gene. Diabetes 1988;37:657–661.

43. Kahn BB, Cushman SW, Flier JS. Regulation of glucose transporter specific mRNA abundance in rat adipose cells with fasting and refeeding. Implications for in vivo control of glucose transporter number. J Clin Invest 1989;83:199–204.

44. Kahn BB. Divergent effects of diabetes and insulin treatment on glucose transporter mRNA levels in rat adipose cells. Clin Res 1988;36:484A.

45. James DE, Brown R, Navarro J, Pilch PF. Insulin-regulatable tissues express a unique insulin-sensitive glucose transport protein. Nature 1988;333:183–185.

46. Horuk R, Matthaei S, Olefsky JM, Baly DL, Cushman SW, Simpson IA. Biochemical and functional heterogeneity of rat adipocyte glucose transporters. J Biol Chem 1986;261:1823–1828.

47. James DE, Strube M, Mueckler M. Molecular cloning and characterization of an insulin-regulatable glucose transporter. Nature 1989;338:83–87.

48. Charron MJ, Brosius III FC, Alper SL, Lodish HF. A glucose transport protein expressed predominantly in insulin-responsive tissues. Proc Natl Acad Sci USA 1989;86:2535–2539.

49. Birnbaum MJ. Identification of a novel gene encoding an insulin-responsive glucose transporter protein. Cell 1989;57:305–315.

50. Fukumoto H, Kayano T, Buse JB, Edwards Y, Pilch PF, Bell GI, Sieno S. Cloning and characterization of the major insulin-responsive glucose transporter expressed in human skeletal muscle and other insulin-responsive tissues. J Biol Chem 1989;264:7776–7779.

51. Kaestner KH, Christy RJ, McLenithan JC, Braiterman LT, Cornelius P, Pekala PH, Lane MD. Sequence, tissue distribution, and differential expression of mRNA for a putative insulin-responsive glucose transporter in mouse 3T3-L1 adipocytes. Proc Natl Acad Sci USA 1989;86:3150–3154.

52. Fukumoto H, Seino S, Imura H, Seino Y, Eddy RL, Fukushima Y, Byers MG, Shows TB, Bell G. Sequence, tissue distribution, and chromosomal localization of mRNA encoding a human glucose transporter-like protein. Proc Natl Acad Sci USA 1988;85:5434–5438.

53. Thorens B, Sarkar HK, Kaback HR, Lodish HF. Cloning and functional expression in bacteria of a novel glucose transporter present in liver, intestine, kidney, and β-pancreatic islet cells. Cell 1988;55:281–290.

54. Hediger MA, Coady MJ, Ikeda TS, Wright EM. Expression cloning and cDNA sequencing of the Na$^+$/glucose co-transporter. Nature 1987;330:379–381.

55. Kahn BB, Cushman SW. Subcellular translocation of glucose transporters: role in insulin action and its perturbation in altered metabolic states. Diabetes/Metab Rev 1985;1:203–227.

CHAPTER 12

Insulin resistance, abnormal free fatty acid metabolism, and fasting hyperglycemia in patients with non-insulin-dependent diabetes mellitus

GERALD M. REAVEN

Department of Medicine, Stanford University School of Medicine and Geriatric Research, Education and Clinical Center, Veterans Administration Medical Center, Palo Alto, CA 94304, U.S.A.

Introduction

Resistance to insulin-stimulated glucose uptake in patients with NIDDM, as well as in those with impaired glucose tolerance (IGT), was first emphasized by reports published from our laboratory approximately 20 years ago [1–3]. Our initial findings have been subsequently confirmed by many investigators [4]. Although it is now generally recognized that resistance to insulin-stimulated glucose uptake is characteristic of patients with either IGT or NIDDM, the role that this defect plays in the pathogenesis of NIDDM remains controversial. In this brief review we shall focus on the physiological events that result from the presence of resistance to insulin-stimulated glucose uptake, based upon the view that the manner in which an individual responds to insulin resistance, irrespective of its cause, determines the degree to which glucose tolerance will deteriorate.

Relationship between insulin resistance and degree of glucose intolerance

The data in Fig. 1 illustrate the relationship between fasting plasma glucose concentration and insulin-stimulated glucose uptake (R_d) in individuals with normal glucose tolerance, IGT and NIDDM [5]. These results demonstrate that insulin-stimulated glucose uptake was lower than normal in patients with either IGT or NIDDM. Since

Correspondence and reprint requests to: G.M. Reaven, M.D. GRECC (182/B), VA Medical Center, 3801 Miranda Avenue, Palo Alto, CA 94304, U.S.A.

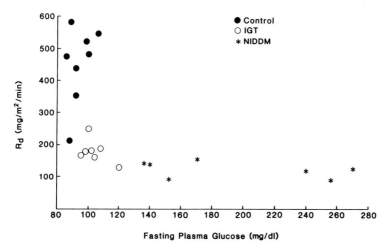

Fig. 1. Relationship between total glucose uptake (R_d) during glucose clamp studies and fasting plasma glucose concentration in control individuals with normal glucose tolerance (●), impaired glucose tolerance (○) or non-insulin-dependent diabetes mellitus (*). Reproduced from Ref. 5 with permission of the journal and the authors.

glucose uptake was reduced to almost the same degree in IGT and NIDDM, these data indicate that there is essentially no relationship between fasting plasma glucose concentration and insulin-stimulated glucose uptake in these patients, i.e., they are all insulin-resistant, whether their fasting plasma glucose concentration is 100 mg/dl (5.6 mmol/l) or 250 mg/dl (13.9 mmol/l). Thus, resistance to insulin-stimulated glucose uptake cannot, by itself, account for differences in the degree to which glucose tolerance deteriorates in patients with IGT or NIDDM, and some other factor must be implicated to explain why fasting plasma glucose is 125 mg/dl (6.9 mmol/l) in one patient with NIDDM and 250 mg/dl (13.9 mmol/l) in another.

Another conclusion from the data shown in Fig. 1 is that insulin-stimulated glucose uptake varies almost three-fold in individuals with normal glucose tolerance, and that some subjects with normal oral glucose tolerance are as insulin-resistant as patients with IGT or NIDDM. In order to define this phenomenon more clearly, we performed glucose clamp studies in 100 non-obese individuals with normal oral glucose tolerance [6]. The 100 subjects were divided into four quartiles on the basis of the glucose clamp results, and the results demonstrated that insulin-stimulated glucose uptake in the quartile of the most insulin-resistant subjects was approximately one-third of the value in the most insulin-sensitive quartile. Thus, the three-fold variation between the most insulin-sensitive and most insulin-resistant normal subjects, seen in Fig. 1, was confirmed when similar measurements were carried out in a large population of individuals with normal oral glucose tolerance. Furthermore, the absolute value for glucose uptake in the subjects in the lowest quartile was comparable in degree to that of patients with IGT and NIDDM shown in Fig. 1. Thus, resistance to insulin-stimulated glucose uptake of a similar degree of severity exists in patients with IGT and NIDDM, irrespective of magnitude of hyperglycemia, and at least one-fourth of the normal population. How can degree of glucose tolerance vary so dramatically in individuals with comparable degrees of resistance to insulin-stimulated glucose uptake?

Beta cell compensation for insulin resistance

Plasma glucose and insulin responses to a 75 g oral glucose load were also determined in the 100 subjects with normal glucose tolerance discussed in the preceding paragraph. The plasma glucose responses of the four groups were essentially identical and within normal limits. In contrast, the insulin responses of the four groups were quite different. The highest insulin levels were seen in individuals with the greatest degree of insulin resistance. At the other extreme, normal individuals who were most insulin-sensitive had the lowest insulin response. The other two groups were intermediate with respect to both insulin response and insulin action, and there was an overall correlation ($r = 0.65$, $p < 0.001$) between degree of insulin resistance and insulin response to the oral glucose challenge.

These data suggest that glucose tolerance is normal in the lowest quartile individuals, despite their severe degree of insulin resistance, because they can secrete enough insulin to compensate for the insulin resistance. Variations in beta cell response also seem to account for the differences in glucose tolerance that occur in patients with IGT and NIDDM, shown previously to have comparable degrees of insulin resistance. Support for this point of view can be seen in Fig. 2. These results display the plasma glucose and insulin responses before and after breakfast (8 a.m.) and lunch (noon) in normal individuals and patients with NIDDM and progressive degrees of hyperglycemia [7]. Patients with NIDDM and the lowest day-long levels of glycemia had the highest insulin levels. The progressive increase in ambient glucose level seen in the patients with NIDDM was associated with a decline in plasma insulin concentration. Thus, patients with NIDDM and a relatively mild degree of hyperglycemia were hyperinsulinemic as compared with normal individuals, and the inability to sustain the hyperinsulinemic state was associated with the development of severe hyperglycemia.

The data presented to this point suggest that the ability of insulin-resistant subjects to compensate for this defect will largely determine the degree to which their glucose tolerance deteriorates. If the beta cell is able to respond to the insulin resistance by secreting large amounts of insulin, gross decompensation of glucose tolerance can

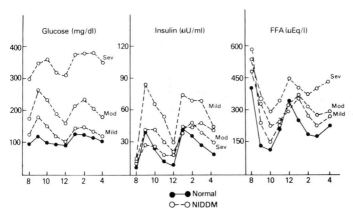

Fig. 2. Mean ($\pm$ SEM) plasma glucose, insulin and FFA concentrations at hourly intervals from 8 a.m. to 4 p.m. in individuals with either normal glucose tolerance ($\bullet$–$\bullet$) or non-insulin-dependent diabetes mellitus ($\bigcirc$-----$\bigcirc$). Patients with non-insulin-dependent diabetes mellitus were divided into three groups on the basis of their degree of glucose intolerance: mild (fasting glucose < 140 mg/dl); moderate (fasting glucose 140–250 mg/dl); and severe (fasting glucose > 250 mg/dl). Meals were eaten at 8 a.m. (20% of daily calories), noon (40% of daily calories) and 6 p.m. (40% of daily calories). Each meal contained (as percent of total calories) 15% protein, 40% fat and 45% carbohydrate. Reproduced from Ref. 7 with permission of the journal and the authors.

be prevented, and individuals will have either normal glucose tolerance, IGT or NIDDM with mild fasting hyperglycemia. However, when hyperinsulinemia cannot be sustained, and circulating insulin levels are 'normal' in absolute terms, severe hyperglycemia develops in individuals who are insulin-resistant.

Abnormal regulation of free fatty acid (FFA) metabolism in NIDDM

If we assume that hyperglycemia develops in patients with NIDDM when hyperinsulinemia cannot be maintained, the next question to be addressed is what regulatory function of insulin has failed when circulating insulin levels are no longer elevated. To answer this question it is necessary to define a process which can be significantly modified by a small change in plasma insulin concentration, since it is apparent from the data in Fig. 2 that relatively small differences in absolute insulin level exist between individuals with NIDDM and markedly different levels of glycemia. In this regard, recent results from our laboratory seem to be relevant [8]. In these experiments the ability of insulin to suppress plasma FFA concentration was quantified in normal subjects, patients with mild NIDDM (fasting glucose < 175 mg/dl: 9.7 mmol/l) and severe NIDDM (fasting glucose > 250 mg/dl: 13.9 mmol/l). These studies were carried out by measuring the fall in plasma FFA concentration seen when plasma insulin concentration was raised by infusing insulin at increasing rates, during a period of time when plasma glucose concentration was maintained constant. The entire study lasted 280 minutes, with the rate of insulin infusion increased every 70 min. The mean ($\pm$ SEM) plasma insulin concentration (μU/ml) achieved at the end of each 70-min period was 6.0 $\pm$ 0.6, 13.5 $\pm$ 0.5, 27.3 $\pm$ 1.1 and 51.2 $\pm$ 0.4. Plasma FFA concentrations fell progressively in all three study groups when plasma insulin concentrations were raised from approximately 6 to 50 μU/ml, while plasma glucose concentration was held constant [8]. Furthermore, relatively small increments in plasma insulin concentration led to substantial falls in plasma FFA concentration, and half-maximal suppression of basal plasma FFA level was achieved at an insulin concentration of approximately 20 μU/ml. The dose-response curve relating plasma insulin concentration to glucose uptake has quite different characteristics and it has been estimated [9] that maximal stimulation of glucose uptake takes place at a plasma insulin concentration of approximately 675 μU/ml, with half-maximal stimulation at an insulin level of 60 μU/ml. Thus, it is unlikely that significant changes in insulin-stimulated glucose uptake can result from the relatively small differences in plasma insulin concentration that exist between subjects with normal glucose tolerance and insulin-resistant patients with diabetes seen in Fig. 2. However, the results in Fig. 2 show that the differences in plasma insulin concentration that exist between the experimental groups with varying degrees of glucose tolerance are associated with profound changes in circulating plasma FFA level.

The results of the studies described above indicate that hyperinsulinemia in patients with mild NIDDM was able to maintain near-normal plasma glucose and FFA levels, whereas insulin levels which were equivalent to those of normal individuals were associated with extreme elevations in plasma glucose and FFA concentrations in patients with severe NIDDM. The fact that both plasma FFA and glucose concentrations rise when hyperinsulinemia cannot be maintained permits us to speculate that patients with NIDDM develop fasting hyperglycemia because they cannot sustain the increased insulin-secretory response needed to prevent elevations of circulating FFA concentration.

Elevated FFA concentration and development of fasting hyperglycemia

There is evidence that elevated plasma FFA levels can inhibit insulin-stimulated glucose uptake [10], and this mechanism may contribute to the development of fasting hyperglycemia. However, we do not believe it is the major pathophysiological effect of high plasma FFA levels. The logic of this decision can be discerned from consideration of the results shown in Fig. 1 indicating that resistance to insulin-stimulated glucose uptake is comparable in patients with IGT and NIDDM over a wide range of fasting plasma glucose concentrations. Thus, it does not seem reasonable to suggest that an increase in insulin resistance, secondary to elevated plasma FFA levels, plays an important role in development of severe fasting hyperglycemia. On the other hand, elevated plasma FFA levels might be responsible for stimulating hepatic glucose production. Thus, an increase in FFA flux to the liver has been shown to augment hepatic glucose production in intact human beings [10] and perfused rat liver [11]. Increased FFA oxidation by the liver has been associated with stimulation of hepatic gluconeogenesis [12], possibly due to the ability of the acetyl CoA generated to activate allosterically pyruvate carboxylase, a key gluconeogenic enzyme. In addition, acetyl CoA appears to reduce the activity of pyruvate dehydrogenase [13]. As a result, an increase in rate of hepatic and muscle fatty acid oxidation in diabetes, secondary to a rise in plasma FFA level, would be expected to lead to a decrease in activity of pyruvate dehydrogenase, resulting in an increase in both conversion of glucose to lactate in muscle and hepatic gluconeogenesis. Finally, we have shown that there is a direct relationship between plasma FFA concentration and both hepatic glucose production and fasting plasma glucose concentration [14]. The presence of significant correlation coefficients between variables does not prove that they are causally related, but the data support the hypothesis that increased hepatic glucose production, secondary to an elevation in circulating FFA concentration, may play a significant role in the development of fasting hyperglycemia in NIDDM.

Conclusions

Resistance to insulin-stimulated glucose uptake is present in the great majority of patients with IGT or NIDDM [1-4]. Furthermore, resistance to insulin-stimulated glucose uptake of a degree comparable to that seen in patients with NIDDM exists in approximately 25% of non-obese individuals with normal oral glucose tolerance [6]. Resistance to insulin-stimulated glucose uptake is also common in overweight individuals with normal glucose tolerance [15], and it has recently been demonstrated to occur in patients with essential hypertension [16]. The difference in the degree to which glucose tolerance is maintained in these various groups appears to be a function of the ability of the beta cell to compensate for the defect in insulin action [17]. Glucose tolerance does not deteriorate significantly in insulin-resistant patients if they are able to increase their insulin-secretory response and maintain a state of chronic hyperinsulinemia. When this goal cannot be achieved, gross decompensation of glucose homeostasis occurs.

We propose that the relationship between insulin resistance, plasma insulin level and glucose tolerance summarized above is mediated to a significant degree by changes in ambient plasma FFA concentration. Although patients with NIDDM are also resistant to insulin suppression of plasma FFA concentration, plasma FFA concentration can be reduced by relatively small increments in insulin concentration [8]. Consequently, elevations of circulating plasma FFA concentration can be prevented if large amounts of insulin can be secreted [5,7]. If hyperinsulinemia cannot be maintained, plasma FFA concentration will not be suppressed normally, and the increase in plasma FFA concentration will result in increased hepatic glucose production. Since these events are taking place in individuals who are quite resistant to insulin-stimulated glucose uptake, it is apparent that even small increases in hepatic glucose production are likely to lead to significant fasting hyperglycemia under these conditions.

We believe that the formulation outlined above provides the best explanation at this time for the development of fasting hyperglycemia in patients with NIDDM and is subject to experimental validation. Whether or not the proposed sequence of events actually occurs remains to be seen.

Acknowledgements

Supported by Research Grants from the National Institutes of Health (NIDDK 30732-06 and RR-00070).

References

1. Shen S-W, Reaven GM, Farquhar J. Comparison of impedance to insulin-mediated glucose uptake in normal subjects and in subjects with latent diabetes. J Clin Invest 1970;49:2151–2160.
2. Ginsberg J, Olefsky JM, Reaven GM. Further evidence that insulin resistance exists in patients with chemical diabetes. Diabetes 1974;23:674–678.
3. Ginsberg H, Kimmerling G, Olefsky JM, Reaven GM. Demonstration of insulin resistance in untreated adult onset diabetic subjects with fasting hyperglycemia. J Clin Invest 1975;55:454–461.
4. Reaven GM. Insulin resistance in noninsulin-dependent diabetes mellitus: does it exist and can it be measured? Am J Med 1983;74:3–17.
5. Golay A, Chen Y-DI, Reaven GM. Effect of differences in glucose tolerance on insulin's ability to regulate carbohydrate and free fatty acid metabolism in obese individuals. J Clin Endocrinol Metab 1986;62:1081–1088.
6. Hollenbeck C, Reaven GM. Variations in insulin-stimulated glucose uptake in healthy individuals with normal glucose tolerance. J Clin Endocrinol Metab 1987;64:1169–1173.
7. Fraze E, Donner CC, Swislocki ALM, Chiou Y-AM, Chen Y-DI, Reaven GM. Ambient plasma free fatty acid concentrations in noninsulin-dependent diabetes mellitus: evidence for insulin resistance. J Clin Endocrinol Metab 1985;61:807–811.
8. Swislocki ALM, Chen Y-DI, Golay A, Chang M-O, Reaven GM. Insulin suppression of plasma-free fatty acid concentration in normal individuals and patients with Type 2 (non-insulin-dependent) diabetes. Diabetologia 1987;30:622–626.

174

9. Rizza RA, Mandarino LJ, Gerich JE. Dose-response characteristics for effects of insulin on production and utilization of glucose in man. Am J Physiol 1981;240 (Endocrinol Metab 3): E630–E639.

10. Ferrannini E, Barrett EJ, Bevilacqua S, DeFronzo RA. Effect of fatty acids on glucose production and utilization in man. J Clin Invest 1983;72:1737–1747.

11. Williamson JR, Kreisberg RA, Felts PW. Mechanism for stimulation of gluconeogenesis by fatty acids in perfused rat liver. Proc Natl Acad Sci USA 1966;56:247–254.

12. Williamson JR, Browning ET, Olson MS. Interrelations between fatty acid oxidation and the control of gluconeogenesis in perfused rat liver. Adv Enzyme Regul 1968;6:67–99.

13. Randle PJ. α-Keto acid dehydrogenase complexes and respiratory fuel utilization in diabetes. Diabetologia 1985;28:479–484.

14. Golay A, Swislocki ALM, Chen Y-DI, Reaven GM. Relationships between plasma free fatty acid concentration, endogenous glucose production, and fasting hyperglycemia in normal and non-insulin dependent diabetic individuals. Metabolism 1987;36:692–696.

15. Reaven GM, Olefsky JM. Role of insulin resistance in the pathogenesis of hyperglycemia. Adv Mod Nutr 1987;II:229–266.

16. Shen D-C, Shieh S-M, Fuh MM-T, Wu D-A, Chen Y-DI, Reaven GM. Resistance to insulin-stimulated-glucose uptake in patients with hypertension. J Clin Endocrinol Metab 1988;66:580–583.

17. Reaven GM. Role of insulin resistance in human disease. Diabetes 1988:37:1595–1607.

Complications of NIDDM

CHAPTER 13

Non-insulin-dependent diabetes and hypertension

ELIZABETH BARRETT-CONNOR

*University of California, San Diego, Department of Community and Family Medicine, La Jolla, CA 92093,
U.S.A.*

Introduction

Diabetes and hypertension, two common chronic diseases associated with age and obesity, are, not surprisingly, often seen together. The well-known clinical association has been confirmed in industrial and population-based cohorts, but its magnitude and etiology remain controversial, despite a very large scientific effort by many investigators [1–5]. After an extensive review of this literature, it seemed increasingly unlikely that it could be covered in its entirety or that important new insights could be produced. Consequently the present review examines the prevalence and consequences of the association of non-insulin-dependent diabetes mellitus (NIDDM) and high blood pressure, using data from the Rancho Bernardo cohort, a geographically defined community of upper-middle-class older Caucasian adults in Southern California. Thereafter a broader database is used to consider briefly the etiology and treatment of these two conditions.

The Rancho Bernardo study

In 1972–74, 82% of residents aged 30 and older were seen for a brief interview and evaluation, which included blood pressure, fasting plasma glucose and lipids, and a medical history with regard to diagnosis and current treatment for diabetes and hypertension. Over 5000 participants of average age 59 years participated. Within 6 months (median interval 100 days), one-third of this group were re-examined in much greater detail, at which time repeat measures of blood pressure and fasting plasma glucose were obtained along with a more detailed medical and behavioral history, lipoproteins and ECG. These two visits, in 1972–74 and 1973–75, were part of a Lipid Research Clinic Prevalence Study, to which we added simple questions about known diabetes and hypertension and measurements of baseline blood pressure and glucose.

Ten to 12 years later (1984–87) all surviving members of this cohort were invited to participate in another evaluation, this one focused on diabetes. The overall response rate for this evaluation was 83%; 79% of those aged 50 and older were able to come to the clinic. At this visit, a 75 g oral glucose tolerance test was performed in the morning on fasting subjects; blood pressure was again measured according to protocol, and additional data were again obtained about medical history, medication use and life-style. In addition, fasting and 2-hour insulin levels were measured in conjunction with the oral glucose tolerance test in two-thirds of participants. Since we wished to distinguish non-insulin-dependent diabetes mellitus (NIDDM) from insulin-dependent diabetes mellitus (IDDM), all those taking insulin were excluded from the analyses presented here. There were in fact only 16 insulin-using subjects aged 50 and older, at least half of whom had insulin-dependent diabetes by C-peptide or age-of-onset criteria.

Coincidence of diabetes and hypertension

At the 1972–74 visit, the prevalence of known diabetes (defined by history) in these older adults was similar to that reported from a U.S. Public Health Survey of a more representative sample of the United States population (Table 1); 'new diabetes' (fasting hyperglycemia) was less common in Rancho Bernardo than in the PHS study, presumably because the national survey diagnosis used post-challenge glucose, which

TABLE 1

Age-specific prevalence of known and new diabetes in U.S. Public Health Service Survey and in Rancho Bernardo, CA, 1972–1974 [6]

Age (years)	Known diabetes (%)		New diabetes* (%)	
	USPHS	RB	USPHS	RB
35–44	0.8	1.2	1.9	1.5
45–54	1.8	3.8	3.7	3.9
55–64	3.7	3.9	7.3	4.6
65–74	5.5	5.9	9.3	3.2
75 +	4.9	6.0	19.9	3.3

*USPHS based on two-hour post-challenge glucose level; Rancho Bernardo (RB) based on fasting plasma glucose value.

rises with age, and we used fasting glucose, which does not [6]. The 20% prevalence of hypertension in Rancho Bernardo was similar to that reported in United States Surveys [7]. With regard to body mass index (BMI), on average Rancho Bernardo women were leaner than United States women while Rancho Bernardo men were very similar to United States men seen in the National Health and Nutrition Examination Survey [6].

When the coexistence of diabetes and hypertension were examined in the 3456 adults aged 50–79 at the 1972–74 visit, a history of hypertension was significantly more common in both men and women with diabetes than in men and women without diabetes [7]. Since some of this excess could reflect ascertainment bias, i.e. persons with diabetes being more exposed to health-care providers and more likely to have high blood pressure diagnosed, it is important to note that the excess of known hypertension was less striking in persons with 'new diabetes', i.e., those who were so classified based only on fasting hyperglycemia first recognized at this visit, who represented nearly half of all diabetic subjects (Fig. 1).

Examining the measured blood pressure in this cohort illustrates another problem that plagues cross-sectional studies of diabetes and hypertension. Many persons identified as diabetic are receiving antihypertensive medication, usually diuretics that can increase blood glucose and probably unmask diabetes. In this population in 1972–74, well before the maximum blood pressure control efforts in the United States, 56% of nondiabetics and 58% of diabetic patients with a history of hypertension were taking antihypertensive drugs, and apparently appropriately so, since people using antihypertensive agents had higher mean systolic and diastolic blood pressure than those not taking such medication [7]. To interpret the association of blood pressures with blood glucose, when both could be modified by antihypertensive agents, analyses are

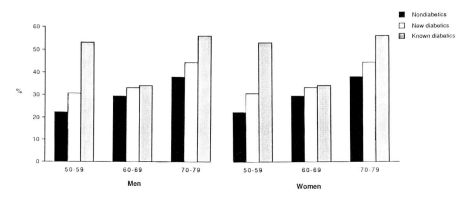

Fig. 1. Prevalence of known hypertension by diabetic status, Rancho Bernardo men and women aged 50–79 years, 1972–1974. Adapted from Ref. 7.

required that exclude subjects taking these drugs. When those having blood pressure treatment, primarily diuretics, in 1972–74 were excluded from analyses, diabetic patients in general showed a two-fold excess risk of categorical systolic and categorical diastolic hypertension. This association was independent of age, but was small after BMI was considered in the analysis (Table 2). Before concluding that the association of diabetes and hypertension independent of obesity is weak, however, it is important to note that individuals with the highest blood pressures were excluded when analyses were restricted to persons not taking antihypertensive drugs. This dilemma regarding the appropriate handling of data so confounded by treatment complicates the interpretation of many investigations of the prevalence of diabetes in hypertensives and vice versa.

In addition, in 1972–74 the diagnosis of diabetes was dependent on history or fasting hyperglycemia. In a more recent survey we have found that two-thirds of the older adults who have diabetes meet only post-challenge glucose criteria. Since a glucose tolerance test was not done at the first visit, they would have been misclassified as nondiabetic, thus minimizing differences between the two groups.

We have just begun to examine the relationship of blood pressure to diabetes using data from over 2000 members of this cohort who had a glucose tolerance test in 1984–1987 when they were aged 50–89 years. Based on World Health Organization criteria, 60% had normal glucose tolerance, 26% had impaired glucose tolerance (IGT) and 14% had NIDDM [8]. Over 40% of those with NIDDM, two-thirds of whom were not known previously to have diabetes, were taking antihypertensive medication, nearly twice the rate for those with normal glucose tolerance. In analyses that did not exclude those so treated, those with IGT or NIDDM had higher mean systolic blood pressure levels than those with normal glucose tolerance; as shown in Table 3, after adjusting for age and obesity these differences were statistically (and

TABLE 2

Age- and obesity-adjusted mean blood pressure (mmHg) by diabetic status: Rancho Bernardo 1972–1974 [7]

	Men		Women	
	SBP	DBP	SBP	DBP
Nondiabetic	139.6	81.2	135.4	79.8
New diabetic	140.5	82.8	136.3	79.1
Known diabetic	144.3	82.0	142.9	82.4

Excludes persons taking antihypertensive drugs. SBP, systolic blood pressure; DBP, diastolic blood pressure.

TABLE 3
Age- and body-mass-index-adjusted mean systolic blood pressure (mmHg) in Rancho Bernardo men and women aged 50–89 years, 1984–1987

	Normal	IGT	New NIDDM	Known NIDDM
Men	136.7	141.4**	148.2**	145.3**
Women	138.1	141.3*	141.0	146.3*

$*p < 0.05$; $**p < 0.001$ compared with normal subjects.
Includes those taking antihypertensive drugs.
Adapted from Reaven, P., Browner, D. and Barrett-Connor, E. Unpublished manuscript.

probably clinically) significant (P. Reaven et al., unpublished results). Furthermore, hypertension antedated the diagnosis of diabetes and of renal disease.

It was suspected that post-challenge hyperglycemia reflected obesity and aging to a greater extent than did fasting hyperglycemia. Blood pressure levels were therefore also compared among diabetics who had fasting hyperglycemia (≥ 140 mg/dl (7.8 mmol/l) regardless of post-challenge levels) with blood pressure in those who had only post-challenge hyperglycemia (≥ 200 mg/dl; 11.1 mmol/l). Contrary to expectation, fasting hyperglycemia was associated with a (non-significantly) higher BMI but similar waist–hip ratios and no significant differences in the mean blood pressure levels, compared with those with post-challenge hyperglycemia alone (Table 4).

TABLE 4
Age-adjusted blood pressure (mmHg) and body mass index by fasting or post-challenge glucose level diagnosis of NIDDM, Rancho Bernardo 1984–1987

	Fasting plasma glucose ≥ 140 mg/dl		2-h plasma glucose ≥ 200 mg/dl, and FPG < 140 mg/dl	
	Men ($n = 52$)	Women ($n = 27$)	Men ($n = 97$)	Women ($n = 114$)
SBP	150.8	147.6	145.6	146.2
DBP	78.2	74.2	78.5	75.3
BMI	27.7	27.0	26.0	25.2
WHR	0.93	0.84	0.93	0.83

WHR, waist–hip ratio.

182

Consequences of hypertension in older adults with NIDDM

In 1983 we reported the seven-year heart disease mortality experience of those aged 40–79 in 1972–1974, comparing 212 men and 131 women who had diabetes defined by history or fasting hyperglycemia with 2104 nondiabetics who had fasting plasma glucose levels less than 110 mg/dl (6.1 mmol/l) and who had no personal or family history of diabetes [9]. The age-adjusted relative risk of death attributed to ischemic heart disease was 2.5 for diabetic men and 3.4 for diabetic women. In a multivariate proportional hazards model, diabetes predicted ischemic heart disease in both sexes, independent of age, systolic blood pressure, BMI, cholesterol and cigarette smoking (Table 5).

The risk of stroke was also examined in those aged 50–79 at baseline [10]. Based on the 12-year follow-up, diabetic subjects had a higher age-adjusted stroke risk than nondiabetics and this risk was greater in those with higher blood pressure. The risk of ischemic heart disease was independent of blood pressure, demonstrating that hypertension does not explain all the increased risk of cardiovascular disease among diabetic people.

We have recently begun to examine the contribution of hypertension to cardiovascular disease risk in people with and without diabetes using the fifteen-year follow-up of this cohort. In this analysis (Langer et al., unpublished), the cardiovascular death rate in people with diabetes alone, hypertension alone or both has been compared with that in subjects with neither diabetes nor high blood pressure at baseline. As shown in Table 6, hypertension was a stronger risk factor for cardiovascular disease than diabetes in men, whereas diabetes was a stronger risk factor than hypertension in women. When both diabetes and hypertension existed together, the relative risk of cardiovascular disease was higher than for either attribute alone.

TABLE 5

Standardized coefficients for ischemic heart disease mortality in Rancho Bernardo men and women aged 40–79 years; 1972–1980

	Men	Women
Diabetes	2.96*	2.53*
Age	3.51*	4.13*
Cholesterol	2.16*	4.24*
Systolic blood pressure	2.13*	1.04
Body mass index	0.16	−0.07
Smoking	0.36	1.51

*$p < 0.05$.

TABLE 6
Age- and BMI-adjusted sex-specific CVD mortality, Rancho Bernardo, 1972-1987

Diabetes mellitus	Hyper-tension	Men ($n = 2060$)		Women ($n = 2276$)	
		Relative risk (C.I.)		Relative risk (C.I.)	
−	+	2.1	(1.6-2.7)	1.9	(1.3-2.7)
+	−	1.3	(0.7-2.2)	2.6	(1.2-5.7)
+	+	3.0	(1.8-5.0)	9.9	5.1-19.0)

Adapted from Langer, R.L. and Barrett-Connor, E. Unpublished manuscript.

The etiology of the diabetes-hypertension association

Several possible causes of hypertension in NIDDM have been proposed, but only one will be discussed here. The association of serum insulin with hypertension was reported in 1966 [11] but it was not until the 1985 report of the association of blood pressure with endogenous insulin in middle-aged Israelis [12] that this concordance attracted considerable attention. The notion that insulin raises blood pressure, and explains the excess of hypertension among diabetics, has been eagerly embraced. Possibly the initial enthusiasm for this hypothesis reflected the prolonged lack of success in elucidating the etiology of such a well-known association. Given the even longer and more spectacular failure to determine the etiology of essential hypertension, it is not surprising that the insulin-causes-hypertension connection was also sought enthusiastically in patients without diabetes. It was exciting to think that insulin could be the cause of the higher blood pressures seen in overweight adults, many of whom also have hyperinsulinemia, and it was biologically plausible, with several mechanisms suggested for such an association, such as insulin-mediated sodium retention and sympathetic or cardiovascular hyperreactivity [13-15].

When the Israeli study [12] appeared, our group, like others, attempted to confirm these provocative findings. The failure has possibly colored my interpretation of the literature. In all fairness, however, the published results are far more contradictory than a casual review of the reviews would suggest.

Our results (Asch et al., unpublished) are based on 784 men and 653 women aged 50-93 years who had a glucose tolerance test and insulin levels measured when seen in 1984-87. Their average age was 68 years and 54% were female. Using a blood pressure of $\geqslant 140/90$ mmHg as the definition of hypertension (to approximate the Israeli Study [12] definition of $\geqslant 143/93$), almost half the subjects had hypertension; 14% had NIDDM by history or OGTT using WHO criteria. Overall, the post-challenge

184

insulin levels were higher in those with hypertension (96.7 vs. 78.1 mU/l), whereas fasting insulin levels did not differ significantly by blood pressure group (14.2 vs. 12.7 mU/l). For comparison with the Israeli study, the contribution of hypertension to the variability of insulin was analysed, rather than the reverse. In this analysis, diabetic status, age and BMI accounted for about one-fifth of the overall variability in post-challenge insulin whereas blood pressure did not account for a significant portion of the variability. After adjusting for age, diabetes and obesity, the difference between mean insulin levels in hypertensive versus normotensive subjects decreased from 18.7 to 4.4 mU/l.

When post-challenge insulin levels were compared in participants without previously diagnosed diabetes (to exclude treatment effects), according to obesity and diabetes status subgroups, hypertensive subjects had higher insulin levels in three subgroups and similar or lower levels in three subgroups (Fig. 2). Only the non-obese diabetic subjects had statistically significantly higher insulin levels in the presence of hypertension (116.6 vs. 92.3 mU/l). The largest difference was in the obese diabetics, where those with hypertension had, on average, a 30.8 mU/l *lower* post-challenge insulin level than those without hypertension. A similar finding was reported by Modan et al. in the Israeli Study [12].

Although the multiple subgroup analysis approach can legitimately be deplored, these represent the groups used in published studies, which generally consisted of even fewer subjects in each category. The many other studies that examined the link between hyperinsulinemia and hypertension in adults used a variety of subject sources and types of diabetes (hypertension and obesity) and analytic design. As shown in Table 7, about half show a positive association between either fasting or

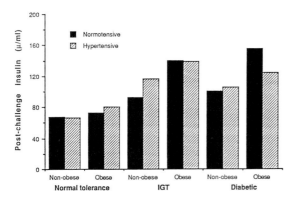

Fig. 2. Mean 2-hour post-challenge plasma insulin level by blood pressure, obesity and glucose tolerance status, Rancho Bernardo men and women, aged 50–93 years, 1984–1987. From Asch, Barrett-Connor, and Wingard (unpublished data).

TABLE 7

Published associations between endogenous insulin and blood pressure in clinical studies

First author (yr) [Ref.]	Association with insulin	
	Fasting	Post-challenge
Non-diabetic non-obese subjects		
Welborn (1966) [11]	+	
Berglund (1976) [16]	+	
Hedstrand (1976) [17]	0	0
Bonora (1987) [18]	0	+
Zavaroni (1989) [19]		+
Obese subjects		
Berglund (1976) [16]	−	
Lucas (1985) [20]	+	
Mancini (1986) [21]	−	0
Manicardi (1986) [22]	0	+
Weinsier (1986) [23]	0	
Bonora (1987) [18]	0	0
Diabetic subjects		
Christlieb (1985) [24]	+	0
Lowenthal (1985) [25]	+	
Uusitupa (1987) [26] Men	0	0
Women	0	+
Mbanya (1988) [27]	+	
Verdecchia (1988) [28]	0	

0 = no association;

− = negative association;

+ = positive association.

post-challenge insulin and hypertension, but neither the insulin variable nor the subgroup is consistent across studies [11,16–28].

Because of the problems of subject selection and the heterogeneity of insulin and blood pressure in the clinical studies, the four non-clinic-based studies merit particular note (Table 8). The Israeli study [11], which used a 100 g glucose load, found no overall association between fasting insulin and hypertension after adjusting for obesity and diabetes. The sum of post-challenge insulin levels was higher in hypertensives than normotensives in all glucose tolerance groups save one. Insulin levels were said to be unrelated to age in the Israeli cohort, so the data were not age-adjusted. This is curious, since age and post-challenge insulin are usually strongly related and were found to be highly correlated in Rancho Bernardo. In the Paris Prospective Study

TABLE 8
Population-based studies of endogenous insulin and blood pressure

First author (yr)	Population	Control variables	Blood pressure		Association	
			SBP > (mmHg)	DBP > (mmHg)	Fasting	Post-challenge
Cambien (1982) [29]	6471 Paris employees	Age, BMI, 2-hour glucose	mean	mean		0
Modan (1985) [12]	1241 Israelis	BMI, glucose tolerance, Rx	145	93	0	− Obese diabetic + All others
Fournier (1986) [31]	248 Miami employees	Age, BMI	mean	mean	+	
Cambien (1987) [30]	2144 Paris employees	Age, BMI, FPG	mean	mean	0	
Asch (unpbl.)	1437 Rancho Bernardo	Age, sex, BMI, glucose tolerance, Rx	SBP ≥ 140	DBP ≥ 90	+ Obese non-diabetic 0 All others	+ Non-obese diabetic 0 All others

[29,30] of middle-aged men without treated diabetes or hypertension, there was no relationship between fasting or post-challenge insulin and hypertension that persisted after adjusting for age, obesity and fasting plasma glucose. In a smaller Miami study [31] of nondiabetic hospital employees, however, fasting insulin levels were associated with mean blood pressure after adjusting for age and obesity.

Although it is far from clear the degree to which glucose challenge, subject selection and analytic approach explain the observed differences in the insulin-blood pressure connection, these data taken together suggest that it is too soon to accept the hypothesis that insulin is independently associated with hypertension, however eagerly a solution to the diabetes–blood pressure conundrum is sought.

Several other small pieces of evidence may also argue against a direct insulin–blood pressure association. In the rat model, streptozotocin-induced diabetes without insulin supplementation is usually followed by a rise in arterial pressure within the first week; blood pressure levels are maximal around the fourth week and remain elevated thereafter [32]. In another animal model, insulin infusion with glucose held constant for 7–28 days raised plasma insulin by 5–10-fold but did not raise blood pressure in dogs [33].

The effect on blood pressure of reducing insulin dosage in 12 women with NIDDM, half of whom were hypertensive, was reported recently [34]. A significant decrease in body weight and urinary sodium was seen in all women, which was correlated directly with a fall in systolic and diastolic blood pressure in hypertensive but not normotensive patients. One explanation for these results is that the insulin–blood pressure association is mediated by the obesity-enhancing effect of insulin. If so, it is noteworthy that no effect was seen in normotensives who also lost weight.

If hyperinsulinemia were a direct cause of hypertension then it could be expected that insulin treatment would raise blood pressure. Surprisingly, in the excitement about the recent studies of blood pressure and insulin, no attention has been paid to the University Group Diabetes Program (UGDP) study, a placebo-controlled randomized clinical trial of exogenous insulin [35]. In that study (of subjects who had IGT or NIDDM by current criteria), placebo recipients gained less weight than those who were treated with standard or variable doses of insulin. Those given insulin gained more weight but had better glucose levels, compared to the placebo group. After five years they also had higher systolic and diastolic blood pressure. As shown in Table 9, the percent classified as hypertensive during follow-up, among those who were not hypertensive at baseline, showed a stepwise increment from placebo to insulin standard (low dose) to insulin variable (higher dose) assignment. This study offers perhaps the strongest evidence to date for an effect of insulin on blood pressure, but does not invoke insulin resistance, as suggested by the elegant studies of Ferranini et al. [36].

Is hyperinsulinemia or insulin resistance causally related to high blood pressure,

TABLE 9

Percent of initially normotensive University Group Diabetes Program study subjects who completed at least one follow-up examination and who were later classified as hypertensive [35]

	Placebo ($n = 128$)	Insulin-standard ($n = 139$)	Insulin-variable ($n = 142$)
SBP $\geq$ 160 and/or DBP $\geq$ 95 mmHg	50	55	56
Treated for hypertension	32	40	46*
Both	23	28	35*

*$p < 0.05$ compared with placebo.

or simply another marker for the well-known blood pressure–obesity association? A dynamic assessment of B-cell function and insulin resistance may help to elucidate the hyperinsulinemia-hypertension link in fat and lean adults with and without NIDDM. It is too soon, however, to accept insulin as the common denominator. Inconsistencies certainly suggest that endogenous insulin is not necessarily the causal factor [37].

The treatment of hypertension in NIDDM

Clinical trials of the treatment of hypertension in diabetics are short in duration, and focus on the efficacy of such treatment on blood pressure and not the prevention of cardiovascular disease. With the recognition that the most commonly used antihypertensive drugs can raise glucose levels and adversely alter plasma lipids [38], a plethora of recent clinical trials have attempted to demonstrate lesser or no such effects with some of the newer antihypertensive agents. In these trials, glucose or lipid variables rather than cardiovascular disease are studied. A recent review concluded that diuretics and beta blockers should be excluded from antihypertensive drug selection because they worsen glucose tolerance [39].

The purpose of blood pressure treatment is, of course, to prevent cardiovascular disease. Diabetes has been a specific exclusion in the protocol of most large randomized clinical trials designed to evaluate the benefit of antihypertensives in the prevention of cardiovascular disease. When diabetic subjects have been included, the number in each primary prevention study is usually too small for analysis. One notable exception is the Hypertension Detection and Follow-up Program (HDFP), where diabetes was not an exclusion criterion [40].

Table 10 shows that participants with either diabetes by history or hyperglycemia had a higher death rate from all causes combined than those without, the difference

TABLE 10

The Hypertension Detection and Follow-up Program five-year mortality by diabetes criteria [40]

| | Criterion | n | Age-sex-race-adjusted rate | | |
			Stepped care	Referred care	% Difference
FPG	< 140	5196	51.8	67.8	−23.6
	≥ 140	255	74.9	104.1	−29.0
1-h plasma glu-cose	< 205	3765	51.6	65.9	−13.4
	≥ 205	1436	43.8	79.1	−45.0
Diabetes Rx	No	5553	56.3	71.2	−20.9
	Yes	307	58.0	78.9	−26.5

being most striking for fasting hyperglycemia, which provides the most unequivocal diagnosis of NIDDM. Further, in every diagnostic category, those who were assigned to the more aggressive antihypertensive treatment group fared better than those who were referred to usual care, which may or may not have included antihypertensive therapy. Because treatment in the stepped-care group began with chlorthalidone, these results are particularly reassuring with regard to the use of diuretics in the management of high blood pressure in patients with diabetes.

Conclusion

Hypertension precedes the diagnosis of NIDDM and the appearance of recognizable renal disease, and carries an increased risk of cardiovascular disease and death. The etiology of the hypertension is obscure, but it is apparently independent of obesity, at least as usually estimated. Hyperinsulinemia is a candidate mechanism, but the data are more inconsistent than definitive. Whatever the mechanism, treatment with common antihypertensive drugs, including diuretics, appears to reduce the risk of cardiovascular disease despite undesirable effects on lipids and glucose.

Acknowledgement

This research was supported by NIDDK Grant PHS DK38801.

190

References

1. Jarrett RJ, Keen H, Chakrabarti R. Diabetes, hyperglycaemia and arterial disease. In: Keen H, Jarrett J, (eds.). Complications of Diabetes, 2nd edn. London: Edward Arnold. 1982;179–204.
2. Drury PL. Diabetes and arterial hypertension. Diabetologia 1983;24:1–9.
3. Fuller JH. Blood pressure and diabetes mellitus. Handbook of Hypertension 1985;6:318–330.
4. Ramos OL. Diabetes mellitus and hypertension: state of the art lecture. Inter-Am Soc Proc (Suppl I, Hypertension) 1988;11:114–118.
5. Sowers JR, Levy J, Zemel, MB. Hypertension and Diabetes. Med Clin North Am 1988;72: 1399–1413.
6. Barrett-Connor, E. The prevalence of diabetes mellitus in an adult community as determined by history or fasting hyperglycemia. Am J Epidermiol 1980;111:705–712.
7. Barrett-Connor E, Criqui MH, Klauber MR, Holdbrook M. Diabetes and hypertension in a community of older adults. Am J Epidermiol 1981;113:276–284.
8. Wingard DL, Sinsheimer P, Barrett-Connor EL, McPhillips JB. The prevalence of non-insulin dependent diabetes mellitus in older adults: a community-based study. Diabetes Care (in press).
9. Wingard DL, Suarez L, Barrett-Connor E. The sex differential in mortality from all causes and ischemic heart disease. Am J Epidermiol 1983;117:165–172.
10. Barrett-Connor E, Khaw K-T. Diabetes mellitus: an independent risk factor for stroke? Am J Epidemiol 1988;128:116–123.
11. Welborn TA, Breckenridge A, Rubinstein AH, Dollery CT, Fraser TR. Serum insulin in essential hypertension and in peripheral vascular disease. Lancet 1966;i:1336–1338.
12. Modan M, Halkin H, Almog S, Lusky A, Eshkol A, Shefi M, Shitrit A, Fuchs Z. Hyperinsulinemia. A link between hypertension, obesity, and glucose intolerance. J Clin Invest 1985;75:809–817.
13. DeFronzo RA. The effect of insulin on renal sodium: Diabetologia 1981;21:165–171.
14. Rowe JW, Young JB, Minaker KL, Stevens AL, Pallotta J, Landsberg L. Effect of insulin and glucose infusions on sympathetic nervous system activity in normal man. Diabetes 1981;30:219–225.
15. Weidmann P, Beretta-Piccoli C, Trost BN. Pressor factors and responsiveness in hypertension accompanying diabetes mellitus. Hypertension 7 (Suppl II) 1985;33–42.
16. Berglund G, Larsson B, Andersson O, Larsson O, Svärdsudd K, Björntrop P, Wilhelmsen L. Body composition and glucose metabolism in hypertensive middle-aged males. Acta Med Scand 1976;200:163–169.
17. Hedstrand H, Aberg H: Detection and characterization of middle-aged men with hypertension. Acta Med Scand 1976;199:273–280.
18. Bonora E, Zavaroni I, Alpi O, Pezzarossa A, Bruschi F, Dall'Aglio E, Guerra L, Coscelli C, Butturini U. Relationship between blood pressure and plasma insulin in non-obese and obese non-diabetic subjects. Diabetologia 1987;30:719–723.
19. Zavaroni I, Bonora E, Pagliara M, Dall'Aglio E, Luchetti L, Buonanno G, Bonati PA, Bergonzani M, Gnudi L, Passeri M, Reaven G. Risk factors for coronary artery disease in healthy persons with hyperinsulinemia and normal glucose tolerance. N Engl J Med 1989;320:702–705.
20. Lucas CP, Estigarribia JA, Darga LL, Reaven GM. Insulin and blood pressure in obesity. Hypertension 1985;7:702–706.
21. Mancini M, Strazullo P, Trevisan M, Contaldo F, Vaccaro O, Cappuccio FP. Pathophysiological interrelations of obesity, impaired glucose tolerance, and arterial hypertension. Prev Med 1985;14:428–435.
22. Manicardi V, Camellini L, Bellodi G, Coscelli C, Ferrannini E. Evidence for an association of high blood pressure and hyperinsulinemia in obese men. J Clin Endocrinol Metab 1986;62:1302–1304.
23. Weinsier RL, Norris DJ, Birch R, Bernstein RS, Pi-Sunyer FX, Yang M-U, Wang J, Pierson RN, Van Itallie TB. Serum insulin and blood pressure in an obese population. Int J Obesity 1986;10:11–17.

24. Christlieb AR, Krolewski AS, Warram JH, Soeldner JS. Is insulin the link between hypertension and obesity? Hypertension 1985;7(Suppl II):54–57.

25. Lowenthal LM, Pim B, Hillson RM, Dhar H, Hockaday TDR. Blood pressure at diagnosis of type 2 diabetes correlates with plasma insulin concentration but not during the next 5 years. Diabetes Res 1985;2:65–69.

26. Uusitupa M, Siitonen O. Pyörälä K, Mustonen J, Voutilainen E, Hersio K, Penttilä I. Relationship of blood pressure and left ventricular mass to serum insulin levels in newly diagnosed non-insulin-dependent (type 2) diabetic patients and in non-diabetic subjects. Diabetes Res 1987;4:19–25.

27. Mbanya J-C N, Thomas TH, Wilkinson R, Alberti KGMM, Taylor R. Hypertension and hyperinsulinemia: a relation in diabetes but not essential hypertension. Lancet 1988;i:733–734.

28. Verdecchia P, Gatteschi C, Benemio G, Guerrieri M, Porcellati C. Hyperinsulinaemia and hypertension in diabetes. Lancet 1988;ii:343–344.

29. Cambien F, Jacqueson A, Richard JL, Rosselin G, Ducimetiere P. Groupe d'Etude sur l'Epidémiologie de l'Athérosclérose. INSERM Symposium No. 22: Advances in Diabetes Epidemiology. Amsterdam: Elsevier, 1982;189–196.

30. Cambien F, Warnet JM, Eschwège E, Jacqueson A, Richard JL, Rosselin G. Body mass, blood pressure, glucose and lipids – does plasma insulin explain their relationships? Arteriosclerosis 1987;7:197–202.

31. Fournier AM, Gadia MT, Kubrusly DB, Skyler JS, Sosenko JM. Blood pressure, insulin and glycemia in nondiabetic subjects. Am J Med 1986;80:861–864.

32. Kohlmann D Jr, Bossolan D, Zanella MT, Ramos OL, Ribeiro AB. Hypertension in experimental diabetes mellitus: role for major vasopressor systems. Hypertension 1987;9:531.

33. Hall JE, Coleman TG, Mizelle HL. Does chronic hyperinsulinemia cause hypertension? Am Hyper 1989;2:171–173.

34. Tedde R, Sechi LA, Marigliano A, Pala A, Scano L. Antihypertensive effect of insulin reduction in diabetic-hypertensive patients. Am Hyper 1988;2:163–170.

35. Knatterud GL, Klimt CR, Goldner MG et al. Effects of hypoglycemic agents on vascular complications in patients with adult-onset diabetes: VIII. Evaluation of insulin therapy: final report. Diabetes 1982;29:1001–1005.

36. Ferrannini E, Buzzigoli G, Bonadonna R, et al. Insulin resistance in essential hypertension. N Engl J Med 1987;7:317–350.

37. O'Hare JA. The enigma of insulin resistance and hypertension. Am J Med 1988;84:505–510.

38. Ames RP. Coronary heart disease and the treatment of hypertension: impact of diuretics on serum lipids and glucose. J Cardiol Pharm 1984;6:S466–S473.

39. Houston MC. Approaches to treatment of hypertension in diabetic patients. Cardiovasc Rev Res 1988;Nov:30–35.

40. The Hypertension Detection and Follow-up Program Cooperative Research Group. Mortality findings for stepped-care and referred-care participants in the Hypertension Detection and Follow-up Program, stratified by other risk factors. Prev Med 1985;14:312–335.

CHAPTER 14

Antiplatelet drugs and the prevention of progression of macrovascular disease in diabetes mellitus

JOHN A. COLWELL

Charleston VA Medical Center, 109 Bee Street, Charleston, SC 29403, and Medical University of South Carolina, 171 Ashley Avenue, Charleston, SC 29425, U.S.A.

Macrovascular disease in diabetes

Scope and impact

In 1987, it was estimated that there were 6.5 million individuals who were known to have diabetes mellitus in the United States. About 5.44 million of these (84%) were aged 45 or over. In that same year 564,868 new cases of diabetes were diagnosed and 620,625 individuals with diabetes were hospitalized because of the chronic complications of diabetes. The majority of these hospitalizations (77%) were for the treatment of cardiovascular complications. In all, the total cost of diabetes in 1987 in the U.S. was $20.4 billion, and a great proportion of this cost can be ascribed to the chronic macrovascular complications of diabetes [1].

Macrovascular disease is a major contributor not only to morbidity, but also to mortality in patients with diabetes mellitus. Diabetes is the seventh leading cause of death in the U.S. and accounted for 1.8% of all deaths in the U.S. in 1982 [2]. Diabetes is a contributing cause of death in an additional 5%. Ischemic heart disease and cerebrovascular disease are involved in about 85% of diabetes deaths. Although these statistics are impressive, it is likely that they are an underestimate, since diabetes is underreported significantly on death certificates [2]. Life expectancy is clearly decreased in diabetes.

We recently analysed the impact of diabetes at the Charleston VA Medical Center, a 313-bed facility which serves a primary service area within a 110-mile radius. The hospital serves about 134,000 veterans, most of whom are males. It is closely affiliated with the Medical University of South Carolina, and its programme includes open-heart surgery, peripheral vascular surgery, cardiology and diabetes services. In 1988, there were 712 discharges recorded in 458 patients in whom diabetes was named as a primary or secondary diagnosis. A large proportion (393 patients = 86%) of these patients exhibited vascular complications of diabetes. Hypertension was found in 49% of these patients. When readmission was necessary, it was usually because of cardiovascular complications.

These national and local figures underscore the impact of the cardiovascular complications of diabetes on medical care in the United States. They reflect the well-known fact that individuals with diabetes mellitus are at an increased risk for cardiac, peripheral vascular and cerebrovascular disease. In view of the large numbers of individuals with diabetes who are newly diagnosed each year, with the yield of diabetes in those over age 65 approaching 20%, and with the great impact these vascular complications in diabetes have upon the patients and upon the economy, it is important to consider primary and secondary preventive strategies for macrovascular disease in diabetes.

Major cardiovascular risk factors

The four classic cardiovascular risk factors are hypertension, hypercholesterolemia, cigarette smoking and diabetes mellitus. Collaborative clinical trials have been performed in which modification of the first three risk factors has been accomplished, and the effect of such intervention on subsequent vascular events has been measured. The majority of these studies have been done in nondiabetic populations, and recommendations for preventive strategies in patients with diabetes, therefore, rest on a data base extrapolated from studies in nondiabetic individuals.

Consensus has been reached regarding the efficacy of hypertension control, cessation of smoking and lowering of plasma cholesterol in preventing future cardiovascular events. Firm recommendations from consensus panels are now in the public domain [3–5], and these preventive efforts are made with increasing frequency by practicing physicians and by their patients. In spite of the absence of collaborative trials in diabetic patients, it has been generally accepted that reduction of these three classic risk factors is a logical preventive approach to take with diabetic subjects.

Controversy still exists, however, about the value of glycemic control in preventing macrovascular complications of diabetes. Previous prospective trials gave no definitive answer to this question [6], and present trials are directed primarily at microvascular disease [7], or are not yet complete [8].

There has also been interest in defining the pathogenesis of atherosclerosis in diabetes, in the hope that a thorough understanding of the pathogenesis could lead to the development of prevention strategies which could arrest that process at an early stage of its development. One such strategy which gives great promise is antiplatelet therapy in diabetes. This paper will review our present state of knowledge in this area.

Pathogenesis of atherosclerosis in diabetes

In the 'response-to-injury' hypothesis of the pathogenesis of atherosclerosis, interaction of platelets with damaged endothelium appears to play a pivotal role [9–11]. According to this hypothesis, endothelial injury from mechanical damage, hypertension, hypercholesterolemia, elevated plasma free fatty acids, immune mechanisms and other factors may occur and initiate the process of atherosclerosis. At an area of endothelial damage, there may be adherence of monocytes, followed by subendothelial migration and lipid accumulation. Counter-regulatory repair processes may arrest the lesion, or progression to further vascular injury may follow. Platelets may adhere to the area of damage and a platelet thrombus may form as platelets aggregate and release vasoconstrictor and pro-aggregatory arachidonic-acid metabolites as well as growth factors which may stimulate smooth muscle cell migration and proliferation at the site of the injury. Lipid-laden macrophages may accumulate and plaque formation and thrombosis occur unless counter-regulation is successful. A series of events which may occur in diabetes is shown in Fig. 1.

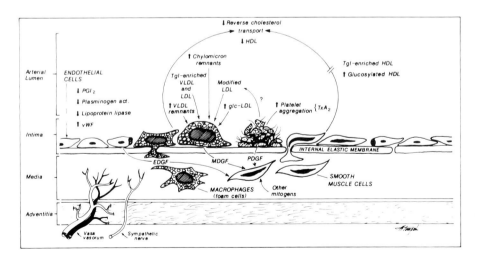

Fig. 1. One concept of the pathogenesis of atherosclerosis in diabetes mellitus. (Reproduced from Ref. 12 with permission from the C.V. Mosby Co.)

Platelets and diabetes mellitus

The response-to-injury hypothesis ascribes a role for the platelet in the pathogenesis of atherosclerosis. This has been one reason for a large number of studies of platelet function in people with diabetes and in animal models of diabetes. Recent reviews have considered this subject in detail, and should be consulted for complete references [12–18]. A summary of alterations of platelet function which have been described in diabetes is shown in Table 1.

There is no clear indication what the precise relationship of these findings is to diabetic vascular disease. Theoretically, altered platelet behavior could be a cause, a result, both a cause and a result, or bear no relationship to diabetic vascular disease. There is general agreement that many of the alterations of platelet behavior shown in Table 1 can be found in diabetic subjects with established vascular disease. Similarly, many of these alterations can be found in nondiabetic subjects with advanced large-vessel disease. These findings have led to the prevailing view that macrovascular disease could alter platelet behavior and by so doing could set up a vicious cycle which would promote progression of that vascular disease.

A more controversial question is whether the diabetic state causes altered platelet function in the absence of vascular disease. Those who support this view point to studies in which platelet hypersensitivity and increased thromboxane release can be demonstrated in IDDM subjects who are free from clinical vascular disease. Since the clinical recognition of vascular disease may be questioned, and since these findings are not always present in IDDM [19], recent studies have focussed on altered platelet function in animal models, shortly after induction of diabetes. Evidence to support the view that the altered metabolic state of diabetes contributes to changes in platelet function in these animal studies is given in Table 2.

These studies support the view that the platelet alterations described in diabetic subjects may not only result from existing vascular disease, but may also result from the altered metabolic state of diabetes mellitus. However, it remains conjectural as

TABLE 1
Alterations of platelet function in diabetes

In vitro	In vivo
↑Adhesiveness	↑Turnover
↑Aggregability	↓Survival
↑Thromboxane release	↑Beta-thromboglobulin
Platelet-plasma interactions	↑Plasma Factor 4
↑vWF fibrinogen	↑Platelet-derived growth factor
↑Immune complexes	↑Circulating platelet aggregates
↑Glycosylated LDL	

TABLE 2
Altered platelet function in animal models of diabetes

In vitro	In vivo
↑Aggregability	↑Turnover
↑Thromboxane release	↓Survival
Non-arachidonic acid pathways	Reversal by insulin

to whether altered platelet function contributes directly to vascular disease in diabetic or nondiabetic subjects. Nevertheless, this has been an attractive hypothesis to many investigators.

Antiplatelet therapy in diabetes mellitus

In view of the possible involvement of platelets in the accelerated atherosclerosis of diabetes mellitus, several primary and secondary prevention trials with antiplatelet agents have been done in patients with diabetes mellitus. The rationale for such studies has been strengthened by the findings of platelet hypersensitivity and increased platelet thromboxane synthesis in diabetes and by the ready availability of cyclo-oxygenase inhibitors such as aspirin with a very low toxic–therapeutic ratio. There has been increasing evidence of the effectiveness of aspirin therapy in a number of secondary prevention trials [20] and in at least one primary prevention trial in non-diabetic subjects [21,22].

The first study in diabetic subjects was a V.A. Cooperative study in which aspirin (325 mg tid) plus dipyridamole (75 mg tid) was compared with placebo therapy in a group of male type II diabetic patients who had gangrene, or who previously had an amputation for gangrene [23]. This was a very late secondary prevention trial in which it was postulated that antiplatelet therapy would prevent vascular death or the amputation of the opposite extremity from occlusive vascular disease. No effect of antiplatelet therapy was seen on either or both of these endpoints. Since the event rates were less than predicted, it is likely that the sample size of 231 patients was too small to provide the power needed to see an effect. Alternatively, antiplatelet therapy may not be effective in far advanced diabetic vascular disease. The study did show protection against stroke or transient ischemic attacks in a subgroup of patients who were at high risk. While these results are supportive of those found in studies in non-diabetic subjects [20], they should be interpreted with some caution, since they represent subgroup analyses after multiple analyses of the data.

A second large study is now underway in which major vascular events are monitored in a group of approximately 4000 IDDM and NIDDM patients who are enrolled in the Early Treatment Diabetic Retinopathy Study (ETDRS). Although the study is primarily one of different forms of photocoagulation for diabetic retinopathy and maculopathy, patients are also randomly assigned to either aspirin (650 mg daily) or placebo therapy. Retinopathy and major vascular events are monitored. This study will provide definitive information on the indications for aspirin therapy as a primary and/or secondary prevention strategy in diabetes. It will be completed in 1989.

One smaller study in diabetic patients with advancing diabetic nephropathy has been reported. In about 25% of patients, the administration of aspirin (325 mg tid) plus dipyridamole (75 mg tid) was associated with a preservation of renal function, while in 75% of patients the expected deterioration occurred [24]. This study had no placebo group, but is suggestive that there may be a subgroup of diabetic patients with nephropathy who could receive benefit from antiplatelet therapy. There are no clear clinical indicators as to which patients with renal failure might benefit from antiplatelet therapy.

Attempts have been made to alter platelet function in diabetes by dietary means, sulfonylureas and insulin therapy. Fish oil supplementation to a diabetic diet has received some attention, and there is some evidence that platelet thromboxane release will decrease on such diets in IDDM patients [25]. Conflicting data on the effects of oral sulfonylurea agents on platelet function have appeared, presumably reflecting heterogeneous diabetic populations, variation between agents and/or variability of platelet aggregation profiles when studied longitudinally in diabetic subjects. In our laboratories, a double-blind crossover study of tolazamide vs. placebo in a group of NIDDM patients showed no effect of this sulfonylurea on platelet aggregation. Several reports have shown that intensive insulin therapy will lower platelet thromboxane release in IDDM [26,27], and intensive insulin therapy will lower platelet-derived growth factor activity in IDDM [28]. Platelet aggregation to ADP and thrombin, however, may not change after insulin therapy in diabetes, suggesting that nonarachidonic acid-related pathways may be important in platelet behavior in diabetes.

Antiplatelet therapy in nondiabetic subjects

A recent review of 25 randomized controlled trials of antiplatelet therapy after stroke or myocardial infarction in nondiabetic subjects revealed the following findings in the 29,000 subjects studied [20]:

1. No effect on non-vascular mortality;
2. Reduction in vascular mortality of 15%;
3. Reduction in subsequent stroke or myocardial infarction of 30%;
4. No significant differences in the effects of different doses of aspirin (300–325 mg once daily or 900–1500 mg/day in divided doses.

Discussion

In spite of evidence of altered platelet function in diabetes, particularly in patients with established vascular disease, few large-scale multicenter trials have been done and results have not been encouraging. At best, one can suggest that aspirin and di-pyridamole therapy may prevent strokes and transient ischemic attacks in a subset of NIDDM diabetic patients after amputation for gangrene [23] and that such combined therapy may also delay the rate of progression of renal failure in a subset of patients with diabetic nephropathy and renal failure [24]. There are a number of possible explanations for this state of affairs. First, the hypothesis that platelets contribute to vascular disease may be in error. This seems unlikely, in view of the encouraging results reported from secondary intervention studies in nondiabetic patients [20]. A more likely possibility is that in the controlled clinical trial in diabetic patients reported to date, the sample size was too small and event rates were less than predicted, compromising the power of the study. It is also likely that vascular disease was too far advanced to be affected by antiplatelet therapy. At this stage of disease in the large vessels, one can postulate that lipid accumulation, smooth muscle cell proliferation, plaque formation and thrombosis are activities that overwhelm the contribution of platelet-endothelial interactions to the process. There will be useful information which bears on this point from the ETDRS, which can be viewed as a mixed primary and secondary intervention trial in IDDM and in NIDDM. The use of aspirin in these subjects is under way, and effects of aspirin vs. placebo on the microvascular endpoint of retinopathy and the macrovascular endpoint of cardiac events and/or vascular death will be known when that trial is completed.

There are other reasons of a theoretical nature why studies have been negative to date. Attention is usually paid to the inhibition of the cyclo-oxygenase pathway by aspirin to suppress thromboxane production. High doses of aspirin have been used in many studies; these doses will also inhibit production of the prostanoid which counterregulates against platelet adhesion: prostacyclin. Theoretically, this could promote thrombosis. There are reasons, however, to speculate that this is not the case. There is compelling evidence from analysis of 25 of the secondary prevention trials in nondiabetic subjects (in which aspirin has been used after a vascular event has occurred) that protection against a subsequent major vascular event is often conferred by doses of aspirin sufficient to suppress prostacyclin synthesis [20]. In these studies, doses of aspirin from 300 to 325 mg or 900 to 1500 mg/day, with or without dipyridamole, have conferred protection against major cardiovascular events. These studies suggest that prostacyclin may not be a critical factor in vascular thrombosis. In any case, many studies have shown diminished prostacyclin release and/or action in diabetes [12,13]; thus, it may well be that further inhibition by aspirin may not be physiologically important.

There are some theoretical reasons to support a higher dose of aspirin and a prolongation of blood levels in patients with diabetes than in nondiabetic individuals. Platelet survival is often shortened in patients with diabetic vascular disease, and relatively frequent aspirin administration or the use of slow-release preparations to give relatively constant blood levels appears to be needed to block cyclo-oxygenase pathways in newly formed and released platelets [29].

Finally, new evidence has indicated that there are platelet pathways which are altered in diabetes which do not involve arachidonic acid conversion to thromboxane. In studies in man, washed platelets from diabetic subjects with retinopathy are hypersensitive to thrombin, even when arachidonic acid conversion to thromboxane is blocked by aspirin [30]. It is interesting to note that this process is accentuated by fibrinogen binding to platelets. In view of high fibrinogen levels and accelerated turnover in diabetes, this process could theoretically be of clinical importance. Such speculation is supported by recent studies which identify plasma fibrinogen level as a significant risk factor for cardiovascular disease [31]. Thrombin sensitivity in the presence of aspirin blockade has been seen in washed platelets from diabetic rats [32]. There is evidence for enhanced ADP-induced primary platelet aggregation of washed platelets from diabetic subjects with retinopathy [33]. Primary aggregation does not require activation of the arachidonic acid pathway. Finally, thromboxane synthetase inhibition in subjects with IDDM will reduce serum thromboxane and platelet aggregability, but does not affect various in vivo indicators of platelet hyperfunction, including plasma beta-thromboglobulin, platelet factor 4 or platelet micro-aggregates [34]. All of these studies indicate that mechanisms independent of products of the arachidonic acid pathway appear to be involved in the hypersensitivity of platelets seen in diabetes mellitus. Pharmacological strategies directed at these mechanisms have not been developed or explored in clinical trials.

Since the precise roles of thromboxane and prostacyclin in thrombosis are not known, it is possible that aspirin may act through its antithrombotic properties. Aspirin is a weak anticoagulant, and reduces the activity of coagulation factors II, VII, XI and X in a dose-dependent manner. Aspirin in doses of 900–1500 mg/day enhances the fibrinolytic activity of blood in a dose-dependent fashion in spite of the fact that it may inhibit the release of tissue plasminogen activator.

Recommendations

In view of the accelerated atherosclerosis of diabetes, and since there appears to be minimal toxicity associated with antiplatelet therapy, diabetic patients who have had a previous stroke, myocardial infarction and/or clinically apparent peripheral vascular disease should be placed on aspirin as a secondary prevention strategy. Because of results in nondiabetic subjects, a dosage of approx. 325 mg once daily is recommended. Because diabetic subjects with clinically evident macrovascular disease may have accelerated platelet turnover, a slow-release preparation of 325 mg of aspirin daily should be used. Higher aspirin doses may be used, but carry the risk of increased bleeding, and do not appear to offer advantages over single-dose therapy.

In diabetic subjects with no evidence of macrovascular disease, a primary prevention approach with aspirin therapy is not indicated. First, the data in nondiabetic populations are fragmentary and incomplete [21,22]. Second, there are no clinical trials reported in diabetes in which aspirin is used as a primary prevention strategy. Knowledge of major vascular event rates in those patients in the ETDRS who are free from macrovascular disease should help resolve this issue.

Recommendations for antiplatelet therapy, either as a primary or a secondary prevention strategy in diabetic subjects with microvascular disease of the eyes and/or kidneys, must be made with caution. The issue regarding secondary prevention in the case of established retinopathy will be resolved by the ETDRS, in which progression of established retinopathy is a primary endpoint in diabetic subjects. It is unlikely that this study will give useful data on nephropathy, which is not a primary endpoint. The one published study in diabetic patients with nephropathy [24] suggests that there is a subgroup of subjects in whom antiplatelet therapy may be useful. One cannot make large-scale recommendations from a pilot study of this type, however.

Thus, the recommendations for antiplatelet therapy in diabetes, like those for the treatment of hyperlipidemia and hypertension in diabetes, are based primarily upon controlled clinical trials in nondiabetic subjects, with some modifications based upon the diabetic state. Metabolic control of glucose, hemoglobin A_{1c} and lipids is an appropriate approach to accompany specific antiplatelet therapy in diabetes mellitus.

Acknowledgement

Supported by Veterans Administration Medical Research Funds.

References

1. Direct and indirect costs of diabetes in the United States in 1987. Center for Economic Studies in Medicine (Pracon, Inc.). Alexandria, VA: American Diabetes Association, Inc., 1988.
2. Harris MI, Entmacher P. Mortality from diabetes. In: Diabetes in America, U.S. Department of Health and Human Services, Public Health Service, National Institutes of Health, National Institutes of Arthritis, Diabetes, and Kidney Diseases, NIH Publication No. 85-1468, 1985; Chapter XXIX, pp. 1–48
3. The 1988 Report of the Joint National Committee on Detection, Evaluation, and Treatment of High Blood Pressure. Arch Int Med 1988;148:1023–1038.

4. Clinical Opportunities for Smoking Intervention. U.S. Department of Health and Human Services, Public Health Service, National Institutes of Health, National Heart, Lung, and Blood Institute, NIH Publication No. 86-2178, 1986.

5. Report of the Expert Panel on Detection, Evaluation, and Treatment of High Blood Cholesterol in Adults. U.S. Department of Health and Human Services, Public Health Service, National Institutes of Health, National Heart, Lung, and Blood Institute, 1988.

6. University Group Diabetes Program: I – Design, methods and baseline results. Diabetes 1970; 19(Suppl.2):747–783.

7. Diabetes Control and Complications Trial (DCCT): Results of Feasibility Study. Diabetes Care 1987;10:1–19.

8. UK Prospective Diabetes Study. Diabetes 1985;34:793–798.

9. Ross R, Glomset JA. The pathogenesis of atherosclerosis. N Engl J Med 1976;295:369–377, 420–425.

10. Ross R. The pathogenesis of atherosclerosis: an update. N Engl J Med 1986;314:488–500.

11. Mustard JF, Packman MA, Kinlough-Rathbone RL. Platelets and atherosclerosis. In: Miller NE, ed. Atherosclerosis: mechanisms and approaches to therapy. New York; Raven Press, 1983;29–43.

12. Colwell JA, Lopes-Virella MF, Winocour PD, Halushka PV. New concepts about the pathogenesis of atherosclerosis in diabetes mellitus. In: Leven ME, O'Neal LW, eds. The diabetic foot. St. Louis, C.V. Mosby Co, 1988;51–70.

13. Winocour PD, Halushka PV, Colwell JA. Platelet involvement in diabetes mellitus. In: Longnecker GL, ed. The platelets: physiology and pharmacology. New York: Academic Press, 1985;341–366.

14. Mustard JF, Packham MA. Platelets and diabetes. N Engl J Med 1987;311:665–666.

15. Ruderman NB, Haudenschild C. Diabetes as an atherogenic factor. Prog Cardiovasc Dis 1984;26:373–412.

16. Osterman H, Van de Loo J. Factors of the hemostatic system in diabetic patients. A survey of controlled studies. Haemostasis 1986;16:386–416.

17. Colwell JA, Lopes-Virella MF, Halushka PV. Pathogenesis of atherosclerosis in diabetes mellitus. Diabetes Care 1981;4:121–133.

18. Colwell JA. Macroangiopathy. In: Alberti KGMM, Krall LP, eds. Diabetes Annual 4. Amsterdam: Elsevier Science Publishers, 1988;355–383.

19. Allesandrini P,McRae J, Feman S, FitzGerald GA. Tromboxane biosynthesis and platelet function in type I diabetes mellitus. N Engl J Med 1988;319:208–212.

20. Antiplatelet Trialists' Collaboration. Secondary prevention of vascular disease by prolonged antiplatelet treatment. Br Med J 1988;296:310–331.

21. Special Report. Preliminary report: findings from the aspirin component of the ongoing physicians' health study. N Engl J Med 1988;318:262–264.

22. Relman AS. Aspirin for the primary prevention of myocardial infarction. N Engl J Med 1988;318:245–246.

23. Colwell JA, Bingham SF, Abraira C, Anderson JW, Comstock JP, Kwaan HC, Nuttall F and The Cooperative Study Group. V.A. Cooperative Study on antiplatelet agents in diabetic patients after amputation for gangrene: II. Effects of aspirin and dipyridamole on atherosclerotic vascular disease rates. Diabetes Care 1986;9:140–148.

24. Donadio JF Jr, Ilstrup DM, Holley KE, Romero JC. Platelet-inhibitor treatment of diabetic nephropathy: a 10-year prospective study. Mayo Clin Proc 1988;63:3–15.

25. Maines AP, Sanders TAB, Imeson JD, et al. Effects of a fish oil supplement on platelet function, haemostatic variables and albuminuria in insulin-dependent diabetics. Thrombosis Res 1986;53:643–655.

26. Mayfield RK, Halushka PV, Wohltmann HJ, et al. Platelet function during continuous insulin infusion treatment in insulin-dependent diabetic patients. Diabetes 1985;34:1127–1133.

27. McDonald JWD, Dupre J, Rodger NW, Champion MC, Webb CD, Ali M. Comparison of platelet thromboxane synthesis in diabetic patients on conventional insulin therapy and continuous insulin infusion. Thromb Res 1982;28:705–712.

28. Hamet P, Sugimoto H, Umeda F, Lecavalier L, Franks DJ, Orth DN, Chiasson J-L. Abnormalities of platelet-derived growth factors in insulin-dependent diabetes. Diabetes 1987;36:667–672.

29. DeMinno G, Silver MJ, Cerbone AM, et al. Trial of repeated low-dose aspirin in diabetic angiopathy. Blood 1986;68:886–889.

30. DeMinno G, Silver MJ, Cerbone AM, Riccardi G, Rivellese A, Mancini M. Platelet fibrinogen binding in diabetes mellitus. Diabetes 1986;35:182–185.

31. Kannel WB, Wolf PA, Castelli WP, et al. Fibrinogen and risk of cardiovascular disease. J Am Med Assoc 1987;258:1183.

32. Winocour PD, Kinlough-Rathbone RL, Mustard JF. Pathways responsible for platelet hypersensitivity in rats with diabetes mellitus. II. Spontaneous diabetes in BB Wistar rats. J Lab Clin Med 1986;107:154–158.

33. Bensoussan D, Levy-Toledano S, Passa PH, Caen J, Canivet J. Platelet hyperaggregation and increased plasma level of von Willebrand Factor in diabetic retinopathy. Diabetologia 1975; 11:307–312.

34. Dallinger KJC, Toop M, Gyde OHB, et al. Specific thromboxane synthetase inhibition and haemostasis in insulin-dependent diabetics. Diabetes Res 1986;3:377–380.

Treatment of NIDDM

What should be controlled in non-insulin-dependent diabetes: the use of insulin and the European consensus

P.J. WATKINS

Diabetic Department, King's College Hospital, London, U.K.

Introduction

Non-insulin-dependent diabetes mellitus (NIDDM) is one of the world's commonest disorders, affecting not only the affluent overweight populations but many others besides. Quite apart from the symptoms directly caused by hyperglycaemia, the disease is responsible for a substantial increase in mortality, chiefly from major arterial disease, and an increased morbidity from the specific complications of diabetes leading to blindness, renal failure, foot sepsis and amputations.

The aims of treatment have always been to eliminate symptoms and improve the quality of life. The introduction of new treatments and techniques means that these aims can now be extended and attempts made on the one hand to prevent complications occurring at all, and on the other to diminish their impact when they do occur. If longevity can be restored to normal then that too must be one of our aims. Finally, since diabetic patients, by the requirements of their disorder, need to attend their doctors on a regular basis, there is a unique opportunity for detecting and treating other disorders, perhaps at an earlier stage then in the non-diabetic population. Observations on this aspect of diabetic care have never been made: its importance is, however, enshrined in the European consensus, and places the care of diabetics very firmly in the hands of well-trained physicians whose interests and practice extend beyond a narrow and over-specialized view of diabetes [1].

Achievement of these aims therefore demands attention to many facets of health, both clinical and biochemical. Reduction of hyperglycaemia is not disputed; clinical attention to weight reduction and treatment of hypertension are clearly important, as is advice on smoking. Attention to lipids, especially with the availability of new treatments, is also becoming an increasingly important part of diabetes care.

Both European and USA groups [1,2] have drawn up a series of measurable criteria by which to assess the adequacy of treatment. Those recommended by the European group are shown in Table 1: they differ in minor aspects from similar recommendations from the USA. However, the criteria are very strict indeed, and as a result the majority of diabetic patients are likely to deviate from the ideal in one or more of the set criteria for 'good control'. Thus, a survey from one of the most distinguished clinics in the UK found that amongst 2046 NIDDM patients, 24% had a random blood glucose of 16 mmol/l or more, and 35% had an HbA_1 of more than 11% [3]. Discussions on management become increasingly difficult, especially with an ageing population [4,5]. This paper will focus on the oldest and still unresolved problems

TABLE 1

Targets for control: European recommendations[a]

		Good	Acceptable	Poor
Blood glucose fasting[b]	mg/dl	80–120	≤ 140	> 140
	mmol/l	4.4–6.7	≤ 7.8	> 7.8
Post-prandial	mg/dl	80–160	≤ 180	> 180
	mmol/l	4.4–9.9	≤ 1 0	> 10
HbA_1[c]	%	< 7.5	7.5–8.5	> 8.5
Urine glucose	%	0	≤ 0.5	> 0.5
Total cholesterol[d]	mg/dl	< 200	< 250	≥ 250
	mmol/l	< 5.2	< 6.5	≥ 6.5
HDL-cholesterol	mg/dl	> 40	≥ 35	< 35
	mmol/l	> 1.1	≥ 0.9	> 0.9
Fasting triglycerides	mg/dl	< 150	< 200	> 200
	mmol/l	< 1.7	< 2.2	> 2.2
Body mass index	kg/m^2	♂ < 25	≤ 27	> 27
		♀ < 24	≤ 26	> 26
Blood pressure	mmHg	≤ 140/90	≤ 160/95	> 160/95

[a]Adapted from Ref. 1.

[b]This is the ideal and may be difficult, impossible or unnecessary to achieve in certain patients.

[c]References ranges for HbA_1 vary greatly depending on the method. Values recommended here obtained with microcolumns. Normal range: 5–7.5% (NB: will vary between laboratories).

[d]Lower targets may be desirable in younger patients.

of controlling hyperglycaemia with special reference to the use of insulin in NIDDM patients.

When to start insulin in NIDDM

Few physicians in Europe use insulin as the first treatment after dietary failure, although this practice may be commoner in the USA. Most physicians recommend oral hypoglycaemic agents if diet alone fails: when these treatments together are judged to be optimal, failure to achieve 'good' control as defined above must lead to a decision whether or not to start insulin treatment. Both USA and European recommendations are vague [1,2]; both draw attention to the distinction between obese and non-obese diabetic subjects. USA guidelines give relatively more specific advice relating to age and fasting blood glucose levels, with a trend towards a diminishing use of insulin with increasing age and weight which might have some dangers in individual cases.

Specific advice on starting insulin needs more exact definition. Poor control in the presence of intercurrent illness or during pregnancy contributes precise and undisputed indications. Patients in whom diabetic symptoms persist usually benefit from insulin administration, although lethargy and tiredness are difficult to gauge and many of them only appreciate their malaise after the improvement in well-being which follows insulin treatment.

The importance of weight change as opposed to actual weight deserves special emphasis. If a poorly controlled patient is gaining weight, insulin is contraindicated, and tightening of dietary measures becomes crucial: administration of insulin to these patients rarely improves control and serves only to increase their weight still further [6]. On the other hand, obesity alone is not an absolute contraindication to the need for insulin. In contrast, if weight is decreasing, a strong case is made for institution of insulin treatment. Serial measurements of weight are therefore crucial in the management of diabetes. The loss of weight can be particularly insidious: in a typical patient it occurred slowly over several years as a result of increasingly stringent dieting used by the patient to maintain adequate control. Before insulin was started, his postprandial blood glucose levels were no higher than 9 mmol/l, yet the effect of insulin treatment on his health and weight were spectacular. Insidious weight loss provides a firm indication for insulin treatment but it may often be overlooked.

Patients whose control remains poor without either symptoms or weight change present physicians with one of the most difficult decisions in diabetes management.

Predictors for insulin treatment

Forecasting the need for insulin can be attempted. Thus, the presence of complement-fixing islet cell antibodies increases the likelihood that insulin will be needed, but even in IDDM only about half of these patients develop diabetes over 9 years [7]. Patients with the lowest serum insulin or C-peptide levels are also more likely to become insulin-requiring, and Tattersall has presented evidence that those with the lowest C-peptide/glucose ratios most often needed insulin [3]. Simple clinical features such as youth or thin physique may also point towards a likely need for insulin, although neither age, diabetes duration, sex nor weight provides reliable indications. None of these measurements, however, either clinical or biochemical, provides exact indications for insulin need in an individual case.

Effectiveness of insulin

There are a number of studies which examine the effects of insulin in NIDDM patients. Although there is ample evidence for insulin resistance in NIDDM [8], insulin will nevertheless increase glucose utilization, even in obese subjects. These effects can also be achieved with sulphonylureas and such studies do not provide a basis for predicting insulin need [9]. Indeed improvements in diabetic control using either insulin or sulphonylureas are not even related to measured insulin-stimulated glucose metabolic clearance rates [10].

Effects of insulin on diabetic control in NIDDM

When insulin is used as the primary treatment in NIDDM, as it was in the UGDP study and is in the UK prospective study [11,12], many patients, perhaps the majority, readily achieve satisfactory diabetic control on quite modest doses of insulin (e.g. in the UGDP study, 89% were well controlled with less than 20 units daily after the first 3 months). These observations do not apply to treatment of patients when diet and oral hypoglycaemic agents have failed. Tattersall has undertaken the best clinical study of this problem: insulin administration to such patients over 6 months led to a significant improvement of blood glucose in only one-third of patients and improved symptoms and well-being in fewer than half [3]. More patients may show improvements in control if larger doses of insulin are used, and one-third of Turner's patients needed over 80 units daily to achieve this [12]. The price of better control by causing severe hyperinsulinaemia is debatable, and has been discussed elsewhere.

Disadvantages of insulin treatment

(a) Hypoglycaemia
The hazards of hypoglycaemia to which all insulin-treated diabetic subjects are prone need no emphasis, and are of course inevitable in an insulin-dependent diabetic pa-

tient. Indeed, in the DCCT trial, achievement of tight control has been fraught with problems from serious hypoglycaemia. To offer this complication to an asymptomatic NIDDM patient must temper the decision regarding the use of insulin in these patients, since the only purpose of doing so is to tighten control. There is little detailed information available on this problem, but in one of Turner's studies using ultralente insulin more than 40% of patients during 2 months treatment suffered episodes of hypoglycaemia sufficiently severe to interrupt their daily activities [12]. Quite apart from the dangers of such episodes, some patients, notably those holding particular types of driving licence, will lose their employment when insulin treatment is started.

(b) Weight gain
The worst situation which can be reached when insulin is used in treating symptomless NIDDM patients is that in which weight gain is promoted without any significant improvement in diabetic control. Even when hyperglycaemia is reduced, weight gain is almost inevitable: this amounted to an average of 2.3 kg in just 2 months insulin treatment in a study by Turner [12], and 4.2 kg in 6 months in that by Tattersall, with a maximum gain of 13 kg in the latter [3]. The advantages of improvements in diabetic control on the one hand must therefore be set against the adverse effects of substantial weight gain on the other.

These problems of hypoglycaemia and weight gain represent the chief reasons why insulin is, with good intentions, so often withheld from indifferently controlled NIDDM patients.

The use of insulin and diabetic complications

Probably the main reason for tightening control in symptomless patients must be the prevention of diabetic complications [13]. Whether primary prevention can be achieved is one of the most extensively studied aspects of diabetes and still lacks certainty. The influence of tight control of diabetes on established complications is even less sure and indeed unlikely once major structural damage has occurred. Thus, there is no evidence for any alteration of the course of nephropathy even if continuous subcutaneous insulin infusion is undertaken at a relatively early stage [14]. No treatment alters established neuropathy or vascular disease sufficiently severe to cause foot ulceration; and at least one study suggested that the effect of tight control was less convincing after 30 years of age than before [15].

These observations are pertinent to management in non-insulin-dependent diabetes, in which complications may be present either at diagnosis or at least within the first five years [16]. Thus, proteinuria and microalbuminuria are often present at diagnosis especially after 50 years of age. In the UK study of renal failure in diabetes, nearly one-third of cases presented within 5 years of diabetes onset [17]. Retinopathy occurs in about one-fifth of patients before five years [18], and is found in as many as 10–20% at diagnosis, if photographs are examined; and foot ulcers in NIDDM may be found very early in the course of diabetes and are sometimes the mode of presentation.

The value of insulin, therefore, in asymptomatic NIDDM patients with established complications may be very limited. However, the knowledge that complications may develop in the very earliest years of known diabetes in these patients may emphasize the need for strenuous efforts to achieve good control, by insulin if need be, at the very beginning.

Treatment regimens

The lack of guidelines which will predict which patients will benefit from insulin treatment means that a novel clinical strategy must be adopted. We frequently recommend a short-term trial of insulin treatment, perhaps for 1 to 2 months, to discover whether advantages outweigh disadvantages. It is our experience that most patients opt to remain on insulin after the trial period is complete. Tattersall found that 60% preferred to return to oral hypoglycaemic agents.

Starting insulin as an out-patient simplifies the establishment of the trial period. Most patients, at least in the UK, will be assisted in this by the diabetic specialist nurse or health visitor. This technique simplifies the procedure and it is also cheap.

The insulin regimens which are used in treating NIDDM patients are similar to those used for IDDM patients. Insulin is most frequently given twice daily, but it can be used from once to four times daily. Once-daily regimens are sometimes more successful in NIDDM than IDDM patients because of the presence of a small amount of basal insulin secretion from the patients' own B cells. Turner's recommendation to use once-daily ultralente insulin has not gained widespread popularity because either its duration of action remains insufficient, or nocturnal hypoglycaemia becomes a serious problem: there are therefore no clear advantages compared with using other more conventional insulins. Combined insulin and sulphonylurea regimens have often been described, but the advantages, if there are any, are slender, and they are little used [19].

Practical recommendations

The decision to start insulin treatment in a NIDDM patient is not an easy one, especially amongst the many older diabetic patients who are overweight and poorly controlled. Many considerations are needed, as follows:

(1) Ensure as far as possible that the recommended diet is kept, that oral hypogly-caemics are being taken, and that medications which exacerbate hyperglycaemia (e.g. thiazide diuretics) are stopped. These aspects require intensive care and edu-cation, and a home visit can be invaluable. Sometimes admission to hospital achieves all these aims and demonstrates to the patient that good control can be achieved.

(2) If diabetic symptoms persist, a patient is more likely to need insulin.

(3) If the weight is decreasing, patients are likely to need insulin: if it is increasing, they are more likely to be over-eating.

(4) Some patients just manage to maintain adequate control by exceptionally rigor-ous dieting: tell-tale signs are a wasting patient whose urine tests show ketonuria. Insulin treatment with an adequate diet has a miraculous effect on such a patient.

(5) Poorly controlled, overweight patients who are not losing weight present a se-rious dilemma: if one is satisfied that they are keeping to their prescribed treat-ment (and frequently they are not) then insulin should probably be tried. Insulin resistance and further weight gain are common problems in this situation. There are times, therefore, when insulin treatment for these patients is not appropriate.

(6) The denial of symptoms should not deter the physician from recommending insu-lin treatment: many patients feel better and at the very least have a boost to their energy reserves.

(7) The obvious dangers of hypoglycaemia together with potential loss of employ-ment must be taken into account if the value of insulin treatment is only border-line.

(8) Established complications are not likely to be affected by insulin treatment; on the other hand, their development very early during the clinical course of NIDDM points to the potential importance of good control, if necessary by insu-lin treatment, at a very early stage.

It is sometimes difficult to persuade NIDDM patients to take insulin. A very practical arrangement whereby insulin is recommended for one month in the first instance can help most patients feel the benefit and opt to continue. If they do not improve, noth-ing has been lost, and oral hypoglycaemic agents can be resumed.

References

1. Alberti KGMM, Gries FA. Management of non-insulin-dependent diabetes mellitus in Europe: a consensus view. Diabetic Med 1988;5:275–281.
2. Rifkin H (ed). Physician's guide to non-insulin dependent (type II) diabetes – diagnosis and treat-ment. Am Diabetes Assoc, 1988.
3. Peacock I, Tattersall RB. The difficult choice of treatment for poorly controlled maturity onset dia-betes: tablets or insulin? Br Med J 1984;288:1956–1959.

4. Tattersall RB. Diabetes in the elderly – a neglected area? Diabetologia 1984;27:167–173.

5. Tattersall RB. When to use insulin in the maturity onset diabetic. Postgrad Med J 1987;63:859–864.

6. Reaven GM. Beneficial effect of moderate weight loss in older patients with NIDDM poorly controlled with insulin. J Am Geriatr Soc 1985;33:93–95.

7. Spencer KH, Bottazzo GF. Aetiology and pathogenesis of type 1 diabetes: immunology. In: Besser GM, Bodansky HJ, Cudworth AG, eds. Clinical diabetes: an illustrated text. Philadelphia: JB Lippincott Company, 1988;9.1–9.16.

8. Reaven GM, Chen Y-DI, Donner CC, Fraze E, Hollenbeck CB. How insulin resistant are patients with non-insulin dependent diabetes mellitus? J Endocrinol Metab 1985;61:32–36.

9. Firth FG, Bell PM, Rizza RA. Effects of tolazamide and exogenous insulin on insulin action in patients with non-insulin-dependent diabetes mellitus. N Engl J Med 1986;314:1280–1286.

10. Hollenbeck CB, Reaven GM. Treatment of patients with non-insulin dependent diabetes mellitus: diabetic control and insulin secretion and action after different treatment modalities. Diabetic Med 1987;4:311–316.

11. UK Prospective Study II. Reduction in HbA$_{1C}$ with basal insulin supplement. Sulphonylurea or biguanide therapy in non-insulin dependent diabetes. Diabetes 1985;34:793–798.

12. Holman RR, Steemson, J, Turner RC. Sulphonylurea failure in type 2 diabetes: treatment with a basal insulin supplement. Diabetic Med 1987;4:457–462.

13. Schiffrin A. Reversibility of diabetic complications. In: Nattrass M, ed. Recent advances in diabetes. Edinburgh: Churchill Livingstone, 1989;195–208.

14. Bending JJ, Viberti GC, Watkins PJ, Keen H. Intermittent clinical proteinuria and renal function in diabetes: evolution and the effect of glycaemic control. Br Med J 1986;292:83–86.

15. Kohner EM, Dollery CT, Bulpitt CJ. Cotton wool spots in diabetic retinopathy. Diabetes 1969;18:691.

16. Watkins PJ, Grenfell A, Edmonds M. Diabetic complications of non-insulin dependent diabetes. Diabetic Med 1987;4:293–296.

17. Joint Working Party on Diabetic Renal Failure. Renal failure in diabetics in the UK: deficient provision of care in 1985. Diabetic Med 1988;5:79–84.

18. Soler G, Fitzgerald MG, Malins JM, Summers ROC. Retinopathy at diagnosis with special reference to patients under 40 years of age. Br Med J 1969;3:567–569.

19. Longnecker MI, Elsenhans VD, Leiman SM, Owen OE, Boden G. Combined therapy with insulin and sulphonylurea in non-insulin dependent diabetes mellitus. Arch Int Med 1986;146:673–676.

© 1989 Elsevier Science Publishers B.V. (Biomedical Division)
Frontiers of diabetes research: current trends in non-insulin-dependent diabetes mellitus
K.G.M.M. Alberti and R. Mazze, editors

CHAPTER 16

Model care 1989: some thoughts from the United Kingdom

P.D. HOME

Freeman Diabetes Unit and Department of Medicine, University of Newcastle upon Tyne, U.K.

Introduction

Model care may be taken as implying the devising of a structure which will deliver optimal care to people with diabetes. In this context the structure includes both people and facilities, but more controversially the organization and processes by which they become more effectively deployed. The existence of such a structure should imply that at least its parts have been put to test against traditional or alternative ideas, but sadly there is an almost universal absence of sound comparisons to bolster the opinions given below.

Quality of life and aims of model care

What is the aim of model care? Diabetes is an unusual condition in that even poorly managed patients are asymptomatic for years, while optimal metabolic management (in particular nutritional modifications and insulin injection) implies significant deterioration in perceived quality of life. The judgement as to what degree of interference with current life-style can be justified by a potential reduction in thrombotic, vascular, infective and microvascular risks is still largely intuitive, and certainly the instruments for quantitation of current versus future quality of life are not yet available. A qualitative statement of the aim of model diabetes care might therefore be: 'To obtain optimal metabolic control with minimal disruption of quality of life.'

Unfortunately this implies that optimal metabolic control cannot be obtained in all patients. We therefore have to add a second aim: 'To ensure regular screening for complications associated with diabetes, so that appropriate treatment is instituted at the optimal time'.

Education

It is assumed that the arguments for good professional education (with continued follow-up), and for a programme of patient education need not be repeated here. The questions of which staff and on what site are addressed below. Education about diabetes does, however, need to reach other professionals with contact with diabetic patients, from cardiologists and vascular surgeons, through primary care physicians, to nurses dealing with diabetic patients on surgical wards. Without such education the care of the person with diabetes can become sub-optimal just at a time when it may be most critical. Any hospital performing procedures on people with diabetes must have a 24-h service of specialist advice.

Education must also reach out to the general population if prejudice in employment is to be avoided, problems at school anticipated, and deviations from social eating norms understood. These roles are best fulfilled by a national patient-based diabetes organization, such as the British Diabetic Association in the UK.

The appropriate diabetologist

Helping patients obtain good metabolic control in their own home environment involves a good deal of listening and understanding, an appreciation of the problems of changing behaviour, and preparedness to accept that failure is not simply the patient's 'fault'. These qualities differ from those of the 'take-it-out-and-cure-it' surgeon, the 'get-a-cannula-in-there' cardiologist, and even the 'diagnose-with-a-battery-of-tests' endocrinologist. The white coat and dark suit do not belong in a diabetes consultation, any more than the desk between doctor and patient. A diabetologist needs to specialize to practise these techniques, although some overlap with similar specialities (lipidology, some aspects of social and family medicine) is not inappropriate.

The appropriate site for diabetes care

To professional medical staff the modern hospital, with its hotel-style foyer and up-to-date architecture, may seem a pleasant and uplifting place to work. The majority of our patients, however, have had psychologically negative experiences of hospitals, if not personally then through visits or admissions of relatives. The anxiety that is engendered in hospital visits by patients with diabetes is generally underestimated, and the likely effect of this on assimilation of advice and education as yet unquantified.

The philosophy of hospital-style care is also alien to the practice of diabetes, the undercurrent of illness-to-be-cured-by-doctor affecting the attitude of both doctor and patient. The corollary of these problems is that diabetes care needs to be delivered elsewhere than the hospital building itself, a conclusion supported by the often fragmentary spread of services contributing to diabetes care within a hospital.

As a result of deliberations of this kind diabetes care in the United Kingdom is being increasingly transferred to purpose-built Diabetes Centres [1], a decision which cannot be taken lightly because of added capital and recurrent costs. In its ideal site such a Diabetes Centre is positioned well away from the hospital itself, but the consequences of this in terms of extra staffing, access to hospital records and efficient deployment of staff with responsibilities to ward patients mean that the compromise of a separate building within the hospital grounds may be necessary.

The team approach

The importance and role of the diabetes specialist nurse are now fully established, and will not be discussed in detail here. Nevertheless it seems clear that the day-to-day functions of the diabetes service, essentially those involving patient contact, are increasingly passing into the hands of nurse specialists, who also play a major role in the education of non-medically qualified staff around the hospital, and in talking to parent and patient groups. Model care also demands that certain forms of patient education are most appropriately given in the home, in particular initiation of insulin therapy, a role readily adopted by nurse practitioners.

The ideal diabetes service therefore rapidly comes to consume considerable amounts of specialist nurse time, but this cannot be in isolation from the activities of doctors or other health care professionals. Indeed it is evident, particularly for people with NIDDM, that many of the educational activities of the diabetes specialist nurse overlap with those of other health professionals, and in particular dieticians (nutritionalists) and chiropodists (podiatrists). Indeed it is clear that to be effective these professionals need to work together as one team on the same site, this providing a further argument for the purpose-designed Diabetes Centre. It certainly cannot be the case that people with diabetes should be expected to expend valuable time (often 90 minutes travel and waiting per consultation) visiting the professionals individually.

218

The resource-centre concept

If it is accepted that diabetes care needs to be provided from a purpose-designed site, and that it needs a team of professionals to obtain optimal care, then clearly these facilities should be available to all who have diabetes, whatever doctor is primarily responsible for their care. For many reasons such patients may remain under the care of a primary health care practitioner (general practitioner, family practitioner), but it cannot be correct that they are therefore denied the expertise of health professionals in diabetes.

In this situation the concept of the separate Diabetes Centre and the care team approach can usefully come together to provide access to optimal care for patients who remain the responsibility of the primary care practitioner, and who are perceived as not requiring specialist medical supervision [2]. However, for the Diabetes Centre to be successful as a Resource Centre for all patients with diabetes, changes in organization of practice may be required. Thus it is important that patient referral to the Resource Centre is not necessarily seen as a referral to the physician in charge of the Centre. In other words it must be possible for health professionals working at the centre to receive referrals themselves, directly from primary medical practitioners. While some interaction between these staff is essential (in the education field for example), even referral among the health professionals at the Diabetes Centre can be problematic with such patients on occasion, and demands sensitive communication with the referring physician.

Aids to model care

Model care of people with diabetes can benefit from a number of simple aids to care, none of which should now need a large investment of funds.

Form-based records
Basing all clinical records on forms is simple in diabetes care, because the basic data set is similar for all patients seen. The advantages of form-based records are surprisingly great, given the reluctance of many physicians to introduce them in the past.
1. The record form acts as a prompt to whoever is filling it in, ensuring that all appropriate tasks are completed at each patient visit.
2. A structured form allows very rapid recall of data from a patient's accumulated notes, as the data fields are similarly placed on each page.
3. Use of different-coloured forms for different health professionals (or rather for different types of visit to the Diabetes Centre) similarly allows rapid access to the most recent data relevant to that aspect. Similarly, different-coloured forms can be used for annual review or new patient visits.

4. If diabetes records are combined with other medical records, data access is improved by having distinct forms.

Electronic data-gathering and output
Four basic kinds of data can be usefully collected onto computer-based systems. Blood glucose recording systems are now well established for patients using blood glucose meters, and are particularly valuable when large numbers of records are collected over long periods of time, together with time and date.

A second use of computers is in questionnaire administration for assessment of knowledge, quality of life and patient satisfaction. For general patient use software must be especially user-friendly, and keyboards may need modification to restrict key presses to a limited number of central keys. Having done this, however, sophisticated marking of questionnaires can be rapid, automatic and highly reliable, and the result logged for use in other data-bases (see below).

If care is to be open to all with diabetes, then some kind of register of such people, at least containing name, address and caring institution or physician, can be used to prompt queries as to delivery of care on a regular basis. Such a system should, however, be more than a simple list of patients, and can be used to improve the quality of care. Evident examples are that appointments for annual review (see below) can be issued on an anniversary or birthday basis, or that patients with particular problems such as microalbuminuria can be contacted when changes in the process of care are thought desirable.

The fourth important use of computers in diabetes care is in medical audit, and analysis of outcomes, discussed further below. This can be linked into the population base and referral pattern as an aid to long-term planning and resource management.

Biochemical data
Model care inevitably places great reliance on measures of diabetic, or rather metabolic, control. Intermittent blood glucose estimation is probably of little value if only performed on the occasion of patient visits to the clinician. Thus it will be affected by the stress of the visit, an abnormal exercise pattern, often an abnormal eating pattern, and is open to manipulation in the short term. Although fasting measurements are advocated by some workers, it is evident from published results that many outpatient estimations are not truly fasting.

Glycosylated haemoglobin estimation should be the basis of assessment of blood glucose control, except in patients with haemoglobin disturbances. To be useful, however, the assay must have a low inter-assay coefficient of variation, and sadly too few laboratories achieve this or make such information available. Serum fructosamine estimation has the advantage of being cheaper and quicker to perform, while being invalidated by conditions disturbing protein rather than haemoglobin turn-

220

over. There is at present little evidence to suggest that either of these measures is a better estimate of the underlying variable of concern, average blood glucose concentration.

Fructosamine estimation does have the advantage, however, of being quick enough to be performed at the time of the patient's visit to the clinic, thus adding impact to the result and saving resources devoted to additional visits. Such a technique can also be used for lipid estimations, which should be a regular feature of care of type 2 diabetic patients [3].

All biochemical tests should only be performed by laboratories which take part in recognized external quality-control schemes.

Organization of care

It is a fallacy to suppose that all aspects of diabetes care can be satisfactorily delivered on the basis of regular but similar visits to a clinician. Even if rather more time is available than most clinicians habitually devote to each patient, and other health professionals are available at the time, the contradictions between a holistic approach to diabetes self-management, the medical approach of screening for complications and managing related problems, and the educational approach to improving knowledge are likely to overwhelm physician and patient alike.

It is also organizationally sound to split the annual review functions of medical review away from other aspects of care, using separate forms and specific procedures to ensure complete review. The annual review should then include:
1. Screening for early signs/symptoms of complications;

TABLE 1

Categories of outcome measures that may be used to assess the quality of diabetes care

Category	Examples
Health outputs	Glycosylated haemoglobin
	Patient knowledge of diabetes
Quality of life measures	Sickness impact profile
Process outcomes	Physician visits
	Screening for retinopathy
True outcomes	Visual impairment
	Myocardial infarction
	Hyperosmolar state

2. Screening for related risk factors, especially in relation to macrovascular disease;

3. A personal audit of medical status, including drug therapy, overall measures of control, etc;

4. An educational/quality of life assessment.

The annual review clinic is also a useful time to collect other data required for audit (see below).

Special 'clinics' should also exist for other visits of a clearly defined nature, such as new patients, or group education sessions, where procedures specific to the occasion are indicated. More particularly patients in special groups may be usefully seen apart from the majority. Thus patients with vascular disorders affecting the feet may benefit from joint surgical-medical consultations, just as pregnant patients should be seen in joint medical-obstetric clinics. Adolescent patients are best managed separately from children and older adults.

Audit and outcomes

No physician should be satisfied that the standard of care given to the patients under care is satisfactory, unless the delivery and outcome are formally reviewed on a regular basis. Diabetes presents particular problems in this respect, as a chronic disease, with erratic outcomes, and with the potential conflict between good control and current quality of life in some patients.

Audit of facilities simply involves confirming that needs and organization of care described above are available to all patients.

Audit of processes is particularly important in diabetes care both for their own sake (screening for retinopathy) and because true health outcomes (amputation, ischaemic heart disease) may occur only after many years in the care process.

Outcome measures (Table 1) therefore have to depend to some extent on surrogates for true outcomes. Thus the physician needs to be aware of the spread of glycosylated haemoglobin concentrations achieved in his patients, in the belief that these have some relationship to later microvascular disease. Similar considerations apply to lipids and macrovascular disease, or knowledge and foot ulcers/amputation. Computer processing allows analysis of results by categorization (good, satisfactory, unsatisfactory) for any variable, and assessments can be made (for the whole care population) of changes from year to year.

Measures of quality of life are as yet unsatisfactory for use in routine care, those developed specifically for diabetes being far too detailed and cumbersome to administer routinely. This aspect of outcome measurement needs further development before it can become a standard feature of model care.

222

Consumer feedback

Lastly, model care cannot be taken as such unless it takes into account the views of the care consumer, usually conveniently disguised under the label 'patient'. The relationship between people with diabetes and their care advisers is still often such that frustrations and ideas go unspoken and unwritten, so that formal opportunity for expressions of views must be given. Computer registers do allow surveys of patients in care to be conducted with ease, to answer such questions as:
1. Is the quality of care perceived as high?
2. Are problems going unanswered?
3. Is the process of care satisfactory?

References

1. Day JL, Spathis M. District diabetes centres in the United Kingdom. Diabetic Med 1988;5:372–380.
2. Roberts S. Developments at North Tyneside Diabetes Resource Centre. Diabetic Med 1989; 6:363–365.
3. Alberti KGMM, Gries FA. Management of non-insulin-dependent diabetes in Europe: a concensus view. Diabetic Med 1988;5:275–281.

CHAPTER 17

Model care of NIDDM: an American perspective

RICHARD BERGENSTAL, DONNELL ETZWILER,
PRISCILLA HOLLANDER, MARTHA SPENCER,
ELLIE STROCK and ROGER MAZZE

*International Diabetes Center, and the University of Minnesota School of Medicine,
Minneapolis, MN, U.S.A.*

Introduction

Non-insulin-dependent diabetes mellitus is increasingly becoming a serious concern in public health and health care delivery. In 1984, in the United States, more than 5 million individuals were diagnosed with NIDDM and an estimated further 5 million were suspected of having undiagnosed NIDDM [1]. Each year over 600,000 individuals are newly diagnosed and more than 300,000 die with diabetes as a contributing factor [2,3]. Based on the current population growth of 3%, the known incidence and prevalence of NIDDM, and a longer life span, it has been estimated that by the end of this century more than 20,000,000 individuals will have NIDDM in the United States, with as many as 25–35% having serious micro- and macro-vascular complications [4–6]. The vast majority of these individuals will be treated for both their diabetes and its complications principally by the 178,000 primary care physicians (internists and family practitioners) in practice [7]. Current projections suggest that as many as 85% of the individuals with diabetes residing in urban and suburban communities and 95% of those with diabetes residing in rural communities will seek both primary and secondary care from these physicians [8]. The concentration of care of NIDDM amongst primary care physicians with varying levels of training and expertise suggests the need for a comprehensive and rational approach to the diagnosis and treatment of diabetes and toward the prevention of its complications.

In 1984, the American Diabetes Association, supported by a grant from the Upjohn Company, attempted to develop a more systematic approach toward the treatment of NIDDM by the general practitioner through its Clinical Education Program (CEP). Using a multi-faceted strategy, encompassing telecommunications, regional symposia and local seminars, along with printed material, over a two-year period the CEP reached an estimated 45,000 primary care physicians [7,8]. Following the educational program an evaluation of both the initial and long-term impact of the CEP was undertaken. This evaluation included direct interviews of more than 600 program participants to ascertain their current knowledge and skills levels, to characterize their current practice patterns and to determine how effective the CEP had been in altering current approaches to the treatment of NIDDM. The overall evaluation revealed that, while able to reach this large number of physicians, the program was unable to significantly alter the principal practice patterns related to the treatment of NIDDM. While the CEP was successful in its ability to reinforce the World Health Organization's system for classifying non-insulin-dependent diabetes as NIDDM (type 2), and while in general the majority of physicians (87%) would begin to rely on such standard measures as glycosylated hemoglobin, the fundamental aspects of treatment (the basis for initiating diet, oral agent or insulin therapies) remained unchanged [7]. Close scrutiny of both the seminar series and the accompanying text, *The Physician's Guide to Type II Diabetes (NIDDM): Diagnosis and Treatment*, revealed that there was no consistency in the educational program with regard to the principles upon which specific treatment strategies related to selection of therapy and evaluation of efficacy should be based. In subsequent interviews with the CEP participants it was suggested that the lack of clear guidelines left them without specific standards to follow in their routine treatment of NIDDM.

Since there is currently a lack of widespread consensus related to specific standards for the treatment of NIDDM which could be followed by the primary care physician, this paper sets out to describe a rational, systematic approach toward the treatment of NIDDM and to examine whether such an approach could be used by primary care physicians as the basis upon which they treat non-insulin-dependent diabetes. Further, it sets out to describe how this approach will rely on computer-assisted clinical decision-making systems.

Establishing a standardized approach to treatment

Because of the wide differences in approaches toward non-insulin-dependent diabetes in America, we set out to examine the treatment of NIDDM from a rational and scientific perspective. Three phases of this examination were planned. In phase I, a team composed of four endocrinologists, a clinical epidemiologist, a family practitioner, three nurse clinician specialists in diabetes and a dietitian was formed for the purpose of investigating current approaches toward treatment of NIDDM. At biweekly conferences over a period of five months each step in the diagnosis and treatment of NIDDM (obese and non-obese) was carefully delineated. For purposes of conceptualization, steps in treatment were divided into three phases: *baseline, therapeutics* and *stabilization. Baseline* referred to the process of collecting appropriate laboratory and ambulatory data upon which to establish the initial therapeutic intervention, i.e., diet only, oral hypoglycemic agents or insulin. The *therapeutic* phase encompassed the period from initial intervention through to stabilization of glycemia. During this phase gross changes in therapy may occur. The third phase, *stabilization*, is marked by fine changes in treatment regimen related to adjustments in dose, changes in caloric intake and exercise. This phase is characterized by a stabilization of glycemia as reflected in glycosylated hemoglobin levels as well as self-monitored blood glucose values within the normal range. By establishing this conceptual framework it is possible to identify the specific criteria for entering and exiting a phase.

Applying computer technologies

Because previous approaches to establishing guides to care for primary care physicians in NIDDM have not succeeded in meeting their objectives, it was decided to employ an innovative approach heretofore not tested in diabetes. Whereas computers have been successfully introduced in the treatment of diabetes in the form of memory-based reflectance meters and computer programs which aggregate and interpret self-monitored blood glucose data, to date their use in assisting clinical decision-making in terms of treatment choices in NIDDM has been lacking [9–19]. We therefore sought a set of computer tools which would enable us to clearly and precisely delineate the steps in the treatment of NIDDM. Easyflow, a computer-based system for assistance in identifying the various elements in clinical decision-making, was selected [20]. Using this program, each step in the treatment of type II diabetes could be abstracted and characterized as: *(a) entry criteria/criteria for changing treatment, (b) clinical decision, (c) action site, (d) treatment modality, (e) added information, (f) documentation, and (g) monitoring. Entry criteria* relates to the raw and interpreted data upon which to base the treatment decision. Thus, the results of a laboratory test, such as HbA_1, would be the basis for moving from a therapeutic phase to stabilization, which in turn would affect self-monitoring practices. *Clinical decisions* associates the current condition of the patient to the various choices. Thus if the patient's blood glucose is lower than 50 mg/dl take action A, while if the blood glucose is between 50 and 150 mg/dl take action B and if more than 150 mg/dl take action C. *Action site* refers to where the actual steps to be taken should occur (e.g., in the hospital, in the office, referral to a subspecialist). Therapeutic steps are to be found in the *treatment module.* The three fundamental therapies, diet only, oral agent and diet, and insulin and diet, are therefore associated with a set of criteria and decisions upon which their choice would be based. *Added information* refers to important details related to any of the decision, treatment, action and criteria modules. *Documentation* establishes the information that would be needed to be collected by either the patient or the physician to evaluate how efficacious the treatment was in meeting the therapeutic goals. *Monitoring* is associated with the schedule of physician and patient data collection, including the timing of laboratory tests and the frequency of self-monitoring of blood glucose.

This clinical decision-making approach, utilizing Easyflow, allows the development of high-level specifications for coding which, in turn, would facilitate use of an expert system. VPExpert was selected as the expert system which would be used to guide the primary care physician through the clinical decisions related to treatment selection [21]. VPExpert enabled us to establish the logic by which each decision would be made and clearly identify the basic assumptions upon which each decision was based. The final program, meant for use in either a micro-computer or a hand-held computer, relies on competency-based interventions. In such a program there exist fail-safe mechanisms permitting the physician to always have control over the clinical decision-making process. The computer program acts as a reminder/model-builder. At each juncture it provides information related to the likely consequences of the clinical decision based on previous data collected and stored in the program. Thus, the program might remind the physician that the maximum allowable dose of an oral agent had been reached and that blood glucose levels had not been significantly improved. It might then suggest alternatives, e.g., a different oral agent, initiation of insulin or re-evaluation of patient compliance. The concept of competency-based intervention is that the physician and not the computer program makes the clinical decision. With the completion of the 'design' we were able to proceed to the next phase.

Phase II of the examination was designed to retrospectively analyse the records of randomly selected patients with NIDDM from a pool of 2340 individuals seen in a diabetes speciality center over the past five years. Since four specific conditions of the approach to treatment had been delineated, *(1) diagnosis, and criteria for (2) diet, (3) oral agents and (4) insulin therapy*, subjects were randomly selected for each category. For each subject, the conditions under which diagnosis was made and the criteria by which treatment was initially selected and then altered were abstracted. Where possible, sequential glycosylated hemoglobin values and verified self-monitored blood glucose data were obtained. On selective patients, ambulatory glucose profiles (AGP) were also used to determine the overall efficacy of a particular treatment approach [11]. The AGP permits comparison of a single patient over time as well as groups of patients using verified self-monitored blood glucose data. These data are processed by a computer program to prepare a graphic profile for each subject which collapses SMBG data collected over a period of two weeks and presents these data as five continuous curves (10th, 25th, 50th, 75th, 90th percentiles glucose value at 15-min intervals) as if they occurred on a single, modal day. Two AGPs are shown in Fig. 1 illustrating the variety of profiles found in NIDDM. The upper cell shows poorly controlled NIDDM, with tighter control shown in the lower graph (showing a well-controlled NIDDM patient with a very narrow blood glucose range). The bar graph along the x axis identifies the time and relative number of self-monitored blood glucose tests. The data as represented in each AGP cover a period of two weeks, with an average of four SMBG tests per day. These data were meant to serve as a basis for corroborating or refuting the assumptions upon which the clinical decision-making model was based.

The last phase of this analysis is a prospective study designed to test whether a systematic rule-based approach to clinical decision-making was feasible in a clinical setting. Seven primary care clinics of a university-based medical center were selected for testing. The clinics collectively have over 70,000 patient visits per year, between 15 and 20% of which are estimated to be complicated by diabetes. The purpose of

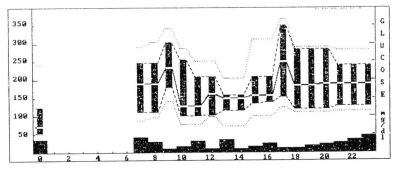

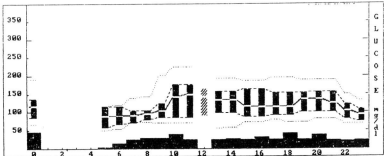

Fig. 1. Ambulatory glucose profiles in NIDDM. The upper AGP has a mean blood glucose of 195 $\pm$ 76 mg/dl. SMBG begins at 6.30 a.m. and ends at 12.30 a.m. Rises in blood glucose are noted following breakfast and dinner. Variability (range of blood glucose between the 25th and 75th percentiles, shown in bars) is highest following dinner. The lower AGP has a mean blood glucose of 112 $\pm$ 22 mg/dl. SMBG begins at 4.30 a.m. and continues to 11.30 a.m., beginning again at 12.30 p.m. The lightly shaded bar over 12 noon is the calculated glucose range based on 11.30 a.m. and 12.30 p.m. data.

this phase is to test whether the introduction of a systematic approach to clinical decision-making in NIDDM, combined with computer-based technologies to assist in the implementation of this approach, would result in significant improvement in metabolic control. The computer-based technologies include use of memory-based reflectance meters for patient data collection, computer analysis of these data and protocolled care using the 'expert' decision-making system. The clinics, operated by family practitioners and composed of a diverse patient mix in terms of ethnicity, age, socioeconomic status and education, represented a clinical research environment in which the impact of this type of approach in chronic care management could be assessed.

Each of seven centers will receive the technology, and primary care physicians at each site will be trained in its use. Patients will be randomly assigned to 'intensified' computer-assisted management or 'conventional' treatment. Comparisons with data collected prior to the introduction of the program will serve as the basis for measuring overall change. Comparison between the control and experimental patients will be the basis for analysis of the contribution of this systematic approach and computer technologies to improved care.

A decision-making model for treatment of NIDDM: establishing standards of care

This paper is limited to the description of the decision-making model developed by the investigators and the subsequent retrospective study. Depicted in Fig. 2 are elements of the overall model divided into four sections: entry criteria, diet, oral agents and insulin.

The entry criteria for confirmed diagnosis of NIDDM are shown in the chart. The patient must meet these criteria (either two fasting plasma blood glucose levels above 140 mg/dl or two random values above 200 mg/dl) to be considered for treatment. The significance of the diamond shape is to indicate a decision. The notation inside the shape provides the conditions, and the notations on the arrows indicate the criteria that have to be met in order to proceed to the next step. Since body mass index is a known risk factor (85% of all NIDDM is paralleled by obesity) it is an added criterion for continuing to treatment and is found in the next diamond shape after age. This is followed by confirmation of the diagnosis of NIDDM and the conditions under which treatment with diet alone would occur. In this model, diet treatment requires the patient to have a fasting plasma blood glucose of less than 300 mg/dl, to be negative to small ketones and to have no acute illness. Unless these criteria are met, diet should not be the choice.

We next examined the conditions under which diet treatment would be deemed a failure and an alternative therapy prescribed. The criteria were established that on

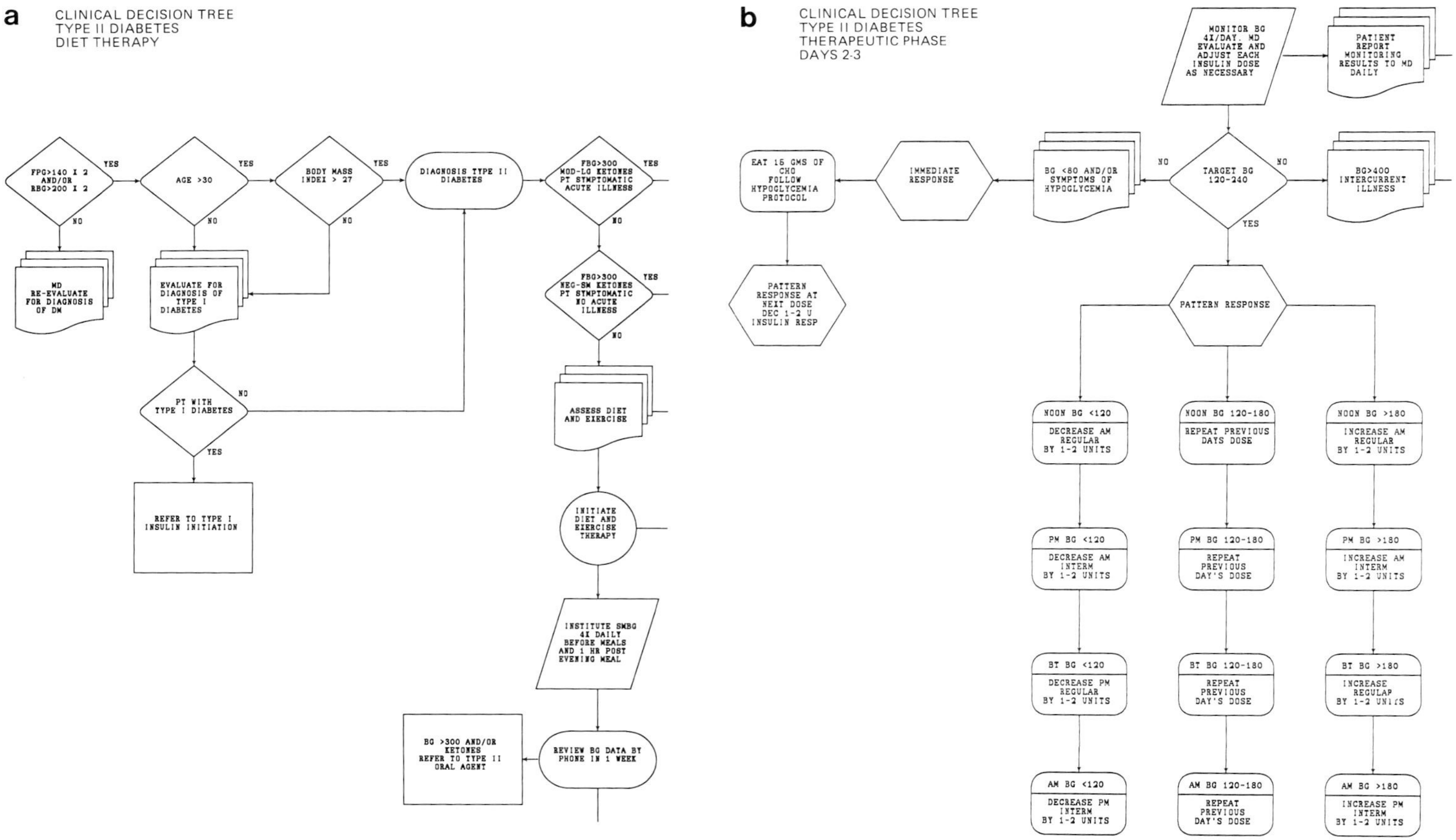

Fig. 2. A staged approach to clinical decision-making. Depicted in this diagram are the steps and conditions for a data-based approach to clinical decision-making. The diamond-shaped boxes signify the decision point. The other shapes relate to the criteria, documentation and action steps.

a monthly basis HbA$_1$ values would be required to drop by at least 1% until they reached to within 1% of the upper limits of normal for a particular HbA$_1$ assay and that verified self-monitored blood glucose values (obtained from a memory-based reflectance meter) would range from 80 to 150 mg/dl. If after two months this target could not be achieved, oral hypoglycemic agents would be initiated.

Depicted also in Fig. 2 are the conditions for discontinuing oral agent use. The same overall criteria of a 1% drop in HbA$_1$ and a concomitant improvement in the range of blood glucose values are used for this therapy. The decisive factor, however, is the requirement that the maximum tolerable dose (MTD) based on both body mass index and patient tolerance should be reached. If after MTD is reached no improvement in HbA$_1$ is found, then data are required upon which a consideration of the specifics of insulin therapy can be based (as noted in Fig. 2).

Once the criteria for initiation of insulin are met, the use of insulin therapy by the primary care physician is guided by a series of prompts and questions (e.g., weight of patient, mean blood glucose, last HbA$_1$ level) to assure safety and efficacy. Two approaches – immediate response and pattern response – are used depending upon whether the patient's blood glucose falls within the preset target range. Immediate response is taken when blood glucose levels fall well outside the preset target on a few occasions and when the therapeutic goal is to re-establish near-normal levels of glycemia. Pattern response is the approach to repeated episodes of, for example, hyperglycemia, for which a permanent solution (increased bedtime intermediate-acting insulin) is sought. As with the other approaches, monitoring of blood glucose with verified data from a memory-based reflectance meter and validation with glycosylated hemoglobin are the principal bases for clinical decision-making.

The guide as outlined above was coded for use in the expert clinical decision-making program. Each element of the decision-making process was transformed into a series of prompts and questions. Based on the answers provided by the primary care physician, the computer program would suggest appropriate treatment modalities and calculate proper doses of insulin based on the phase of treatment (e.g., baseline, therapeutic or stabilization).

To date our findings from a retrospective review of randomly selected cases from among 2600 patients indicate that an approach based on this type of model will result in: (1) a substantially higher proportion of patients treated with insulin (ranging from 40 to 60%); (2) an overall level of metabolic control for 67% of the patients within 1% of normal HbA$_1$, independent of type of treatment, and consistent with patient-generated verified self-monitored blood glucose data; (3) a consistent pattern of lowered blood glucose induced by exercise.

Discussion

Since it has been all but impossible to find an agreed-upon set of specific standards for the treatment of the individual with NIDDM in the United States, we reviewed current approaches and then devised an innovative program for primary care physicians. The method of clinical decision-making proposed in this paper is a far departure from the current ad hoc and inconsistent organization of health care services provided to the individual with NIDDM treated by the general internist or family physician. It depends on systematic collection of data, assumes a rational basis for decision-making, validates each decision with added data and documents each step. The latter is then used as a basis for testing the underlying assumptions concerning this approach.

While currently data are still being collected to validate this system, evidence already exists that this approach is a feasible system for the primary care physician. It provides generally acceptable standards and guides for treatment. Because of its reliance on computer-aided data collection, transmission, aggregation and analysis, it potentially permits the establishment of a network of primary care physicians who communicate via computer with each other and a medical center where expertise in diabetes can be used to enhance the co-management of the individual with diabetes between the primary care physician and the diabetes specialist. Such a system would permit rapid transfer of information, on-line medical expertise for consultation and a means of ensuring a region-wide high level of diabetes care.

With the introduction and widespread application of computer technologies to medicine, it is reasonable to expect that within the next decade diabetes management will be greatly enhanced by the newer technologies. The primary care physician is likely to benefit most, since computer-based technologies are designed to optimize communications and to provide desk-top expert systems. The program described here is one of many innovations that will eventually serve to benefit the individual with diabetes as well as those involved in their treatment

Acknowledgements

The authors gratefully acknowledge the contributions of Diane Reader, R.D., Janet Davidson, R.N., and Judith Joynes, R.N., and the support of the Becton Dickinson Company.

232

References

1. Herman WH, Sinnock P, Brenner E, Brimberry J, Langford D, Nakashima A, Sepe S, Teutsch S, Mazze R. An epidemiological model for diabetes mellitus: incidence, prevalence and mortality. Diabetes Care 1984;7:367–371.
2. Mazze R, Sinnock P, Deeb L, Brimberry J. An epidemiological model of diabetes mellitus in the United States: five major complications. Diabetes Res Clin Pract 1985;(1)185–191.
3. National Center for Health Statistics, National Health Interview Survey, unpublished data, 1980–1987.
4. Centers for Disease Control, Committee for Distribution of the Physicians' Guide, Atlanta, GA, unpublished data, 1986.
5. Eschwège E, ed. Advances in diabetes epidemiology. New York: Elsevier, 1982;135–157.
6. Report of the National Commission on Diabetes to the Congress of the United States, US Department of Health, Education and Welfare, NIH Publication No. (NIH) 76–1020,1975.
7. Mazze R, Deeb L, Palumbo P. Altering physician practice patterns. Diabetes Care 1986;9:420–426.
8. On site surveys of Clinical Education Program participants (unpublished). The American Diabetes Association, 1986.
9. Mazze R, Matsuoka K. Computer applications in diabetes care, research and education. In: Alberti KGGM, De Fronzo R, Keen H, Zimmet P, eds. International Textbook of Diabetes Mellitus. New York: J. Wiley, 1989; (in press).
10. Zimmet P, Lang A, Mazze R, Endersbee R. Computer-based patient monitoring systems: use in research and clinical practice. Diabetes Care 1988;11:62–66.
11. Mazze R, Lucido D, Langer O, Hartmann K, Rodbard D. The ambulatory glucose profile: a representation of verified self-monitored blood glucose data. Diabetes Care 1987;10:111–117.
12. Mazze R, Zimmet P. Computers in diabetes care and patient education: an overview. Pract Diabetes 1987;4:8–11.
13. Shamoon H, Mazze R, Pasmantier R, Lucido D, Murphy J. Assessment of long-term glycemia in type I diabetes using multiple blood glucose values stored in a memory-containing reflectometer. Am J Med 1986;80:1086–1092.
14. Allen L, Yarborough M, Hastedt P, Molter D, Surwit R, Feinglos M. Enhancement of intensive insulin therapy using a hand held computer with remote communications capabilities. Presented at the WHO Conference on Computers in Diabetes Care and Research, American Diabetes Association 46th Meeting, Anneheim, CA, 1986;1–19.
15. Atsumi Y, Matsuoka K. A computer communication system for the diabetics with self-monitoring of blood glucose. Presented at the WHO Conference on Computers in Diabetes Care and Education, American Diabetes Association 46th Meeting, Anneheim, CA, 1986;1–12.
16. Pernick N, Rodbard D. Personal computer programs to assist with self-monitoring of blood glucose and self-adjustment of insulin dosage. Diabetes Care 1986;9:61–69.
17. Zimmet P, Gerstman M, Raper L, Cohen M, Crosbie C, Kuykendall V, Michaels D, Hartmann K. Computerized assessment of self-monitored blood glucose results using a glucometer reflectance photometer with memory and microcomputer. Diabetes Res Clin Pract 1985;1:55–63.
18. Schultz G, Beyer J. A computerized program for diabetes self-adjustment and its application to in- and outpatients. Computer Systems for Insulin Adjustment in Diabetes Mellitus, First International Symposium on Computer Systems for Insulin Adjustment in Diabetes Mellitus (Panscienta-Verlag) 1985:111–117.
19. Schiffrin A, Albisser A, Mihic M. Optimizing conventional insulin therapy using an insulin dosage computer. Diabetes 1984;33:34A.
20. Interactive Easyflow, HavenTree Software Limied, Kingston, Ontario, Canada, 1988.
21. V-P Expert. Berkeley, CA: Paperback Software, 1985.

CHAPTER 18

Diet USA

AARON I. VINIK

Department of Internal Medicine and the Department of Surgery, University of Michigan Medical Center,
Ann Arbor, MI 48109-0331, U.S.A.

Introduction

In the recent past much new information has emerged which is pertinent to nutritional management of the patient with diabetes. Awareness of differences in types of carbohydrate, a reevaluation of the caloric content of food exchanges and the glycemic potential of starchy foods are but a few. The relative freedom of certain populations from coronary artery disease despite extremely high intake of fat has led to reinvestigation of the nature of fats consumed and new data have emerged on their diversity and significant differences in impact on glycemic control and hyperlipidemia. Even proteins have not escaped attention, and recent focus upon their possible role in accentuating the progressive decline in renal function that accompanies diabetes has become a target of energetic research endeavors. Before delving into the realms of specific issues, it is appropriate that we briefly recapture the exciting events that have preceded us.

Historical perspectives

Modern concepts of the role of nutrition in diabetes mellitus have evolved from rationalization of the thinking and controversies of the past [1,2]. To place current philosophies and principles in perspective, a brief historical synopsis is given in Table 1. This survey indicates that current controversies on the relative proportions of carbohydrate and fat in the meal-planning for people with diabetes have perplexed clinicians for centuries.

TABLE 1

Vicissitudes in nutritional recommendations for diabetes

Authors	Year	Recommendation		Comment
		Carbohydrate	Fat	
Papyrus Ebers	1500 BC	Wheat grain, fruit	–	Drive away
		Sweet beer		the passing
Araetus Cappedoca		Starch fruit, sweet wines		of too much wine
Sanskrit	600 AD	Decrease of rice, flour sugar		Madhumeha
Willis	1675	Increase in carbohydrate		Replace urine losses
Rollo	1797	Blood pudding, rancid meat	Low	(high protein)
Pile	1860	Animal foods		
Bouchardat	1870	Low carbohydrates	High	(intermittent fasts)
Naunyn	1870	Low carbohydrates	–	(intermittent fasts)
Allen	1912	Low carbohydrates	Low	Starvation
Von During, Mosse	1889–1902	High carbohydrates	Low	Potatoes, oatmeal
Van Noorden		High carbohydrates		
Geyetin	1923	Moderate carbohydrates	Low	+ insulin
Rabinovich	1930s	High carbohydrates		
Himsworth	1935 [3]	High carbohydrates		Type of carbohydrate
Jenkins, Anderson, Levitt	1970	High carbohydrates		High fiber
ADA (US)	1940–1970	Limited carbohydrate	Moderate	
ADA (US)	1971–1979	Liberalized	Lower	
ADA (US)	1986	Liberal	Low	

The notion that high-carbohydrate, high-fiber, low-fat diets are beneficial for people with diabetes has gained much support and sparked off more than five decades of investigations into the role of dietary fiber in the management of diabetes. Between 1940 and 1970 the American Diabetes Association (ADA) recommended carbohydrate restriction, a view that was reversed with the 1971 revisions which were reaf-

TABLE 2

Recommended daily intake (% of total calories)

Carbohydrate	Protein	Fat			Cholesterol	Fiber
55–60	12–20[a]	< 30			< 200	40[b]
		PUS	S	MS		
		6–8	< 10	remainder		

If the total fat is reduced, all components, polyunsaturated (PUS), saturated (S) and monounsaturated (MS), should be reduced proportionally.

[a]The recommended dietary allowance for protein is 0.8 g/kg. Patients with incipient renal failure may require lower protein intakes. [b]In people taking low-kcal diets 25 g/1000 kcal. Of primary importance has been the recent recognition of the need for new approaches to the implementation of dietary intervention and ways and means of applying strategies for the promotion of adherence to meal planning, a euphemistic term for what was known as the diabetic diet.

firmed with the 1979 and 1986 Principles of Nutrition and Dietary Recommendations for Individuals with Diabetes Mellitus. In essence, the revised recommendations were to restrict fat, limit protein intake to the recommended daily intake (RDI) and fill the void with carbohydrates. These principles are based upon new information and knowledge pertinent to a growing concern for the role of lipids in macrovascular disease and of protein intake upon renal integrity. Table 2 is a summary of the current recommendations.

First and foremost, however, is the need to define caloric needs for diabetes management.

Importance of total caloric intake

The most important dietary objective for obese patients with NIDDM is weight reduction. Weight loss results in improved carbohydrate metabolism and often allows for reductions or withdrawal of insulin or oral medication [4–9]. Weight loss also improves general health, and specifically reduces coronary heart disease risk factors. Weight loss may also improve life-expectancy, since patients who have diabetes and are 20% above average weight have a mortality ratio 2.5–3.0 times that of normal-weight diabetics, while those who are 40% or more above ideal weight have a mortality ratio 5.2–7.9 times that of normal-weight diabetic patients [10].

Weight loss results in reductions in both fasting glucose levels, associated with reduced hepatic glucose output, and postprandial glucose [4,9,11]. However, glucose tolerance does not become entirely normal with weight loss [7,11]. Weight loss also improves insulin resistance [4,8,10,12]. Fasting and postprandial insulin levels decrease in patients who are initially hyperinsulinemic, and fasting and postprandial insulin levels rise in those who are initially hypoinsulinemic [13]. However, despite marked improvements in insulin resistance and B-cell function, the latter remains impaired [4,8], with no change in the first-phase insulin response, testifying to the intrinsic nature of the B-cell defect in NIDDM.

Weight loss is important for NIDDM patients not only because it improves glycemic control, but also for its beneficial effects on other coronary heart disease risk factors. Weight loss in NIDDM patients results in lowering of blood pressure levels [14,15], reductions in LDL cholesterol and triglycerides [16,17], and increases in HDL cholesterol [4,17]. Thus, the overall coronary heart disease risk profile of a NIDDM patient can be greatly improved by weight reduction. Weight reduction also produces a sustained reduction in proteinuria, and may therefore slow the development of clinical nephropathy or end-stage renal disease [18].

Patients with diabetes should be encouraged to lose even small amounts of weight, since modest reductions, without achieving ideal body weight, will result in improved

TABLE 3
A simple method to calculate caloric needs

Build	Women	Men
Medium	Allow 100 lb (45.5 kg) for first 5 ft (1.52 m) of height, plus 5 lb (2.3 kg) for each additional inch	Allow 106 lb (48.2 kg) for first 5 ft (1.52 m) of height, plus 6 lb (2.7 kg) for each additional inch
Small	Subtract 10%	Subtract 10%
Large	Add 10%	Add 10%

For adults:
  Basal kilocalories equals desirable body weight (lb) × 10
  Add activity calories:
    Sedentary add 10% of estimated basal calories
    Moderate add 20% of estimated basal calories
    Strenuous add 40–100% of estimated basal calories

glycemic control and CHD risk profiles. Weight losses of 15–30 pounds in patients who weigh over 200 lb result in both short-term and long-term changes in glycemic control [17]. Although the immediate effects of caloric restriction are greater than the long-term effects of weight loss, maintenance of a 15–30 pound loss produced significant improvements in fasting glucose and insulin, glycosylated hemoglobin and serum lipid levels for at least one year after weight loss. Larger weight losses, averaging 50 lb, produced even greater benefits for patients, although again patients had not attained ideal body weight.

While weight reduction has clear benefits for obese patients with NIDDM, the problem remains that it is difficult for patients to maintain their losses. Studies, such as the University Group Diabetes Program (UGDP), found that patients treated with placebo and diet lost only 2.4% of their body weight at 3 months and 1.6% at $4\frac{3}{4}$ year follow-up [19]. Other long-term studies with diabetic patients similarly show minimal weight losses at follow-up [20]. Recent controlled studies have shown that including training in behavior modification improves outcome in weight control programs [21–24].

Caloric intake versus weight reduction

Improvements in glycemic control occur rapidly after starting a diet, with maximal responses within several days or weeks after initiation of diet. Thus, the improved glycemic control seems to be related to caloric restriction, rather than weight loss per se. However, recent studies have shown that the improvements in glucose homeostasis may be maintained when patients are reassessed after a period of weight loss followed by weight maintenance [11]. Repeated short-term fasts may well be the answer to the problematic over-indulger.

Despite a great deal of research on diet and weight loss, it remains unclear what patients should eat or how much they should eat to produce the best long-term outcome. The goal of weight-reduction programs is usually gradual, sustained weight loss. A weight reduction of 2 lb/week seems most appropriate. To produce a weight loss of 2 lb/week, it is necessary for patients to reduce their current intake by 7000 kcal/week or 1000 kcal/day. A guide to caloric needs is given in Table 3.

More stringent dietary restriction, as accomplished by fasting or very low calorie diets, can also be of benefit to obese NIDDM patients. Davidson [25] has had excellent results using a dietary program which includes one-week periods of in-hospital or outpatient fasts. These fasts are used as part of an intensive program of dietary instruction, involving up to 25 hours of group and individual counseling over a one-year period.

Very low calorie diets have also been recommended [26,27] for obese patients with NIDDM. These diets involve 400–600 kcal/day and are designed to produce rapid weight loss while preserving lean body mass by the provision of dietary protein or protein plus carbohydrates. Current very low calorie diets, which involve high-quality protein and include vitamin and mineral supplementation, are considerably safer than the early liquid protein diets, which produced cardiac dysfunction [28–31]. There remains a great deal of controversy regarding the ideal format of very low calorie diets. Diets which contain a high proportion of protein (called protein-sparing fasts) have been shown to provide better nitrogen balance than diets containing a more balanced distribution of calories from protein, fat and carbohydrates [32]. However, carbohydrate-containing diets produce better maintenance of muscle glycogen, greater exercise tolerance and less ketosis [33]. Some investigators recommend the use of animal protein (lean meat, fish or fowl) served in its food form, but most use milk- or egg-based liquid protein formulas. Vitamins and mineral supplements must be provided with the former, but are usually included within the formula preparations.

Very low calorie diets are usually limited to patients who are 50% or more over their ideal body weight. Contraindications to treatment with very low calorie diets include recent myocardial infarction, hepatic disease, renal failure, IDDM and cerebrovascular disease [31]. Patients must be monitored closely while on the very low calorie diet to ensure that no electrocardiographic changes or electrolyte disturbances result. Oral medications are usually stopped before starting the very low calorie diet and NIDDM patients on insulin are hospitalized initially while insulin is withdrawn.

When used with close medical monitoring, the very low calorie diets appear safe and effective in the treatment of both diabetic and nondiabetic obese individuals. Patients lose approximately 20 kg during a 12-week period on the very low calorie diet. Diabetic patients treated with very low calorie diets achieve rapid reductions in glucose, insulin and serum lipid levels [28–30]. However, maintenance of weight loss has been more problematic. Using the very low calorie diet in combination with behavior modification appears to improve its effectiveness [34].

While the very low calorie diet clearly increases initial rates of weight loss, it remains unclear whether the use of this diet will improve long-term outcome compared with that which can be obtained with a balanced diet involving only moderate calorie reduction (1000–1500 kcal/day). However, very low calorie diets may be of use with certain patients, especially those who are heavier (> 50% above ideal body weight) and have experienced repeated failure at previous efforts to lose weight with balanced diets.

Carbohydrate content of the diet

Debate about the amount of carbohydrate that individuals with diabetes should consume has continued over several centuries. In recent years, the trend has been toward a liberalization of total carbohydrate intake, although some dissension persists [35]. After a review of the data available at that time, the Food and Nutrition Committee of the American Diabetes Association stated in 1971: 'Important dietary concepts have developed during the last decade which require some alteration in long-held precepts. There no longer appears to be any need to restrict disproportionately the intake of carbohydrate in the diet of most diabetic patients. Increase of dietary carbohydrate, even to extremes, without increase of total calories, does not appear to increase insulin requirement in the insulin-treated diabetic patient.' However, the committee acknowledged that 'there are obvious gaps in our knowledge' and that 'there are no controlled prospective studies which provide evidence for choosing the optimal portions of dietary carbohydrate and fat with regards to long-term complications' [36].

In spite of some continued skepticism, the American Diabetes Association [37] reiterated in 1979 and 1986 its stand on the liberalization of the carbohydrate content of the diabetic's diet and has recently been joined in this advocacy by the British and Canadian diabetes associations [38,39]. In addition, diabetologists in Australia [40] and South Africa [41] echo the same majority opinion that the intake of carbohydrate-containing foods by persons with diabetes should equal or even exceed that of nondiabetic individuals.

Those who question this trend toward diets containing 50–60% of total calories as carbohydrate voice specific concerns [42]. Preliminary data involve patients with relatively good regulation of their diabetes, so that little information is available with regard to an increased carbohydrate intake in the diabetic who is poorly controlled. Moreover, the nature of the carbohydrate to be prescribed for the diabetic remains undefined; there are no studies that define the 'ideal' ratio of complex to simple carbohydrates. It is furthermore apparent that, in certain people with diabetes, a high carbohydrate intake may aggravate hypertriglyceridemia [43]. A summary of supportive and contrary studies is given in Table 4.

There are no experimental findings based upon long-term clinical trials using mortality and morbidity statistics to support a firm policy on the issue of carbohydrate content of the diet. There is, however, sufficient circumstantial evidence from both epidemiological and short-term metabolic studies to support the view that diets containing 45–70% of total calories as carbohydrate are beneficial and not harmful [44]. The recommendation that dietary carbohydrate should account for 50–60% of the total energy intake of the insulin-dependent diabetic seems appropriate [37]. Whereas a similar percentage of total calories is appropriate for most non-insulin-dependent diabetics, the amounts of carbohydrate in the diets of such patients are secondary to total caloric intake. Persons with NIDDM and an accompanying hypertriglyceridemia may require lesser amounts of carbohydrate.

Dissertations on the topic 'How much carbohydrate should the person with diabetes consume?' rarely consider that the term carbohydrate is a generic one. Foods contain several types of carbohydrate: monosaccharides such as glucose and fructose; disaccharides such as sucrose, table sugar; and polysaccharides or complex carbohydrates such as starches and glycogen.

Sucrose: disaccharides [57]

Within the last decade, a number of studies have indicated that equimolar amounts of 'carbohydrate' in different foods yield different excursions in postprandial glucose levels. Objections to the glycemic index concept were raised early [58] and have not been resolved [59,60]. These objections resulted in a statement by the consensus conference at the National Institute of Health that recommended against the use of the glycemic index in dietary management of diabetes [61].

Furthermore, there is a lack of agreement between different centers, and dissimilarities have been observed between the glycemic responses to certain foods tested in different centers [62–67]. It is apparent that these differences may be explained by the choice of the food examined, the nature of the preparation of the food, for example baking vs. boiling or par-boiling, differences in the weight of the food fed due to the use of different food tables, and thus these differences may not be due to lack of reproducibility but represent true differences in physical and other as yet undetermined factors between foods that have been considered to be the same. Even rice, when prepared differently, can yield vastly different glycemic properties [68]. Further

TABLE 4
Response to high-carbohydrate high-fiber diets

Investigator	No. of subjects/type DM	Type diet/weeks	% change			
			Insulin dose	FBG	Total chol.	TG
Anderson et al. [45] 1980	14/IDDM, NIDDM	HCHF/3 weeks	-56*	-15	-32*	-11
	11/IDDM, NIDDM	HCHF/2 weeks	-45*	-6*	-22*	-1
Anderson and Ward [46] 1979	20/IDDM, NIDDM	HCHF/2 weeks	-58*	-7	-20*	-2
Kiehm et al. [47] 1976	13/IDDM, NIDDM	HCHF/2 weeks	-36	-26*	-24*	-15
Ney et al. [48] 1982	20/IDDM, NIDDM (subjects pregnant)	HCHF/17 weeks	+ +	-27*	NR	NR
Simpson et al. [49] 1981	9/IDDM	HCHF/6 weeks	NA	-15*	-14*	NR
	18/NIDDM	HCHF/6 weeks				
Simpson et al. [50] 1979	11/IDDM	HCHF/6 weeks	-6	-20*	NR	-9
Simpson et al. [51] 1979	14/NIDDM	HCHF/6 weeks	NA	-12*	-14*	-6
Karlstrom et al. [52] 1984	14/NIDDM	SCHF/3 weeks	NA	-14*	+2	+11
Kinmonth et al. [53] 1982	10/IDDM	SCHF/6 weeks	-7	-35*	NR	NR
Coulston et al. [54] 1987	9/NIDDM	HCLF/2 weeks	NA	0	0	↑
Hollenbeck et al. [55] 1987	NIDDM	HCLF/6 weeks	NA	0	0	+ 30%
Hollenbeck et al. [56] 1986	6/NIDDM	SCHF(11-27 g fiber)	NA	0	0	0

*$p < 0.05$.
NR = not reported.
NA = not applicable.
HCHF = high (70%) carbohydrate, high fiber.
SCHF = standard carbohydrate (50-55%), high fiber.
+ + = Insulin dose and weight gain lower with HCHF diet compared with control during pregnancy.
HCLF (60% CHO) = high carbohydrate, low fat.

factors include the ripeness of foods [69] and the degree of gelatinization of starch [70,71], and many such factors are now emerging as relevant in determining postprandial glycemia and the insulin response [72].

The last major concern with regard to the glycemic index is that there is a lack of difference between mixed meals containing foods of vastly different indices. Several studies have now been reported which fail to show any difference in a glycemic response to mixed meals [59,73,74] and, although there are some studies that show good predictive ability using the index [75–78], others do not concur. A principal reason for this discrepancy appears to be the lack of pretesting of the individual carbohydrate components of the mixed meal at the institute at which the mixed meals have been used, utilizing reference values for the individual components derived from the tables of Jenkins [79].

The key issue pertinent to the implementation of glycemic properties of foods to nutritional management is the clinical gains to be expected through improved control of postprandial glycemic excursions. Unfortunately, very few studies have been published on the effects of incorporating carbohydrate foods that cause relatively low rises in postprandial glucose into the meal plan. Although suggesting improved glucose tolerance and a fall in serum cholesterol after standard meals in diabetic children [53] and a fall in triglyceride and low density lipoprotein cholesterol in hypertriglyceridemic subjects [79], this issue remains to be resolved. Thus, currently it might be in order to establish the glycemic properties of individual foods in a given individual, and to facilitate optimum management of that individual by identification of the foods that cause the least perturbation of blood glucose. It has been further suggested that the glycemic response should be indexed to a standard, for example, white bread, to allow comparisons to be made between the glycemic index of foods tested at different times. The scope of application of this principle is subject to further investigation and may expand the range of possibly useful starchy foods for trial in the nutritional management of patients with diabetes.

The several factors that account for the differences in blood glucose response observed after the ingestion of polysaccharide-containing foods require further delineation. One element that does play a role in the glycemic response of a carbohydrate-containing meal is its fiber content.

Dietary fiber

Since Burkitt, Trowell and Cleave [80–82] suggested that diabetes mellitus, as well as other common disorders, results in part from the modern tendency to consume excessive quantities of refined sugar and simultaneously to eat less unrefined carbohydrates and fiber, an enormous quantity of experimental work has examined the effects of dietary fiber on glucose and insulin kinetics in normal and diabetic subjects.

In summary, these studies show that glucose tolerance improves and insulin secretion diminishes when fiber-enriched diets or meals are consumed by normal and NIDDM subjects [83,84]. Mean levels of glucosuria and glycemia decrease when patients with IDDM consume similar meals [47,85–87]. While the preliminary nature of these studies and lack of a mechanistic process preclude a definite place for fiber-enriched foods in the menu of all diabetics, they are so encouraging that some permanent role for them seems certain. Much of the controversy which surrounds the use of fiber derives from a lack of awareness of differences between fibers and their biological effects.

For convenience, fibers have been divided into two broad classes: the so-called soluble and insoluble. The soluble consists of the gums, gels, mucilages, pectic substances and a portion of what used to be called the hemicelluloses. The insoluble consist of the non-carbohydrate fiber component, lignin, cellulose and some of the hemicelluloses, especially those combined with lignin. In general, it is the soluble fibers that have been demonstrated to have effects on carbohydrate and lipid metabolism. They are fermented to gas and short-chain fatty acids in the colon and contribute little to fecal bulk because the acids are cleared rapidly. The insoluble fibers, on the other hand, are largely responsible for increasing the bulk of the feces but have little metabolic effect.

A number of studies, mainly those of Anderson and colleagues [85–91], have devised high-fiber diets that have been successful in improving diabetic control. These diets contain 70% carbohydrate and 35 g of dietary fiber/1000 kcal. Both IDDM and NIDDM patients on this ratio for short periods of 60–80 days have shown significant decreases in both fasting and postprandial glucose concentrations. A majority of patients have decreased or discontinued insulin or sulphonylurea therapy [91,92] and those patients who followed the high-fiber maintenance diet with 60% carbohydrate for up to 15–21 months have shown additional reduction in fasting glucose levels, allowing reduction or discontinuation of their oral hypoglycemic medication. Contrasting with these effects are studies in which the carbohydrate source was kept constant but the fiber content was either low (11 g/1000 kcal) or high (27 g/1000 kcal) [56,93], in which case no significant effects were found on glucose control, postprandial glucose, hemoglobin A_1 or the insulin requirements in adult patients with NIDDM. Studies by Riccardi and colleagues [94] and Mann [95] have shown that increasing carbohydrate content of the diet has deleterious effects on fasting and postprandial blood glucose as well as the lipid profile but, if the fiber content is increased sufficiently to the region of 44 g or more, then the harmful effects of the high-carbohydrate diet may certainly be mitigated.

The concern that high-fiber diets may impair mineral or vitamin absorption is not borne out by observations in diabetic patients [96]. Meals enriched with fiber have an important potential role in the management of the hyperlipidemia frequently encountered in diabetics [97]. Investigative efforts will better define the specific types of plant fiber and how these should be incorporated into cultural and social customs of the diabetic population. In the meantime, the recommendations of Anderson and Chen [88], Jenkins et al. [98] and Monnier et al. [87] warrant consideration.

Recommendations for the use of fiber
Estimates of the current dietary fiber intake of adults in the United States range from 13 to 30 g/day, with men averaging 19.1 g/day and women 13.4 g/day. A practical goal would be to establish the current intake and gradually increase it twofold. Fiber should be taken in a range of foods to include both soluble types, such as oats, fruits and legumes, and insoluble forms, such as wheat products and bran. Fiber supplementation appears to provide benefit only if given with a diet comprising at least 50% of calories as carbohydrate. Foods should be selected with moderate to high amounts of dietary fiber. The 1986/1987 exchange lists compiled by the American Diabetes Association in conjunction with the American Dietetic Association use a symbol to indicate foods with a fiber content of at least 3 g per serving. These foods include legumes, roots, tubers, green leafy vegetables, all types of whole-grain cereal (including wheat, barley, oats, corn and rye) and fruits. Fruits and vegetables should be eaten raw and not pureed, which causes loss or reduction of the fiber effect. Abdominal cramping, discomfort and flatulence can be minimized by starting with small servings and increasing gradually. Insufficient data are available on the long-term safety of very high fiber diets or fiber supplements, although, to date, there are no reports of serious deficiencies arising from the use of high-fiber diets. People at risk of deficiencies, e.g., postmenopausal women, the elderly, and growing children, may require supplements of calcium and trace minerals. Subjects with upper gastrointestinal dysfunction are at risk of bezoar formation and should be cautioned against a diet high in leafy vegetables such as cabbage. Careful attention must be paid to insulin dose, because hypoglycemia can result if the dose is not reduced appropriately. Children may also benefit from an increase in the fiber content of their diets but may not tolerate large amounts. Pregnant diabetic women appear to tolerate fiber well, but there are too few studies to advise for or against its use in pregnancy. Care must be exercised in the use of novel fibers, because little is known of their safety or efficacy.

Fat content of the meal plan

Hypertriglyceridemia

Elevated plasma levels of triglycerides occur frequently in patients with the diabetic syndromes. The relationship between hypertriglyceridemia and hyperglycemia is complex, and often palindromic [99].

Concern that diets that are restricted in fat but high in carbohydrate may induce elevations of plasma triglyceride concentrations has been voiced [100] and diets of this nature may alter the pathways by which VLDL triglyceride synthesis, apo-B production and VLDL conversion to LDL occurs. It appears that if the high-carbohydrate diet is enriched with guar gum, reductions in serum cholesterol [101] and the ability to blunt the hypertriglyceridemic response induced by the high-carbohydrate, low-fat, low-fiber diet are observed [102]. Furthermore, these diets induce a significant reduction in LDL cholesterol, improvements that are not observed with high-carbohydrate diets alone [103], but these findings have been contested by others [56,104].

Garg and associates recently reported [105] that replacement of carbohydrates by monounsaturated fats does not increase LDL levels and may improve glycemic control and the levels of plasma triglycerides and HDL cholesterol. These diets required 33% of the total energy to be given as olive oil, i.e. the addition of $\frac{1}{4}$ to $\frac{1}{3}$ cup of olive oil as a daily food additive, which may not be acceptable to most people. It does, however, seem prudent to replace polyunsaturated and saturated fats in the diet with kcals derived from the monounsaturated. Table 5 is provided to assist in the selection of oils and foods.

Research into the long-term sequelae of these diets is clearly needed. Whereas it may decrease the saturated fat intake it is not clear that replacement of carbohydrate kcals with fat kcals is beneficial in all forms of NIDDM with different prevailing glucose and lipid levels.

The addition of cholesterol to the diet causes an increase in total cholesterol and LDL cholesterol [106] and the effect depends on the polyunsaturated-to-saturated (P/S) fat ratio in the diet [107]. Cholesterol-restricted diets can produce up to a 15–20% reduction in plasma cholesterol in both normal and hypercholesterolemic patients [108]. Increases in polyunsaturated fatty acids to maintain a dietary P/S ratio of > 0.8 have pronounced hypocholesterolemic effects [109]. Concern has been raised that a diet high in polyunsaturated fatty acids not only reduces total cholesterol and LDL but decreases HDL cholesterol as well. In contrast, dietary trials comparing monounsaturated fatty acids with the polyunsaturated fatty acids demonstrate comparable reduction in LDL but less of an HDL-lowering effect of the monounsaturated oil [110] in both normo- and hypercholesterolemic individuals [111]. There is further concern that the polyunsaturated fatty acids may promote carcinogenesis in experimental animals [112]. Therefore it has been recommended that the percentage of polyunsaturated fatty acids should be confined to 6–8% of total calories and replacement with monounsaturated fats is not unreasonable.

Because plasma cholesterol concentrations in some diabetic individuals may remain raised even after optimal glycemic control is obtained, even more fat-restricted diets comparable to the American Heart Association Phase I, fat 25% cholesterol

TABLE 5
Monounsaturated fatty acid content of selected dietary fats[a]

Dietary fat	Cholesterol (mg/tbsp)	Monounsaturated fatty acid[b]	Polyunsaturated fatty acid[b]	Saturated fatty acid[b]
Oils				
Canola oil[c]	0	62	32	6
Corn oil	0	25	62	13
Olive oil	0	77	9	14
Peanut oil	0	49	33	18
Safflower oil	0	13	77	10
Soybean oil	0	24	61	15
Sunflower oil	0	20	69	11
Fats				
Beef fat	14	44	4	52
Butter fat	33	30	4	66
Chicken fat	11	47	22	31
Lard	12	47	12	41
Margarine	0	49	34	18
Nuts				
Cashew	0	62	17	21
Hazelnut	0	82	10	8
Macadamia[d]	0	83	2	15
Peanut	0	52	33	15
Pistachio	0	74	17	13
Other				
Avocado	0	75	10	15
Peanut butter	0	51	32	17

[a]Reference: Composition of Foods, Agricultural Handbooks. Washington DC: USDA, 1979.
[b]Percent of fatty acid content.
[c]Reference data on file, Proctor and Gamble.
[d]Macadamia nuts are frequently roasted in coconut oil.

200–250 mg/day, or Phase III fat 20% of calories, cholesterol 100–150 mg/day, with or without appropriate hypolipodemic drugs may be prescribed. The rationale for this action and the specifics of this recommendation have been reported [113]. Any unusual circumstances in which extreme hypertriglyceridemia develops (1000–2000 mg/dl), a fat-restricted diet of < 20% of the total calories together with appropriate anti-diabetic therapy and possibly a hypotriglyceridemic agent may be indicated. There is, however, evidence to suggest that ingesting certain fatty acids may have the ability to lower triglyceride levels.

Omega — 3 fatty acids

Recently it has been recognized that certain essential fatty acids of the omega — 3 class ($n - 3$), found in fish oils, particularly icosapentaenoic acid ($20:5n - 3$) and docosahexaenoic acid ($20:6n - 3$), may potentially reduce the coronary vascular risk in diabetes. Their effects include: (1) reduction of plasma VLDL triglyceride concentrations in both normolipemic and hypertriglyceridemic subjects by decreasing VLDL production [114–116]; (2) lowering blood pressure [117]; (3) prolonging platelet aggregation and bleeding time by depressing thromboxane A_2 formation [118,119]. The association between diabetes-increased VLDL production, elevated blood pressure and platelet hyperaggregability with increased thromboxane A_2 formation [120] has suggested that dietary supplementation with fish or fish oil would appear to have the potential to influence these risk factors favorably.

The low prevalence of atherosclerosis among Eskimos in Greenland and mortality from myocardial infarction, despite a diet as high in fat and cholesterol as that of Danes or Americans [117,121,122], may be related to the striking difference between the dietary composition of the fats consumed. Eskimos consume 5–10 g of the long-chain $n - 3$ polyunsaturated fatty acids per day. These observations have stimulated a number of biochemical and physiological studies as well as clinical studies which suggest that $n - 3$ fatty acids have potentially antiatheromatous effects. Humans are unable to synthesize fatty acids with double bonds more distal from the carboxyl end of the fatty acid than the ninth carbon atom. Thus, linoleic acid ($18.2n - 6$) is an essential fatty acid that must be ingested since it cannot be synthesized and is the principal polyunsaturated fatty acid in oil from plant seeds, for example corn oil and safflower oil. Another important dietary class of polyunsaturated fatty acid is alpha-linolenic acid ($18:3n - 3$), which in humans is slowly elongated and desaturated to icosapentaenoic acid and docosahexaenoic acid. Whereas some plant oils, notably linseed, rape seed and soybean oils, contain significant quantities of alpha-linolenic acid, marine animals and phyto- and xeroplankton are rich sources of the longer $n - 3$ polyunsaturated fatty acids, icosapentaenoic and docosahexaenoic acids.

The synthesis of the long-chain $n - 3$ polyunsaturated fatty acids is slow in humans and decreases with aging and certain disease states [123], possibly related to a loss of or decrease in desaturase activity required for the conversion of dietary linolenic acid to icosapentaenoic and docosahexaenoic acids. Since the $n - 6$ fatty acids compete for the desaturase and elongase enzymes, large amounts of the $n - 6$ fatty acids in conventional Western diets interfere with the formation of icosapentaenoic acids and docosahexaenoic acids. This may be altered by increased consumption of fish.

Dyerberg found that levels of total cholesterol and LDL cholesterol were significantly lower and HDL cholesterol higher among Eskimos than among Danes in all age groups of both sexes [121]. The principal effects of fish oil and fish oil supplements were found to be a reduction in the levels of triglycerides and VLDL cholesterol [116] and, since VLDL is a precursor of LDL, this leads to a reduction in LDL cholesterol as well. Fish oils appear to be the most effective means currently known to lower the levels of triglycerides and VLDL, which has been achieved in short-term 1–3 month studies using 4.5–30 g of the $n-3$ fatty acids [124,125]. LDL cholesterols may also be affected by fish oil. There is a blunted rise in total cholesterol and LDL cholesterol levels after a cholesterol-enriched meal in people who have been ingesting fish oil [125]. In patients with hypercholesterolemia but normal triglyceride levels, however, the effects of consumption of fish oil and LDL and HDL cholesterol are inconsistent. Because of differing results, further study of the effects of fish oils and LDL and HDL cholesterol and lipoprotein in the patients with and without hyper-triglyceridemia and with or without diabetes are clearly needed.

In epidemiological studies in Japanese coastal fishing villages compared with inland farming villages, there was reduced mortality from coronary artery disease in the fish-eaters [126]. Kromhout reviewed the Zutphen dietary study, in which 852 middle-aged men who did not have coronary artery disease were followed for 20 years. An inverse relationship was found between the amount of fish eaten and the mortality from coronary artery disease. As little as 35 g of dietary fish per day was associated with a 50% reduction in mortality from coronary artery disease [127]. Similarly, the Western Electric study [128] revealed an inverse relation between the ingestion of fish and mortality from coronary artery disease. A large Swedish study [129] also found less coronary artery disease among subjects consuming large amounts of fish. However, no such relationship has been found in two similar studies [125,126]. The relatively small amounts of fish ingested in the Zutphen and Western Electric studies are unlikely to have provided sufficient icosapentaenoic acid to have been effective and other factors may have been important in this reduction in coronary disease. It has also been reported that $n-3$ fatty acids lower lipid levels at the expense of deterioration in diabetes control [130]. These have, however, been short-term studies in mild diabetes.

Studies are needed to determine whether an increase in dietary $n-3$ fatty acids will reduce the mortality and morbidity from coronary artery disease and, in addition, whether ingestion or supplementation of the diet with $n-3$ fatty acids is safe from the point of view of possible adverse affects. Whereas Greenland Eskimos ingest 5–10 g of $n-3$ fatty acids daily presumably for a life-time, most reported studies have used large quantities for short periods of time. It is possible that small amounts given over a life-time may have beneficial effects.

The most commonly available supplements are capsules containing approximately 0.3 g icosapentaenoic acid and docosahexaenoic acid, and capsules containing up to 50% $n-3$ polyunsaturated fatty acids are marketed. Cod liver oil is about 20% $n-3$ fatty acid but the high content of vitamin A and D limits the quantities that can be safely ingested.

248

Despite the claims that $n-3$ fatty acids can help prevent atherosclerosis, recommendations to the public on diet are conservative and people have been advised to increase their consumption of fish by replacing 2 or 3 meals a week containing red meat with meals containing fish [131]. The $n-3$ fatty acid content of commonly consumed fish is shown in Table 6.

TABLE 6
Omega -3 fatty acid content of fish and fish-oil supplements

Item	Portion (raw weight)	IPA (g)	DHA (g)	Total omega -3 fatty acids (g)
Higher-fat fish				
Bluefish	$3^1/_2$ oz	0.4	0.8	1.2
Halibut, Greenland	$3^1/_2$ oz	0.5	0.4	0.9
Herring, Pacific	$3^1/_2$ oz	1.0	0.7	1.7
Mackerel, Atlantic	$3^1/_2$ oz	0.9	1.6	2.6
Salmon, Pink	$3^1/_2$ oz	0.4	0.6	1.0
Smelt, Rainbow	$3^1/_2$ oz	0.3	0.4	0.8
Trout, Lake	$3^1/_2$ oz	0.5	1.1	2.0
Trout, Rainbow	$3^1/_2$ oz	0.1	0.4	0.6
Tuna, Bluefin	$3^1/_2$ oz	0.4	1.2	1.6
Lower-fat fish				
Cod, Atlantic	$3^1/_2$ oz	0.1	0.2	0.3
Flounder	$3^1/_2$ oz	0.1	0.1	0.2
Haddock	$3^1/_2$ oz	0.1	0.1	0.2
Halibut, Pacific	$3^1/_2$ oz	0.1	0.3	0.4
Perch, Ocean	$3^1/_2$ oz	0.1	0.1	0.2
Pike, Northern	$3^1/_2$ oz	trace	0.1	0.1
Pike, Walleye	$3^1/_2$ oz	0.1	0.2	0.3
Sole, European	$3^1/_2$ oz	trace	0.1	0.1
Tuna, Skipjack	$3^1/_2$ oz	0.1	0.3	0.4
Shellfish				
Clam	$3^1/_2$ oz	trace	trace	0.1
Crab	$3^1/_2$ oz	0.2	0.2	0.4
Lobster, European	$3^1/_2$ oz	0.1	0.1	0.2
Oyster, Pacific	$3^1/_2$ oz	0.4	0.2	0.6
Shrimp	$3^1/_2$ oz	0.2	0.1	0.3
Fish oils				
Cod-liver oil	1 tsp (4.5 g)	0.4	0.4	0.9
Herring oil	1 tsp (4.5 g)	0.3	0.2	0.5
Mehaden oil	1 tsp (4.5 g)	0.6	0.4	1.0
Salmon oil	1 tsp (4.5 g)	0.4	0.5	0.9

TABLE 6 (continued)

Item	Portion (raw weight)	IPA (g)	DHA (g)	Total omega − 3 fatty acids (g)
Other oils				
Canola oil	1 tsp (4.5 g)	0	0	0.5
Fish-oil concentrates				
EPA and DHA™ (Schiff)	1 g capsule	0.110	0.090	0.200
Friendly Fats™ (Twin Lab®)	1 g capsule	0.180	0.107	0.327
MaxEPA™ (Kal®)	1 g capsule	0.180	0.120	0.300
Max EPA™ (Tyson)	1 g capsule	0.180	0.120	0.300
Maximum Potency EPA and DHA™ (Schiff)	1 g capsule	0.180	0.120	0.300
Omega-3™ (Schiff)	1 g capsule	0.300	0.200	0.500
Promega™ (Parke-Davis)	1 g capsule	0.350	0.150	0.500
Proto-chol™ (Squibb®)	1 g capsule	0.180	0.120	0.300
Super EPA® 300 (Futurebiotics)	1 g capsule	0.180	0.120	0.300
New and Improved TwinEPA (TwinLab®)	1 g capsule	0.700	0.155	0.855

IPA, icosapentaenoic acid; DHA, docosahexaenoic acid.

It must be noted, however, that fish caught in coastal waters or lakes may have accumulated large quantities of mercury and chlorinated hypocarbons. There is also the problem of autooxidation and lipid peroxidation products, which may be incriminated in an excess cancer rate, the reduction in the inflammatory and immune response by modifying the production by icosanoids of interleukin 1, and the prolongation of bleeding time which has been observed with ingestion of large quantities of icosapentaenoic acid. Thus, this form of intervention may not be one of the most benign forms available and at this point in time increasing fish intake to 7 ounces of fish per week or 1–3 half-portions twice a week seems prudent.

Uncertainty prevails about the diet-lipid hypothesis and its relationship to atherogenesis [132,133]. Most surveys indicate that increased intake of cholesterol is accompanied by higher levels of total serum cholesterol. Yet this relationship is affected by a number of factors, including the ratio of saturated to polyunsaturated fats in the diet as well as the total caloric intake. Total serum cholesterol levels are often elevated in diabetic subjects, especially those with poor metabolic control [134,135]. Yet it is uncertain whether individuals with IDDM or NIDDM handle dietary cholesterol differently from nondiabetics. As a general principle, it is advisable to restrict both cholesterol (to 300 mg daily) and saturated (animal) fats in the formulation of meal plans. Caloric restriction and weight loss remain the best weapons against hyperlipemia in the diabetic [136].

Protein intake

The recommendation for protein intake must consider the potential impact of dietary protein on diabetic complications. Although a low-protein diet has been the standard approach for treating end-stage renal disease associated with diabetes [137], the role of protein in the development and progression of diabetic nephropathy has not been clearly defined. Fully one-third of individuals with IDDM and 20% of those with NIDDM have diabetic nephropathy 15 years after the diagnosis of diabetes [138]. It has been well established that in the majority, although not all, of patients with renal disease, glomerular filtration rates deteriorate inexorably often to end-stage renal disease, even though the primary inciting injury has subsided spontaneously. Because of the widespread belief that the alteration in renal hemodynamics contributes at least in part to the progressive nephron loss in both animal and human models of renal disease, there has been a surge of interest in attempting to reduce hyperfiltration by dietary manipulation. The hypothesis first suggested by Addis in 1984 and now termed the 'Brenner hypothesis' [139–142] suggested that a high protein intake increases the workload by increasing renal blood flow and renal plasma flow, and the glomerular filtration rate ultimately accelerates glomerulosclerosis. With time, however, renal function begins to deteriorate progressively and it has been suggested that the compensatory increase in GFR and intraglomerular pressure becomes maladaptive and in the long term causes damage to the kidney.

At the time of diagnosis of diabetes there is already hyperfiltration and renal hypertrophy which is usually reversed on insulin therapy institution [18] but may persist for years if metabolic control is poor [143], although it appears that the reduction in proteinuria may be the result of improved glycemic control or possibly a low protein intake.

In the second or subclinical stage of diabetic nephropathy, there are structural lesions within the kidney but not clinical or laboratory signs of renal disease. There is clinical absence of albuminuria, which can be provoked with exercise [144]. There have, unfortunately, been no studies on the evaluation of the role of dietary protein at this stage. The third stage, or incipient diabetic nephropathy, which is now considered to be the forerunner of overt diabetic nephropathy, is characterized by abnormally elevated urinary albumin excretion as measured by radioimmunoassay. The normal albumin excretion is 10 mg/day, with a range of 2.5–25. Viberti suggests that albumin excretion rates of > 30 μg/min, and Mathiesen rates of > 70 μg/min, represent incipient diabetic nephropathy, and a range of 15–300 μg/min [145] is a reasonable estimate. A gradual increase in albuminuria occurs at this stage over a period of years. A prospective study by Viberti and colleagues demonstrated that in IDDM patients an albumin excretion rate of > 30 μg/min predicted the later development of clinical nephropathy. The remnant kidney hypothesis suggests a compensatory mechanism to reduce the number of nephrons to establish the hemodynamic forces in the glomerulus resulting in structural changes to produce proteinuria and hypertension [146–148]. It appears that high protein may increase the workload of the diabetic kidney and protein restriction could restore glomerular hemodynamics before structural changes have advanced to overt diabetic nephropathy [146]. In the fourth stage with overt diabetic nephropathy, these structural changes are associated with altered kidney function. This stage is characterized by persistent proteinuria of > 0.5 g/day, with an estimated fall in glomerular filtration rate of around 1 ml/min/month, but may be reduced by antihypertensive therapy up to 60% with a delay in the progression to end-stage renal disease. Protein restriction may delay the progression of overt diabetic nephropathy to end-stage renal disease.

The average American consumes approximately 1.4 g protein/kg/day. Adults with chronic renal failure take in this quantity, if not more, and the great majority exceed the recommended allowance of 0.8 g/kg/day. The RDA was arrived at as follows: average protein nitrogen lost (0.45 g/kg/day) by healthy adult individuals on a protein-free diet plus two standard deviations (0.15 g/kg/day) plus an increment (0.2 g/kg/day) to cover the less efficient use of dietary protein when caloric intake is inadequate.

Giovanetti in 1905 was the first to demonstrate that a low-protein diet caused a dramatic reduction in urinary nitrogen excretion. This was followed in the '30s and '40s by the clinical observation that a low-protein diet could ameliorate uremic symptoms and slow the rate of rise in creatinine and nitrogen in patients with chronic renal failure. Subsequently it was shown in 1963 that uremic patients on a very low protein diet could be brought into positive nitrogen balance if the diet was supplemented with essential amino acids, which has now led to the Giorodano/Giovanetti diet in the treatment of patients with advanced renal failure.

It is well established that a protein meal or amino acid infusion acutely elevates RPF and GFR. Similarly, chronic ingestion of high-protein diet leads to sustained elevation in RPF and GFR and renal hypertrophy, while a low-protein diet has the opposite effect. A number of studies in animals have demonstrated that a high-protein diet accelerates, while a low-protein diet slows, the rate of progression of chronic renal failure. These observations in animals have provided impetus for the reevaluation of low-protein diets in man. In the 1970s Walser et al. [149] reported that progression of renal failure could be favorably influenced by protein restriction. In the '80s a number of uncontrolled studies have appeared, which also indicate that intervention with low-protein diet slows the rate of progression of renal function deterioration in patients with nondiabetic renal disease. Maschio and colleagues [150] suggested that a protein-restricted diet is equally effective in ameliorating renal deterioration in patients with creatinine clearances above 30 ml/min as well as those below 30 ml/min. These studies have generally been retrospective and have lacked appropriate controls.

A diet with 0.6 g protein/kg has been shown to delay the progression of nephrotic syndrome to end-stage renal disease in a group of patients with mean serum creatinine of 2.3 mg/dl [150–152]. Only three of 25 patients had deterioration of renal function during a five-year period compared with 40% of patients who received 70 g protein/day. In another study, 24 patients with chronic renal failure were fed a diet of 20–30 g of mixed-quality protein supplemented with amino acids and their keto analogues, which was associated with the slowing or arresting of the predicted rise of serum creatinine [153]. While these studies are mainly retrospective in nature, and not well-controlled, a prospective randomized study of 228 patients showed that early moderate protein restriction retarded the development of ESRD. Patients were stratified on the basis of creatinine clearance and were randomized into four groups. The protein restrictions were 0.6 g/kg for a creatinine clearance of 31–60 and 0.4 g/kg for a creatinine clearance of 10–30 [151]. One hundred and forty-nine of the patients were followed for 18 months. The patients on the protein-restricted diet showed a fall in serum protein, urea and phosphorus. Regression analysis of the reciprocal of serum creatinine against time revealed a rate of progression three to five times lower in the protein-restricted groups than in the control group with a free diet.

Other investigators have demonstrated that dietary protein restriction of 0.58–0.96 g/kg per day favorably alters the course of diabetic kidney disease [154]. Yue and colleagues studied only seven diabetic subjects. Because severe protein restriction in previous studies was unpalatable and required supplementation with amino acids, they examined the effects of an isocaloric low-protein diet (0.6 g/kg ideal body wt per day, representing a reduction of $43 \pm 11\%$ from previous protein intake) [155].

Patients were observed for 2 months on their usual diet before they began 3 months of protein restriction. Key findings were that protein restriction was associated with a consistent and significant reduction in albumin excretion in microalbuminuric patients and a fall in daily urinary protein excretion in proteinuric patients of 67, 42 and 50% at 1, 2 and 3 months, respectively. The filtration fraction of albumin dropped by 73%. Dietary protein restriction induced a fall in five of seven diabetic patients (from 104 to 100, 69 to 67, 147 to 107, 133 to 86, and 115 to 79 ml/min). Of interest was the observation that protein restriction resulted in a significant drop in systolic and diastolic blood pressure.

The weight of evidence suggests that dietary protein restriction can slow the progression of chronic renal failure of diverse etiology and this has generated enormous enthusiasm among nephrologists and diabetologists.

Long-term compliance with any dietary regimen is difficult to accomplish [156]. There is reason to doubt whether diabetic Americans – especially adolescents – raised on Big Macs and milk shakes will accept a protein-restricted diet superimposed on repetitive finger-stick glucose testing for most of their lives. Designing a palatable, acceptable diet for such a low-protein intake can be difficult. The American Diabetes

Association encourages a protein intake coinciding with the RDA and an increased carbohydrate and decreased fat intake. It is unclear if and when a low-protein diet should be initiated in persons with diabetes.

One could envisage potentially advantageous as well as deleterious effects of protein restriction on carbohydrate and lipid metabolism. In order to maintain energy balance, a protein-restricted diet must be high in both carbohydrate and fat content. It is well established that when the dietary carbohydrate content is increased even slightly in the presence of pancreatic B-cell insufficiency, marked glucose intolerance ensues. Fasting hyperglycemia is worsened, meal tolerance deteriorates and hyperglycemia is exacerbated. This is true for both IDDM and NIDDM individuals. Institution of an isocaloric diet low in protein content may also have profound effects on lipid metabolism in patients with renal insufficiency. High refined carbohydrate diets augmented triglyceride synthesis in normal, NIDDM and IDDM patients. Although it is agreed that LDL cholesterol is the principal factor predisposing to coronary disease, there is no doubt that hypertriglyceridemia with hyperinsulinemia and a reduction in plasma HDL cholesterol are potential side-effects of this type of diet. High-fat diets are known to increase both LDL cholesterol and triglyceride levels and decrease HDL cholesterol. Thus, a high carbohydrate diet in combination with an increased fat intake would be expected to exacerbate markedly the preexisting hypertriglyceridemia, decreased HDL and increased LDL cholesterol, certainly in NIDDM, and to a lesser extent in IDDM. One must therefore have serious concerns about the institution of a diet that has potential to promote a more atherogenic plasma lipid profile. There is a need for prospective information concerning the impact of these low-protein, high-carbohydrate, high-fat diets on plasma lipid levels in both diabetic and nondiabetic subjects with chronic renal insufficiency. It is also possible that the institution of low-protein diets in diabetic patients may be hazardous, since insulin is a key regulator of protein metabolism, and accelerated gluconeogenesis, impaired branched-chain amino acid metabolism and accelerated rates of protein degradation with negative nitrogen balance and muscle wasting occur in patients with diabetes. This picture becomes more evident in patients with end-stage renal disease, and institution of low-protein diets may be particularly deleterious in diabetic individuals with advanced renal insufficiency.

It is, therefore, with considerable reserve that a recommendation is made for dietary protein intake of 12–20% of the total calories, which provides flexibility in food selection but exceeds the actual need for individuals with diabetes who do not have evidence of renal complications. The daily adult recommended dietary allowance (RDA) for protein is 0.8 g/kg weight, with an additional 30 g for pregnancy and lactation [157]. Extra protein is also needed during acute catabolic states associated with physiological stress such as surgery and wound-healing. Patients who have evidence of malnutrition or who need parenteral nutrition support are likely to have increased protein requirements. Efforts to increase the soluble dietary fiber may increase vegetable protein intake, which can substitute for animal protein, but no data are available as to whether protein from animal sources increases the workload of the kidney more than that from vegetable sources. Reducing protein intake to the RDA may be helpful at the preclinical stage. In incipient diabetic nephropathy there is growing evidence that restriction of protein intake may prevent or delay progression of nephropathy. In overt diabetic nephropathy in which albumin excretion exceeds 500 mg/day, protein restriction may vary from 0.4 to 0.8 g/kg depending on the patient's willingness to modify dietary intake, the impact upon quality of life and other nutritional considerations. If protein restriction is to < 40 g/day, serum albumin should be monitored and essential amino acids may need to be supplemented. If the daily protein intake is 20–30 g/day, keto analogue supplementation should also be considered. The use of protein restriction as the primary mode of treatment or in combination with dialysis in uremia-induced diabetic nephropathy may not be desirable if renal transplant is feasible. The hazards of high protein intake on the newly transplanted kidneys have not been resolved.

References

1. Wood FC Jr, Bierman EL. New concepts in diabetic dietetics. Nutr Today 1972;7:4–12.
2. Christakis G, Miridjanian A. In: Ellenberg M, Rifkin H (eds). Diabetes mellitus: theory and practice. New York: McGraw-Hill, 1970;594–623.
3. Himsworth HP. Dietetic factors determining glucose tolerance and sensitivity to insulin of healthy men. Clin Sci 1935;2:67–94.
4. Hughes TA, Gwynne JT, Switzer BR, et al. Effects of caloric restriction and weight loss on glycemic control, insulin release and resistance, and atherosclerotic risk in obese patients with type II diabetes mellitus. Am J Med 1984;77:7–17.
5. Hadden DR, Montgomery DAD, Skelley RJ, et al. Maturity onset diabetes mellitus: response to intensive dietary management. Br Med J 1975;3:276–278.
6. Genuth SM. Insulin secretion in obesity and diabetes: an illustrative case. Ann Intern Med 1977;87:714–716.
7. Savage PJ, Bennion LJ, Bennett PH. Normalization of insulin and glucagon secretion in ketosis-resistant diabetes mellitus with prolonged diet therapy. J Clin Endocrinol Metab 1979;49:830–833.
8. Savage PJ, Bennion LJ, Flock EV, et al. Diet-induced improvement of abnormalities in insulin and glucagon secretion and in insulin receptor binding in diabetes mellitus. J Clin Endocrinol Metab 1979;48:999–1007.
9. Henry RR, Wallace P, Olefsky JM. Effects of weight loss on mechanisms of hyperglycemia in obese non-insulin-dependent diabetes mellitus. Diabetes 1986;35:990–998.
10. Lew EA, Garfinkel L. Variations in mortality by weight among 750,000 men and women. J Chron Dis 1978;32:563–576.
11. Henry RR, Scheaffer L, Olefsky JM. Glycemic effects of intensive caloric restriction and isocaloric refeeding in noninsulin-dependent diabetes mellitus. J Clin Endocrinol Metab 1985;61:917–925.
12. Greenfield M, Kolterman O, Olefsky JM, et al. The effect of ten days of fasting on various aspects

of carbohydrate metabolism in obese diabetic subjects with significant fasting hyperglycemia. Metabolism 1978;27:1839–1852.

13. Stanik S, Marcus R. Insulin secretion improves following dietary control of plasma glucose in severely hyperglycemic obese patients. Metabolism 1980;29:346–350.

14. Reisin E, Abel R, Modan M, et al. Effect of weight loss without salt restriction on the reduction of blood pressure in overweight hypertensive patients. N Engl J Med 1978;298:1–6.

15. Manicardi V, Camellini L, Bellodi G, et al. Evidence for an association of high blood pressure and hyperinsulinemia in obese man. J Clin Endocrinol Metab 1986;62:1302–1304.

16. Kannel WB, Gordon T, Castelli WP. Obesity, lipids, and glucose tolerance: the Framingham study. Am J Clin Nutr 1979;32:1238–1245.

17. Wing RR, Koeske R, Epstein LH, et al. Long-term effects of modest weight loss in type II diabetic patients. Arch Intern Med 1987;147:1749–1753.

18. Vasquez B, Flock EV, Savage PJ, et al. Sustained reduction of proteinuria in type 2 (non-insulin dependent) diabetes following a diet-induced reduction of hyperglycemia. Diabetologia 1984;26:127–133.

19. University Group Diabetes Program. Effects of hypoglycemic agents on vascular complications in patients with adult-onset diabetes. JAMA 1971;218:1400.

20. Wing RR: Improving dietary adherence in patients with diabetes. In: Jovanovic L, Peterson CM, eds. Nutrition and diabetes. New York: Liss, 1985;161–168.

21. Wing RR, Jeffery RW: Outpatient treatments of obesity: a comparison of methodology and clinical results. Int J Obesity 1979;3:261.

22. Ferguson JM. Habits, not diets: the real way to weight control. Palo Alto: Bull, 1976.

23. Mahoney M, Mahoney K. Permanent weight control: a total solution to the dieter's dilemma. New York: Norton, 1976.

24. Brownell KD: The LEARN program for weight control. University of Pennsylvania, 1985.

25. Davidson JK. Educating diabetic patients about diet therapy. Int Diab Fed Bull 1975;20:1.

26. National Institutes of Health. Consensus development conference on diet and exercise in non-insulin-dependent diabetes mellitus. Diabetes Care 1987;10:639–644.

27. American Diabetes Association. The Physician's guide to type II diabetes (NIDDM), 1984.

28. Bistrian BR, Blackburn GL, Flatt JP, et al. Nitrogen metabolism and insulin requirements in obese diabetic adults on a protein-sparing modified fast. Diabetes 1976;25:494–504.

29. Fitz JD, Sperling EM, Fein HG. A hypocaloric high-protein diet as primary therapy for adults with obesity-related diabetes: effective long-term use in a community hospital. Diabetes Care 1983;6:328–333.

30. Genuth S: Supplemented fasting in the treatment of obesity and diabetes. S Am J Clin Nutr 1979;32:2579–2586.

31. Wadden TA, Stunkard AJ, Brownell KD. Very low calorie diets: their efficacy, safety, and future. Ann Intern Med 1983;99:675–684.

32. Hoffer LJ, Bristian BR, Young VR, et al. Metabolic effects of very low calorie weight reduction diets. J Clin Invest 1984;73:750–758.

33. Bogardus C, LaGrange BM, Horton ES, et al. Comparison of carbohydrate-containing and carbohydrate-restricted hypocaloric diets in the treatment of obesity. J Clin Invest 1981;68:399–401.

34. Wadden TA, Stunkard AJ. Controlled trial of very low calorie diet, behavior therapy, and their combination in the treatment of obesity. J Consult Clin Psychol 1986;54:482–488.

35. Bernstein R. Diabetes: the glucograph method for normalizing blood sugar. New York: Crown, 1981.

36. Bierman EL, Albrink MJ, Arky RA, et al. Diabetes 1971;20:633–634.

37. American Diabetes Association's Committee on Food and Nutrition. Principles of nutrition and die-

tary recommendations for individuals with diabetes mellitus: 1979. Diabetes Care 1979;2:520-523.

38. British Diabetes Association: Final draft on the nutrition subcommittee of the Medical Advisory Committee's report of dietary recommendations for diabetics in 1980s. British Diabetes Association (undated).

39. Canadian Diabetes Association: 1980 guidelines for the nutritional management of diabetes mellitus. J Can Dietetic Assoc 1981;42:110–118.

40. Taft P. Diet in the management of diabetes. Why restrict carbohydrate? Med J Aust 1976;1:838–840.

41. Walker ARP. S Afr J Sci 1977;73:74–77.

42. Reaven GM. How high the carbohydrate? Diabetologia 1980;19:409–413.

43. Bierman EL, Hamlin JT III. The hyperlipemic effect of a low-fat, high-carbohydrate diet in diabetic subjects. Diabetes 1961;10:432–437.

44. Ensinck JW, Bierman EL. Dietary management of diabetes mellitus. Annu Rev Med 1979;30:155–170.

45. Anderson JW, Chen WJL, Sieling B. Hypolipidemic effects of high carbohydrate, high fiber diets. Metabolism 1980;29:551.

46. Anderson JW, Ward K. High carbohydrate, high fiber diets for insulin-treated men with diabetes mellitus. Am J Clin Nutr 1979;32:2312.

47. Kiehm TG, Anderson JW, Ward K. Beneficial effects of a high carbohydrate, high fiber diet in hyperglycemic diabetic men. Am J Clin Nutr 1976;29:895–899.

48. Ney D, Hollingsworth DR, Cousins L. Decreased insulin requirement and improved control of diabetes in pregnant women given a high carbohydrate, high fiber, low fat diet. Diabetes Care 1982;5:529.

49. Simpson HCR, Simpson RW, Lousley S, Carter RD, Geekie M, Hockaday TD, Mann JI. A high carbohydrate leguminous fiber diet improves all aspects of diabetic control. Lancet 1981;i:1.

50. Simpson RW, Mann JI, Eaton J, Carter RD, Hockaday TDR. High-carbohydrate diets and insulin-dependent diabetes. Br Med J 1979;2:523.

51. Simpson RW, Mann JI, Eaton J, Carter RD, Hockaday TDR. Improved glucose control in maturity onset diabetes treated with high carbohydrate, modified fat diet. Br Med J 1979;1:1753.

52. Karlstrom B, Vesseby B, Asp NG, Boberg M, Gustaffson IB, Lithell H, Werner I. Effects of an increased content of cereal fiber in the diet of type II (non-insulin dependent) diabetic patients. Diabetologia 1984;26:272.

53. Kinmonth AL, Angust RM, Jenkins PA, et al. Whole foods and increased dietary fiber improve blood glucose control in diabetic children. Arch Dis Child 1982;57:187–194.

54. Coulston AM, Hollenbeck CB, Swislocki ALM, et al. Deleterious metabolic effects of high-carbohydrate, sucrose-containing diets in patients with noninsulin-dependent diabetes mellitus. Am J Med 1987;82:213–220.

55. Hollenbeck C, Swislocki A, Coulston A. Persistence of the deleterious metabolic effects of high-carbohydrate, low-fat diets in patients with noninsulin-dependent diabetes mellitus (NIDDM). Diabetes 1987;36:12A.

56. Hollenbeck CB, Coulston AM, Reaven GM. To what extent does increased dietary fiber improve glucose and lipid metabolism in patients with noninsulin-dependent diabetes mellitus (NIDDM)? Am J Clin Nutr 1986;43:16–24.

57. Nuttall FQ, Gannon MC. Sucrose and disease. Diabetes Care 1981;4:305–310.

58. Coulston AM, Hollenbeck CB, Reaven GM. Utility of studies measuring glucose and insulin responses to various carbohydrate-containing foods. Am J Clin Nutr 1984;39:163–165.

59. Coulston AM, Hollenbeck CB, Liu GC, et al. Effect of source of dietary carbohydrate on plasma glucose, insulin, and gastric inhibitory polypeptide responses to test meals in subjects with non-insulin-dependent diabetes mellitus. Am J Clin Nutr 1984;40:965–970.

60. Hollenbeck CB, Coulston AM, Reaven GM. Glycemic effects of carbohydrates: a different perspective. Diabetes Care 1986;9:641–647.

61. Kolata G. Diabetics should lose weight, avoid fad diets. Science 1987;235:163–164.

62. Crapo PA, Reaven G, Olefsky J. Plasma glucose and insulin responses to orally administered simple and complex carbohydrates. Diabetes 1976;25:741–747.

63. Crapo PA, Reaven G, Olefsky J. Postprandial plasma-glucose and insulin responses to different complex carbohydrates. Diabetes 1977;26:1178–1183.

64. Crapo RA, Kolterman OG, Waldeck N, et al. Postprandial hormonal responses to different types of complex carbohydrate in individuals with impaired glucose tolerance. Am J Clin Nutr 1980;33:1723–1728.

65. Crapo PA, Insel J, Sperling M, et al. Comparison of serum glucose, insulin, and glucagon responses to different types of complex carbohydrate in non-insulin-dependent diabetic patients. Am J Clin Nutr 1981;34:184–190.

66. Jenkins DJA, Wolever TMS, Taylor RH, et al. Glycemic index of foods: a physiological basis for carbohydrate exchange. Am J Clin Nutr 1981;34:362–366.

67. Jenkins DJA, Wolever TMS, Jenkins AL, et al. The glycemic index of foods tested in diabetic patients: a new basis for carbohydrate exchange favoring the use of legumes. Diabetologia 1983;24:257–264.

68. Goddard MS, Young G, Marcus R. The effect of amylase content on insulin and glucose responses to ingested rice. Am J Clin Nutr 1984;39:388–392.

69. Englist HN, Cummings JH. Digestion of the polysaccharides of banana in the human small intestine (abstract). 13th Int Congr Nutr, Brighton, UK 70, 1985.

70. Booher CE, Behan I, McNeans E. Biologic utilization of unmodified and modified food starches (Abstract). J Nutr 1951;45:75.

71. Collings P, Williams C, MacDonald I. Effect of cooking on serum glucose and insulin responses to starch. Br Med J 1981;282:1032–1033.

72. Throne MJ, Thompson LU, Jenkins DJA. Factors affecting starch digestibility and the glycemic response with special reference to legumes. Am J Clin Nutr 1983;38:481–488.

73. Ernest I, Linner E, Svanborg A. Carbohydrate-rich, fat-poor diet in diabetes. Am J Med 1965;39:594–600.

74. Laine DC, Thomas JW, Bantle JP. Comparison of the predictive capabilities of the diabetic exchange lists and the glycemic indices of foods (Abstract). Diabetes 1986;35(Suppl 1):43A.

75. Parillo M, Giacco R, Riccardi G, et al. Different glycaemic responses to pasta, bread, and potatoes in diabetic patients. Diabetes Med 1985;2:374–377.

76. Slama G, Bornet F, Blayo A, et al. Insulinogenic and glycaemic indexes of various starch-rich foods taken in a mixed meal or alone by type 2 diabetics (Abstract). Diabetes 1985;34(Suppl 1):48A.

77. Bornet FRJ, Costagliola D, Blayo A, et al. Insulinogenic and glycemic indices of six starch-rich foods taken alone and in a mixed meal by type 2 diabetics. Am J Clin Nutr 1987;45:588–595.

78. Collier GR, Wolever TMS, Wong GS, et al. Prediction of glycemic response to mixed meals in non-insulin-dependent diabetic subjects. Am J Clin Nutr 1986;44:349–352.

79. Jenkins DJA, Wolever TMS, Kalmusky J, et al. Low glycemic index foods in the management of hyperlipidemia. Am J Clin Nutr 1985;42:604–617.

80. Burkitt DP, Trowell HC (eds). Refined carbohydrate foods and disease: Some implications of dietary fiber. Academic Press, New York; 1975.

81. Trowell HC. Diabetes mellitus and dietary fiber of starchy foods. Am J Clin Nutr (Suppl) 1978;10:53–57.

82. Cleave TL. The saccharine disease. Bristol: Keats Publishing, Inc., 1974.

83. Monnier L, Pham TC, Aguirre L, et al. Influence of digestible fibers on glucose tolerance. Diabetes Care 1978;1:83–88.

84. Kay RM, Grobin W, Track NS. Diets rich in natural fiber improve carbohydrate tolerance in maturity-onset noninsulin dependent diabetics. Diabetologia 1981;20:18–21.

85. Anderson JW, Ward K. Long-term effects of high-carbohydrate, high-fiber diets on glucose and lipid metabolism: a preliminary report on patients with diabetes. Diabetes Care 1978;1:77–82.

86. Simpson HCR, Simpson RW, Sousley S, et al. A high carbohydrate leguminous fibre diet improves all aspects of diabetic control. Lancet 1981;i:15.

87. Monnier LH, Blotman MJ, Colette C, et al. Effects of dietary fibre supplementation in stable and labile insulin-dependent diabetics. Diabetologia 1981;20:12–17.

88. Anderson JW, Chen WL. Plant fiber: carbohydrate and lipid metabolism. Am J Clin Nutr 1979;32:346–363.

89. Anderson JW, Midgeley WR, Wedman B. Fiber and diabetes. Diabetes Care 1979;2:369–379.

90. Anderson JW. The role of dietary carbohydrate and fiber in the control of diabetes. Adv Intern Med 1980;26:67–96.

91. Anderson JW, Ward K. Long-term effects of high-carbohydrate, high-fiber diets on glucose and lipid metabolism: a preliminary report on patients with diabetes. Diabetes Care 1978;1:77–82.

92. Anderson JW, Sieling B. High fiber diets for obese diabetic patients. Obesity Bariatric Med 1980;9:109–117.

93. Brunzell JD, Lerner RL, Hazzard WR, et al. Improved glucose tolerance with high carbohydrate feeding in mild diabetes. N Engl J Med 1971;284:521–524.

94. Riccardi G, Rivellese A, Pacioni D, et al. Separate influence of dietary carbohydrate and fibre on the metabolic control in diabetes. Diabetologia 1984;26:116–121.

95. Mann JI. Lines to legumes: changing concepts of diabetic diets. Diabetic Med 1984;1:191–198.

96. Cummings JH: In: Spiller GA, Amen RJ, eds. Fiber in human nutrition. New York: Plenum Press, 1976.

97. Anderson JW. High-fibre diets for diabetic and hypertriglyceridemic patients. Can Med Assoc J 1980;123:975–979.

98. Jenkins DJA, Wolever TMS, Taylor RH, et al. Rate of digestion of foods and post-prandial glycaemia in normal and diabetic subjects. Br Med J 1980;2:14–17.

99. Fredrickson DS. In: Fajans SS, Sussman KE, eds. Diabetes mellitus: diagnosis and treatment. Vol. III. New York: American Diabetes Association, 1971;377–382.

100. Coulston AM, Liu GC, Reaven GM. Plasma glucose, insulin and lipid responses to high-carbohydrate low-fat diets in normal humans. Metabolism 1983;32:52–56.

101. Jenkins DJ. Dietary fibre, diabetes and hyperlipidaemia. Lancet 1979;ii:1287–1290.

102. Anderson JW, Chen WL, Sieling B. Hypolipidemic effects of high carbohydrate, high-fiber diets. Metabolism 1984;29:116–121.

103. Nuttall FQ, Mooradian D, DeMarais R, et al. The glycemic effect of different meals approximately isocaloric and similar in protein, carbohydrate, and fat content as calculated using the ADA exchange lists. Diabetes Care 1983;6:432–435.

104. Simpson HC, Carter RD, Lousley S, et al. Digestible carbohydrate-an independent effect on diabetic control in type 2 (non-insulin-dependent) diabetic patients? Diabetologia 1982;23:235–239.

105. Garg A, Bonanome A, Grundy SM, et al. Comparison of a high-carbohydrate diet with a high-monounsaturated-fat diet in patients with non-insulin-dependent diabetes mellitus. N Engl J Med 1988;319:829–834.

106. Anderson JT, Grande F, Keys A. Independence of the effects of cholesterol and degree of saturation of fat in the diet on serum cholesterol in man. Am J Clin Nutr 1976;29:1184–1189.

107. Schonfeld G, Patsch W, Rudel LL, et al. Effect of dietary cholesterol and fatty acids on plasma lipoproteins. J Clin Invest 1982;69:1072–1080.

108. Connor WE, Connor SL. Dietary treatment of hyperlipidemia: rationale, technique and efficacy. Med Clin N Am 1982;66:485–518.

109. Grundy SM. Effects of polyunsaturated fats on lipid metabolism in patients with hypertriglyceride-mia. J Clin Invest 1975;55:269–282.
110. Mattson FH, Grundy SM. Comparison of effects of dietary saturated, monounsaturated, and po-lyunsaturated fatty acids on plasma lipids and lipoproteins in man. J Lipid Res 1985;26:194–202.
111. Grundy SM. Comparison of monounsaturated fatty acids and carbohydrates for lowering plasma cholesterol. N Engl J Med 1986;314:745–748.
112. Gammal EB, Carroll KK, Plunkett ER. Effect of dietary fat on mammary carcinogenesis by 7,12-di-methylbenzalphaanthracene in rats. Cancer Res 1967;27:1737–1742.
113. Grundy SM, Gotto AM Jr, Bierman EL, et al. Recommendations for the treatment of hyperlipide-mia in adults: a joint statement of the Nutrition Committee and the Council on Arteriosclerosis of the American Heart Association. Arteriosclerosis 1984;4:445–68A.
114. Bang HO, Dyerberg J, Nielsen AB. Plasma lipid and lipoprotein pattern in Greenlandic west-coast Eskimos. Lancet 1971;i:1143–1145.
115. Nestel PJ, Connor WE, Reardon MF, et al. Suppression by diets rich in fish oil of very low density lipoprotein production in man. J Clin Invest 1984;74:82–89.
116. Phillipson BE, Rothrock DW, Connor WE, et al. Reduction of plasma lipids, lipoproteins and apo-proteins by dietary fish oils in patients with hypertriglyceridemia. N Engl J Med 1985;312: 1210–1216.
117. Bang HO, Dyerberg J, Hjorne N. The composition of food consumed by Greenland Eskimos. Acta Med Scand 1976;200:69–73.
118. Goodnight SH Jr, Harris WS, Conner WE: The effects of dietary omega 3 fatty acids on platelet composition and function in man: a prospective, controlled study. Blood 1981;58:880–885.
119. Driss F, Vericel E, Lagarde M, et al. Inhibition of platelet aggregation and thromboxane synthesis after intake of small amounts of icosapentaenoic acid. Thromb Res 1984;36:389–396.
120. Halushka PV, Mayfield R, Colwell JA. Insulin and arachidonic acid and metabolism in diabetes mellitus. Metabolism 1985;34(Suppl 1):32–36.
121. Dyerberg J, Bang HO, Hjorne N. Fatty acid composition of the plasma lipids in Greenland Eski-mos. Am J Clin Nutr 1975;28:958–966.
122. Kromann N, Green A. Epidemiological studies in the Upernavik district, Greenland: incidence of some chronic diseases 1950–1974. Acta Med Scand 1980;208:401–406.
123. Lands WEM. Fish and human health. Orlando, FL. Academic Press, 1986; 103–106.
124. Sanders TAB, Sullivan DR, Reeve J, et al. Triglyceride-lowering effect of marine polyunsaturates in patients with hypertriglyceridemia. Arteriosclerosis 1985;5:459–465.
125. Nestel PJ. Fish oil attenuates the cholesterol induced rise in lipoprotein cholesterol. Am J Clin Nutr 1986;43:752–757.
126. Hirai A, Terano T, Saito H, et al. Eicosapentaenoic acid and platelet function in Japanese. In: Lo-venburg W, Yamori Y, eds. Nutritional prevention of cardiovascular disease. New York: Academic Press, 1984;231–239.
127. Kromhout D, Bosschieter EB, de Lezenne Coulander C. The inverse relation between fish consump-tion and 20-year mortality from coronary heart disease. N Engl J Med 1985;312:1205–1209.
128. Shekelle RB, Missell LV, Paul O, et al. Fish consumption and mortality from coronary heart dis-ease. N Engl J Med 1985;313:820.
129. Norell SE, Ahlbom A, Feychting M, et al. Fish consumption and mortality from coronary heart disease. Br Med J 1986;293:426.
130. Friday KE, Childs MT, Tsunehara CH, Fujimoto WY, Bierman EL, Ensinck JW. Elevated plasma glucose and lowered triglyceride levels from omega-3 fatty acid supplementation in type II diabetes. Diabetes Care 1989;12:276–281.

131. Grundy S. Summaries, conclusions and recommendations. Session III – lipoproteins and atheroscle-rosis. In: Simopoulos AP, Kifer RR, Martin RE, eds. Health effects of polyunsaturated fatty acids in seafood. Orlando, FL: Academic Press, 1986;14–17.

132. Keys A. Seven Countries: a multivariate analysis of deaths and coronary heart disease. Cambridge, MA: Harvard University Press, 1980.

133. Mann GV. Diet-heart: end of an era. N Engl J Med 1977;297:644–650.

134. Chance GW, Alloutt EG, Eakins SM. Serum lipids and lipoproteins in untreated diabetic children. Lancet 1969;i:1126–1128.

135. Kaufman RL, Assal JPH, Soeldner JS, et al. Plasma lipid levels in diabetic children. Effect of diet restricted in cholesterol and saturated fats. Diabetes 1975;24:672–679.

136. Howard BV, Savage PJ, Nagulesparan M, et al. Changes in plasma lipoproteins accompanying diet therapy in obese diabetics. Atherosclerosis 1979;33:445–456.

137. Levine SE. Nutritional care of patients with renal failure and diabetes. J Am Diet Assoc 1982;81:261–267.

138. Herman WH, Teutch SM. Kidney diseases associated with diabetes. In: Harris MI, ed. Diabetes in Americans. Washington DC: U.S. Govt. Printing Office, NIH publ. No. 85-1468, 1985.

139. Brenner BM, Meyer TW, Hostetter H. Dietary protein intake and the progressive nature of kidney disease: the role of hemodynamically medicated glomerular injury in the pathogenesis of progressive glomerular sclerosis in aging, renal ablation and intrinsic renal disease. N Engl J Med 1982;305:652–658.

140. Meyer TW, Lawrence WE, Brenner BM. Dietary protein and the progression of renal disease. Kidney Int 1983;24(Suppl 16):S243–247.

141. Mitch WE. The influence of the diet on the progression of renal insufficiency. Annu Rev Med 1984;35:249–264.

142. Sumpio BE, Hayslett JP. Renal handling of proteins in normal and disease states. Q J Med 1985;57:611–635.

143. Ditzel J, Brochner-Mortensen J. Tubular reabsorption rates as related to elevated glomerular filtra-tion in diabetic children. Diabetes 1983;32(Suppl 2):28–33.

144. Morgensen CE, Christensen CK, Vittinghus E. The stages in diabetic renal disease with emphasis on the stage of incipient diabetic nephropathy. Diabetes 1983;32(Suppl 2):64–75.

145. Mogensen CK. Renal function changes in diabetes. Diabetes 1976;25:872–879.

146. Laouri D, Kleinknecht C, Gubler MC, et al. Importance of proteins in the deterioration of the rem-nant kidneys, independent of other nutrients. Int J Pediatr Nephrol 1982;3:263–269.

147. Mathiesen ER, Oxenboll B, Johansen K, et al. Incipient nephropathy in type I (insulin dependent) diabetes. Diabetologia 1984;26:406–410.

148. Hans-Henrik P, Andersen AR, Smidt UM, et al. Diabetic nephropathy and arterial hypertension: the effect of antihypertensive treatment. Diabetes 1983;32(Suppl 2): 83–87.

149. Walser M. Nutritional management of chronic renal failure. Am J Kidney Dis 1982;1:261.

150. Maschio G, Oldrizzi L, Tessitore N, et al. Effect of dietary protein and phosphorus restriction on the progression of early renal failure. Kidney Int 1982;22:371–376.

151. Rossman JB, TerWee PM, Meijer S, et al. Prospective randomized study of early protein restriction in chronic renal failure. Lancet 1984;ii:1291–1296.

152. Maschio G, Oldrizzi L, Resitore N, et al. Early protein and phosphorus restriction is effective in delaying progression of chronic renal failure. Kidney Int 1983;24(Suppl 16):S273–277.

153. Mitch WE, Walser M, Steinman TI, et al. The effect of a keto-acid-amino acid supplement to a restricted diet on the progression of chronic renal failure. N Engl J Med 1984;311:623–628.

154. Cavarella A, Di Mizio G, Stefoni S, Borgnino LC, Vannini P. Reduced albuminuria after dietary

protein restriction in insulin-dependent diabetic patients with clinical nephropathy. Diabetes Care 1987;10:407–413.

155. Yue SK, O'Dea K, Stewart P, Conigrave AD, Hosking M, Tsang J, Hall B, Dale N, Turtle JR. Proteinuria and renal function in diabetic patients fed a diet moderately restricted in protein. Diabetes Spectrum 1989;2:112–114.

156. Lockwood L, Frey ML, Gladish NA, Hiss RG. The biggest problem in diabetes. Diabetes Educ 1986;12:30–33.

157. Food and Nutrition Board. Recommended Dietary Allowances, 9th edn. Washington DC: National Academy of Sciences, 1980.

Frontiers of diabetes research: current trends in non-insulin-dependent diabetes mellitus
K.G.M.M. Alberti and R. Mazze, editors

CHAPTER 19

Diet and NIDDM: a view from the Old World

ROBERT TATTERSALL

University Hospital, Nottingham, U.K.

Introduction

One thing on which all diabetologists agree is that NIDDM is a serious disorder with a high mortality and morbidity [1,2]. Although defined in terms of blood glucose concentrations, it is a multimetabolic disorder. From the ambitious U.K. Prospective Study of Maturity-Onset Diabetes [3] and other sources we are beginning to get a clear picture of the typical patient in England. There is a male-dominated sex ratio of 1.54. Both sexes are overweight, although not massively so, with men weighing in at an average of 123% of ideal body weight and women 142% [4]. Nearly half the patients have hypertension at diagnosis [5] and many have dyslipidemia with high serum triglycerides and low levels of HDL cholesterol, particularly the HDL_2 subfraction which is thought to protect against ischemic heart disease [6,7].

As would be expected from this constellation of risk factors, nearly half those with newly diagnosed NIDDM already have macrovascular disease [8]. There is an increased mortality within the first year after diagnosis and in a cohort study in East Germany 44% were dead within ten years [9]. As Panzram [10] says, "the future strategy against premature mortality in type 2 diabetes requires multifactorial approaches. At present we are doing too little too late, if anything can be done at all. The potential improvement of prognosis calls for early and comprehensive measures against the entire complex of known metabolic and vascular risk factors".

In non-diabetic populations many atherogenic risk factors, especially if only one is present per patient, can be modified by diet and the questions are whether (1) this is true in NIDDM, and (2) if so, whether all risk factors can be beneficially affected by a single tolerable diet.

264

Weight

Total energy intake must be reduced to avoid and correct excessive weight [2] and
it has been claimed that "by preventing obesity, the incidence of NIDDM might be
reduced by up to 50%" [11]. Nevertheless, one of the most striking findings in any
long-term study is how well weight is maintained [12] apart from unusual clinics and
particular individual initiatives. In the United Kingdom, the unusual clinic is Belfast,
where patients with newly diagnosed NIDDM lose an average of 9.2 kg by six
months, and maintain it for up to 6 years [13]. In Nottingham [14] we found that
group education was more effective in causing and maintaining weight loss and concluded that the relative success of some clinics and the abject failure of others in
weight control is not related to the diet prescription per se but depends on how diet
is taught and the importance attached to it by those who care for the patient. Psycho-
logy may be as important as dietary principles, and Wood and Bierman [15] question
whether we might "create unhappy patients by badgering them about their diets but
may also create disregulated 'restrained eaters' who will overeat in response to internal and external food-related cues, such as time, fear, or recent eating, irrespective
of whether they actually lose weight or not". If we cannot achieve our primary objective of ideal body weight, perhaps arguing about the glycemic index of foods is the
dietetic equivalent of fiddling while Rome burns?

How much and what sort of carbohydrate?

An Englishman, John Rollo (1797), is credited with having ushered in a long era of
avoidance of carbohydrate in the diabetic diet when he recommended "animal food
and confinement, with an entire abstinence from every kind of vegetable matter..."

Historians [16] remind us that high-carbohydrate (CHO) diets made intermittent
comebacks during the next hundred years with the rice diet (1868), the potato diet
(1903) and the famous oatmeal diet (1912) of Van Noorden. However, these initiatives were stifled by the success of Frederick Allen's 'starvation treatment' and, after
the introduction of insulin and, much later, sulphonylureas and biguanides, physicians tended to de-emphasize the importance of diet. The wheel has now come full
circle and the British Diabetic Association recommends a high-carbohydrate, high-
fibre, low-fat diet for *all* diabetics, although this is tempered by the advice that "any
dietary strategy which is effective in reducing energy intake in the obese non-insulin-
requiring diabetic is acceptable, provided that it is nutritionally sound" [17]. The rationale for the recommendation that a minimum of 55% of energy should be obtained
from carbohydrate is:
(1) Because it approximates to the diet of primitive people and the Japanese, who
    have very low rates of ischaemic heart disease.

(2) Any reduction in carbohydrate inevitably means that the energy has to be made up by fat, and in the traditional English diet this has been saturated fat.

(3) It has been known for decades that a high carbohydrate intake improves glucose tolerance and increases insulin sensitivity.

Published evidence of the benefit of high-CHO diets in NIDDM is not as clear-cut as many believe [18]. These diets do increase insulin sensitivity in normal subjects, leading to a modest [10%] improvement in glucose tolerance. However, as Reaven [19] points out, Himsworth showed quite different effects of a high-CHO diet in IDDM as opposed to NIDDM. In Himsworth's words [20]:

"In the case of the sensitive (i.e. insulin-dependent) diabetic, increase of the carbohydrate content of the diet causes no increase in glycosuria, no rise in the fasting blood sugar level, but produces improvement of sugar tolerance and sensitivity to insulin. In the case of the insensitive diabetic (i.e. NIDDM) increase of dietary carbohydrate causes increase in glycosuria, a tendency to high fasting blood sugar levels, impairment of sugar tolerance and little or possibly no increase in sensitivity to insulin".

As far as I am aware, no subsequent long-term study of a high-carbohydrate diet has contradicted this conclusion, and the nutrition subcommittee of the British Diabetic Association [17] summed it up by saying: "The well-documented adverse effect of carbohydrate in the *untreated* [my italics] diabetic is only to be expected, but *when treatment is adequate* carbohydrate handling is restored to a state which is similar to that in normal subjects". In other words, if a patient with NIDDM is well controlled, whether on diet, sulphonylureas or insulin, high-CHO diets will not lead to a deterioration of diabetic control whereas they will do in poorly controlled and/or untreated patients with NIDDM.

One criticism of many studies of high-CHO diets is that they are short-term and use diets which vary in more than just carbohydrate content. One important variable is the amount of fibre, and my interpretation of 'the fibre story' is as follows.

In 1880 an English physician, Dr. T.R. Allinson (whose 100% stoneground wholemeal flour is still available) wrote, "One great curse of this country is constipation, which is caused in great measure by white bread. From this constipation come piles, varicose veins, headaches, miserable feelings, dullness and other ailments" [20]. For his pains, Dr. Allinson was struck off the Medical Register and only in the late 1960s was the idea that many 'Western' diseases are due to a deficiency of dietary fibre resurrected and popularized by Cleave, Burkitt and Trowell.

Their hypothesis was that the increased frequency of constipation, appendicitis, cancer of the colon and diabetes in Europeans as compared to Africans was due to a deficiency of dietary fibre. This, at least in relation to bowel disorders, is now well accepted but, even if a lack of fibre also causes diabetes (which I doubt), it does not necessarily follow that eating it in normal or exaggerated quantities will be beneficial in treating the established disease. Nevertheless, many diabetologists and dietitians believe this to be the case. In Oxford in the mid-1970s Jenkins and colleagues showed that adding the unabsorbable polysaccharides, guar and pectin, reduced post-prandial glycemia in both normal and diabetic subjects, with a flattening of the insulin response in the former and a need for less insulin in the latter [21]. Not all fibres were equal. To reduce blood glucose, the fibre had to be a high viscosity and incorporated into the food. This differential effect of various fibres and the difficulty in defining exactly what is being fed to patients has led to many problems in evaluating clinical studies. It is easy to define fibre as "components of plant material which resist human digestive enzymes" but interpretation becomes difficult when one is warned that "fibre-rich foods contain a variety of fibres and the effect of each cannot be determined using natural foods. On the other hand, when fibres are extracted from natural foods, their actions may not resemble those of the same fibres when fed as an integral part of the intact food. The fibre-nutrient relationship in foods is disrupted by cutting, cooking and chewing: the actions of fibres are altered further by environmental factors in the gut" [22].

Clinical studies of high-fibre diets in diabetic patients began in the late 1970s, and one in Oxford [23] was particularly influential in the U.K. A six-week crossover study in 18 patients with NIDDM compared a standard HCO diet with a "high HCO diet containing leguminous fibre". The patients, most of whom were on sulphonylureas, were already well controlled, with a fasting blood glucose of 6.7 mmol/l which was reduced to 5.7 mmol/l by the test diet. What was not appreciated at the time (because most people knew little about fibre) was that the test diet contained 96.6 g fibre/day of which "64% was derived from leguminous sources, most of the remainder being cereal fibre in the form of wholemeal bread... beans were consumed twice daily, usually at breakfast and supper". In retrospect it was difficult to know whether the improved diabetic control, such as it was, was due to the high HCO intake, the slow digestion of the legumes or the fibre.

In the more typical less well controlled patient with NIDDM, the effects of a high-CHO, high-fibre diet are conflicting. In Oxford NIDDM patients who completed the trial (11 of 15) had a fasting plasma glucose of 9.6 mmol/l on their usual diet (26 g/day fibre), 8.4 mmol/l after six weeks on a low-CHO diet (12.7 g/day fibre) and 6.8 mmol/l on a high-HCO diet (67 g/fibre day) [24]. However, in Nottingham we treated 33 outpatients with poorly controlled NIDDM with a high-fibre diet for six months and found a rise in fasting plasma glucose from 10.8 to 12.6 mmol/l with no change in lipid levels [25]. The deterioration in control was greatest in those with the highest fibre intake. In Sheffield newly diagnosed overweight patients with NIDDM were treated with a low-energy, high-CHO, low-fat diet supplemented with either cereal fibre or guar gum [26]. There were no differences between the groups in weight or glycemic control after 20 weeks and the only measurable effect of the guar gum was an increase in diarrhoea and flatulence.

The effects of high-fibre diets on glycaemic control and lipids in ordinary patients with NIDDM also seem to be unimpressive in California [27,28], and I agree with Reaven et al. that, even if fibre intakes over 60 g/day work under metabolic ward conditions, it is not possible to persuade most ordinary middle-aged people to eat such a diet as outpatients [28]. If patients with NIDDM are advised to increase their fibre intake, there are difficulties in knowing which foods to eat. For example, only bread which contains whole grains reduces the glycemic response [29] whereas bread advertised as wholegrain may not contain the intact grain but merely flour milled from whole grains (explaining this to a patient would tax even the most experienced dietitian!). A similar problem arises with breakfast cereals advertised as 'high in bran or natural fibre'. Most do not contain enough fibre, even of the right sort, to make any difference to diabetic control and some contain the wrong sort of fibre.

The most influential figure in shaping the 'modern' diabetic diet in the U.K. has been Mann [16], who asks (1): are all starchy carbohydrate foods rich in dietary fibre equally suitable for diabetics? and (2) is restriction of sucrose of critical importance? To the first question his answer is that foods rich in gel-forming fibre (found particularly in various types of cooked dried bean) are especially good and a better source of protein than meat, which is often high in saturated fat. However, this effectively means becoming vegetarian, which may have its attractions to the young but is not acceptable to most middle-aged Englishmen. In answer to the second question the conclusion is that most studies have shown that sucrose in a mixed meal does not produce a greater glycemic response than equivalent amounts of potato or wheat starch. Nevertheless, in U.K. diabetic clinics the heart rules the head and most dietitians advise total avoidance of sucrose on the grounds that, if given an inch, most diabetic patients will take a mile and abuse it.

Hyperlipidemia

It is generally accepted that optimal insulin treatment in IDDM corrects the abnormalities in plasma lipoprotein concentrations and has a favorable influence on the HDL-to-LDL cholesterol ratio [30]. It is also clear that in England many outpatients with NIDDM have hypertriglyceridemia, hypercholesterolemia and decreased HDL cholesterol concentrations [31]. Several prospective studies in varied populations (e.g. ordinary people in Framingham, civil servants in London and policemen in Paris) have suggested that hypertriglyceridemia is a potent risk factor for coronary artery disease and I share the concern that some diets being recommended may aggravate this. When obese NIDDM patients are treated with diet alone, changes in lipoproteins depend on the degree of weight loss and are moderately impressive if a weight loss of 10% or more can be achieved and sustained [30]. However, low-fat high-carbohydrate diets alone (i.e. without weight loss) adversely affect the cardiovascular risk profile in patients with NIDDM, with an increase in VLDL triglyceride and a decrease in HDL cholesterol [27,32]. Indeed, as Reaven points out [19], this is exactly what one would have predicted from studies in normal subjects. One way round this problem is simply to replace saturated fat with poly- and monounsaturated fat, which seems to be successful [27,32]. It is also worth noting that insulin treatment in patients with NIDDM usually lowers triglycerides dramatically and modestly increases HDL cholesterol [30].

Hypertension

Thiazides and beta blockers are themselves diabetogenic and the idea of treating hypertension with diet rather than drugs is theoretically attractive. Pacy et al. [33] showed that a low-fat, high-fibre, low-sodium diet is as effective in lowering blood pressure in NIDDM as bendrofluazide. As with all other dietary strategies the only question is whether people will be sufficiently disciplined in the long term to cut both salt and sugar out of their diet.

Practical considerations

Most of us would agree with the late Kelly West's understatement that "the practical effectiveness of diet therapy leaves something to be desired" [34] and that this is not due to a lack of authoritative guidance. Of 1018 articles on the diabetic diet in the world literature between 1966 and 1982 [35] most began with a statement to the effect that "most patients with NIDDM can be controlled by diet alone" and then detailed the author's dietary beliefs. Almost all these articles are entirely theoretical; a few report short-term effects of the diet in small groups of patients on a metabolic unit, but it is quite exceptional to find any which have tested a diet in substantial numbers of patients under field conditions for 6 months or more. What is also striking in the U.K. and elsewhere is that broadly similar diets appear to be successful in some clinics and not in others, which I believe can only be explained by differences in the methods of teaching and the overall importance attached to diet. Kelly West [34] believed that much of the fault lay with physicians and said "I suspect that a major reason for the de-emphasis of diet is the insecurity of physicians with a method of therapy concerning which they know little. The need here is for devising and continuously modifying a prescription that best fits the propensities of the patient and the therapeutic goals. Few physicians are highly proficient in this although the skills required are not very complex". Teaching a diet is simple in theory but many of us fail to get the message across because we neglect the psychological aspects. Hilde Bruch [37] reminds us that: "For normal people food is never restricted to the biological aspects alone. There is no human society that deals rationally with food in its environment, that eats according to the availability, edibility and nutritional value alone. Food is endowed with complex values and elaborate ideologies, religious beliefs and prestige systems... Obesity although a faulty adaptation may serve as a protection against more severe illness. These individuals cannot function unless the underlying problems are clarified or resolved".

References

1. Tattersall RB. Diabetes in the elderly – a neglected area. Diabetologia 1984;27:167–173.
2. Alberti KGMM, Gries FA. Management of non-insulin dependent diabetes mellitus in Europe: a consensus view. Diabetic Med 1988;5:275–281.
3. U.K. Prospective Study of therapies of maturity onset diabetes. I. Effect of diet, sulphonylurea, insulin or biguanide therapy on fasting plasma glucose and body weight over one year. Diabetologia 1983;24:404–411.
4. U.K. Prospective Diabetes Study. IV. Characteristics of newly presenting type 2 diabetic patients: male preponderance and obesity at different ages. Diabetic Med 1988;5:154–159.
5. U.K. Prospective Diabetes Study. III. Prevalence of hypertension and hypotensive therapy in patients with newly diagnosed diabetes Hypertension 1985;7(Suppl 2):8–13.
6. Barrett-Connor E, Witztum JBL, Holbrook MA. A community study of high density lipoproteins in adult non-insulin dependent diabetics. Am J Epidemiol 1983;117:186–192.
7. Walden CE, Knopp RH, Wahl PW, Beach KW, Strandness E. Sex differences in the effect of diabetes mellitus on lipoprotein triglycerides and cholesterol concentrations. N Engl Med J 1984;311:953–959.
8. Uusitupa M, Siltonen O, Ard A, Pyorala K. Prevalence of coronary heart disease, left ventricular failure and hypertension in middle-aged, newly diagnosed type 2 diabetic subjects. Diabetologia 1985;28:22–28.
9. Panzram G, Zabel-Langhennig R. Prognosis of diabetes in a geographically defined population. Diabetologia 1981;20:587–591.
10. Panzram G. Mortality and survival in type 2 (non insulin dependent) diabetes mellitus. Diabetologia 1987;30:123–131.
11. The Carter Center of Emory University. Closing the gap: the problem of diabetes mellitus in the United States. Diabetes Care 1985;8:391–406.
12. Goodner CJ, Ogilvie JT. Homeostasis of body weight in a diabetes clinic population. Diabetes 1973;22:318–326.
13. Hadden DR, Blair ALT, Wilson EA, et al. Natural history of diabetes presenting at age 40–69 years: a prospective study of the influence of intensive dietary therapy. Q J Med 1986;59:579–598.
14. Heller SR, Clarke P, Daly H, et al. Group education for obese patients with type 2 diabetes: greater success at less cost. Diabetic Med 1988;5:552–556.
15. Wood FC, Bierman EL. Is diet the cornerstone in the management of diabetes? N Engl J Med 1986;315:1224–1227.

16. Mann JI. Lines to legumes: changing concepts of the diabetic diet. Diabetic Med 1984;1:191–198.
17. Nutrition Subcommittee, British Diabetic Association Medical Advisory Committee. Dietary recommendations for diabetes for the 1980s. Hum Nutr Appl Nutr 1982;36a:378–394.
18. Reaven GM. How high the carbohydrate? Diabetologia 1980;19:409–413.
19. Reaven GM. Dietary therapy for non-insulin dependent diabetes mellitus. N Engl J Med 1988;319:862–864.
20. Kellock B. The Fibre Man: the life story of Dr Denis Burkitt. Lion Publishing, 1985.
21. Jenkins DJA, Leeds AR, Gassull MA, et al. Unabsorbable carbohydrates and diabetes: decreased postprandial hyperglycaemia. Lancet 1976;ii:172–174.
22. Anderson JW, Midgley WR, Wedman B. Fiber and diabetes. Diabetes Care 1979;2:369–379.
23. Simpson HCR, Simpson RW, Lousley S, et al. A high carbohydrate leguminous fibre diet improves all aspects of diabetic control. Lancet 1981;i:1–5.
24. Lousley SE, Jones DB, Slaughter P, Carter RD, Jelfs R, Mann JI. High carbohydrate, high fibre diets in poorly controlled diabetics. Diabetic Med 1984;1:21–25.
25. Scott AR, Attenborough Y, Peacock, I, Fletcher E, Jeffcoate WJ, Tattersall RB. Comparison of high fibre diets, basal insulin supplements and flexible insulin treatment for non-insulin dependent (type II) diabetics poorly controlled with sulphonylureas. Br Med J 1988;297:707–710.
26. Beattie VA, Edwards CA, Hosker JP, Cullen DR, Ward JD, Read NW. Does adding fibre to a low energy, high carbohydrate, low fat diet confer any benefit to the management of newly diagnosed overweight type II diabetics? Br Med J 1988;296:1147–1149.
27. Coulston AM, Hollenbeck CB, Swislocki ALM, Chen Y-D I, Reaven GM. Deleterious metabolic effects of high-carbohydrate sucrose containing diets in patients with non-insulin dependent diabetes mellitus. Am J Med 1987;82:213–220.
28. Hollenbeck CB, Coulston AM, Reaven GM. To what extent does increased dietary fibre improve glucose and lipid metabolism in patients with non-insulin dependent diabetes mellitus (NIDDM)? Am J Clin Nutr 1986;43:16–24.
29. Jenkins DJA, Wesson V, Wolever TMS, et al. Wholemeal versus wholegrain breads: proportion of whole or cracked grain and the glycaemic response. Br Med J 1988;297:958–960.
30. Kissebah A, Schectman G. Polyunsaturated and saturated fats, cholesterol and fatty acid supplementation. Diabetes Care 1988;11:129–142.
31. Reckless JDP, Betteridge DJ, WU P, Baynes B, Galton DJ. High-density and low-density lipoproteins and prevalence of vascular disease in diabetes mellitus. Br Med J 1978;1:883–886.
32. Garg A, Bonanome A, Grundy SM, Zhang Z-J, Unger RH. Comparison of high-carbohydrate diet with a high monounsaturated fat diet in patients with non-insulin dependent diabetes mellitus. N Engl J Med 1988;319:829–834.
33. Pacy PG, Dodson PM, Kubicki AJ, Fletcher RF, Taylor KG. Comparison of the hypotensive and metabolic effects of bendrofluazide therapy and a high fibre, low fat, low sodium diet in diabetic subjects with mild hypertension. J Hypertension 1984;2:215–220.
34. West KW. Diet therapy of diabetes: an analysis of failure. Ann Int Med 1973;79:425–434.
35. Tattersall RB, McCulloch DK. Modern aspects of conventional insulin therapy. Ann Clin Res 1984;16:107–117.
36. Bruch H. Eating disorders: obesity, anorexia nervosa and the person within. London: Routledge & Keegan Paul, 1974.

CHAPTER 20

Exercise and non-insulin-dependent diabetes mellitus

EDWARD S. HORTON and JOHN T. DEVLIN

Division of Endocrinology and Metabolism and Nutrition, Department of Medicine, University of Vermont, Burlington, VT, U.S.A.

Introduction

Regular physical exercise was first recognized as an important part of the treatment of diabetes mellitus in ancient times [1] and was frequently prescribed during the pre-insulin era for patients that would now be diagnosed as having non-insulin-dependent diabetes mellitus (NIDDM). With the advent of insulin therapy for patients with IDDM it became apparent that exercise potentiated the action of insulin, resulting in lower insulin requirements and an increased risk of hypoglycemic reactions. In recent years, much has been learned about the role of insulin and other hormones in the regulation of metabolic fuels during and after exercise, and the role of exercise in the treatment of diabetes has been reexamined [2]. It is now clear that in patients with IDDM or insulin-requiring NIDDM physical exercise may create significant problems in blood glucose regulation. These include hypoglycemia during or following exercise, hyperglycemia in response to strenuous exercise and the rapid development of ketosis or ketoacidosis in patients with IDDM when exercise is superimposed on a state of severe insulin deficiency. This has led to the development of strategies for the management of exercise in insulin-treated patients to make it possible for them to participate in a wide range of physical activities as safely as possible, and thus to lead a normal or near-normal lifestyle.

In patients with NIDDM, on the other hand, regular physical exercise may play an important therapeutic role in the management of the disease and is often prescribed along with diet and oral hypoglycemic agents for this purpose. If exercise is to be used as a therapeutic intervention, its effectiveness, the mechanism by which it is beneficial in NIDDM and the associated risks of exercise must be examined. In this paper, current knowledge of the benefits, risks and metabolic effects of exercise in NIDDM will be reviewed.

Benefits of exercise in NIDDM

Many real and potential benefits of regular physical exercise have been identified for patients with NIDDM (Table 1). Whereas exercise in normal individuals has little impact on blood glucose concentrations, moderate-intensity exercise in patients with NIDDM and hyperglycemia is usually associated with a decrease in blood glucose concentrations towards normal. This may be used by patients to help regulate blood glucose on a day-to-day basis and may be a mechanism by which regular physical exercise results in improved long-term diabetic control [3]. In addition to the acute blood-glucose-lowering effect of exercise, it has been recognized for many years that physical training is associated with lower fasting and post-prandial insulin concentrations and apparent increased insulin sensitivity [4,5]. Since NIDDM is characterized by insulin resistance in skeletal muscle, adipose tissue and the liver [6,7], there has been considerable interest in the use of physical training as a means of improving

TABLE 1

Benefits of regular exercise for patients with NIDDM

1. Lower blood glucose concentrations during and following exercise

2. Lower basal and post-prandial insulin concentrations

3. Improved insulin sensitivity

4. Lower glycosylated hemoglobin levels

5. Improved lipid profile
   decreased triglycerides
   slightly decreased LDL cholesterol
   increased HDL cholesterol

6. Improvement in mild-to-moderate hypertension

7. Increased energy expenditure
   adjunct to diet for weight reduction
   increased fat loss
   preservation of lean body mass

8. Cardiovascular conditioning

9. Increased strength and flexibility

10. Improved sense of well-being and quality of life

insulin sensitivity and, thus, ameliorating one of the major abnormalities of NIDDM.

A third benefit of regular exercise is a reduction in cardiovascular risk factors through improvement of the lipid profile and reduction of hypertension. It is now well documented that physical training is associated with a lowering of serum triglycerides, particularly very-low-density lipoproteins, and an increase in HDL_2 cholesterol [8]. There is also a slight decrease in LDL cholesterol with training [9]. Recent studies on the mechanism by which physical training results in lower VLDL and increased HDL_2 concentrations have shown that physically trained skeletal muscle has increased lipoprotein lipase activity compared with untrained muscle. This results in greater extraction of circulating VLDL and increased release of HDL_2 resulting from a transfer of VLDL surface proteins to HDL_3 particles [10]. This improvement in the lipid profile with physical training is observed with running a minimum of 10–12 miles per week and increases in a dose–response fashion up to distances of approximately 40 miles per week [11]. Lower levels of physical activity have little if any effect on lipid profiles.

A less commonly known effect of physical training is improvement in mild to moderate hypertension. This occurs independently of weight loss or change in body composition and can result in a decrease in both systolic and diastolic blood pressure of 5 to 10 mmHg [12,13]. Although the mechanism for this effect is not known, it is correlated with a decrease in serum insulin and triglyceride concentrations [14] and may be related to an effect of chronic hyperinsulinemia on renal sodium retention.

In addition to improvement in cardiovascular risk factors, regular physical exercise may be an effective adjunct to diet for weight reduction. Combined with caloric restriction, exercise has been shown to result in greater loss of adipose tissue mass and relative preservation of lean body mass [15,16]. In some studies, however, particularly with very low calorie diets, exercise may not have any significant effect beyond that of diet alone [17,18].

Finally, physical training in patients with NIDDM results in the same general benefits as in non-diabetic individuals. These include increased fitness and physical working capacity, decreased resting heart rate, increased stroke volume and decreased cardiac work. In addition, there may be psychological benefits including increased sense of well-being and improved overall quality of life.

Risks of exercise in NIDDM

In addition to the benefits of exercise, a number of significant risks for patients with NIDDM have been recognized (Table 2). In patients taking insulin or oral hypoglycemic agents, exercise may result in symptomatic hypoglycemia either during or following exercise. In insulin-treated patients, the increased risk of hypoglycemia may persist for up to 24 hours following prolonged strenuous exercise [19]. In addition, extremely strenuous exercise of short duration may result in a rapid increase in blood glucose concentration which persists for several hours after the exercise is stopped [20]. Another risk of exercise in people with NIDDM is precipitation or exacerbation of underlying cardiovascular disease, which may not have been previously diagnosed. This includes the development of angina pectoris, myocardial infarction or cardiac arrhythmias. Therefore, adults with NIDDM should have a thorough cardiac evaluation before initiating an exercise program. Degenerative joint disease is more common in obese individuals and may be exacerbated by weight-bearing exercising. Also, patients with sensory neuropathy may experience joint and soft-tissue injuries while participating in exercise.

A number of complications of diabetes may be aggravated by exercise and patients with NIDDM should be screened for these before being advised to undertake an ex-

TABLE 2

Risks of exercise for patients with NIDDM

1. Hypoglycemia if treated with insulin or oral agents
    exercise-induced hypoglycemia
    late-onset, post-exercise hypoglycemia

2. Hyperglycemia following very strenuous exercise

3. Precipitation or exacerbation of cardiovascular disease
    angina pectoris
    myocardial infarction
    arrhythmias
    sudden death

4. Worsening of long-term complications of diabetes
    proliferative retinopathy:
        vitreous hemorrhage
        retinal detachment

    nephropathy:
        increased proteinuria

    peripheral neuropathy:
        soft-tissue and joint injuries

    autonomic neuropathy:
        decreased cardiovascular response to exercise
        decreased maximum aerobic capacity
        impaired response to dehydration
        postural hypotension

ercise program. The most important of these is proliferative retinopathy, in which exercise may result in retinal or vitreous hemorrhage. Extremely strenuous exercise or types of exercise associated with Valsalva-like maneuvers are particularly dangerous and should be avoided by patients with proliferative retinopathy. Also, exercise resulting in jarring or rapid head motion may precipitate hemorrhage or retinal detachment. Physical exercise is also associated with increased proteinuria in patients with diabetic nephropathy [21,22]. This is probably the result of changes in renal hemodynamics associated with exercise and it is not known whether this has any effect on the progression of renal disease. As mentioned above, peripheral neuropathy increases the risk of soft-tissue and joint injuries and may be a contraindication to certain types of exercise such as running, jogging or similar activities in which localized trauma may occur. If autonomic neuropathy is present, the capacity for high-intensity exercise may be impaired due to decreased maximum heart rate and aerobic capacity. In addition, there may be impaired response to dehydration and problems with postural hypotension. With proper planning and selection of exercise, most of these complications can be avoided, although in some circumstances physical exercise programs may be contraindicated for the patient with NIDDM.

Exercise and insulin sensitivity

A possible role for physical exercise as a means of treating the insulin resistance associated with obesity and NIDDM was first suggested by Björntorp et al. in the early 1970s [26]. They observed that physically active middle-aged men had significantly lower fasting insulin concentrations and lower insulin responses to oral glucose when compared with untrained men of the same age and body weight [4]. This finding suggested that regular physical activity was associated with increased insulin sensitivity and led them to study the effects of 12 weeks of physical training on glucose tolerance and insulin responses in a group of obese patients with normal glucose tolerance but insulin resistance. Following the period of physical training there was no change in the blood glucose curves, but insulin levels were significantly lower, both fasting and following glucose administration [5]. Subsequently, numerous investigators have demonstrated increased insulin sensitivity and responsiveness in physically trained subjects using a variety of techniques. For example, both normal control subjects and patients with NIDDM have been shown to have a 30–35% increase in insulin-stimulated glucose disposal after physical training, when studied by the hyperinsulinemic-euglycemic clamp technique [6,27]. This increase in insulin sensitivity correlates closely with the training-induced increase in VO_2max [28,29] and is thought to be due primarily to increased glucose uptake in skeletal muscle, since no changes have been observed in hepatic glucose production rates.

It was soon learnt, however, that the increase in insulin sensitivity and responsiveness associated with physical conditioning is rapidly lost when exercise is discontinued. Burstein et al. [30] found that much of the effect is gone within 60 hours, and others have demonstrated that the effect is no longer present after 5–7 days without exercise. In a study by Bogardus et al. [17] comparing the effects of a very low calorie diet with the same diet plus a physical training program on weight loss and blood glucose regulation in NIDDM, the physically trained group had a significant increase in insulin-stimulated glucose disposal rates whereas the group treated by diet alone had no change after 3 months of treatment. The increase in insulin-stimulated glucose disposal in the group treated by diet and physical training was due entirely to an increase in non-oxidative glucose disposal, presumably reflecting increased glycogen synthesis. In this study, the glucose clamp procedures were done 5–7 days after the last exercise session and would, therefore, appear to demonstrate a true effect of physical training rather than a carryover effect from the last bout of exercise.

In recent studies, Mikines et al. [31] have shown that a single bout of exercise increases the sensitivity and responsiveness of insulin-stimulated glucose uptake in untrained individuals. This effect lasts for at least 2 days, but is not observed after 5 days. In addition, physically trained subjects have increased insulin action when studied 15 hours after their last training session when compared with untrained subjects. When studied 5 days after the last training session, insulin responsiveness remains increased compared with untrained subjects, suggesting that there is a long-term adaptive increase in whole body responsiveness to insulin with training [32]. Although the mechanism of this is not yet known, it may be related to increased capillary density in skeletal muscle, an increase in oxidative capacity of skeletal muscle or to other adaptations to training.

Despite the increase in insulin-stimulated glucose uptake that can be demonstrated for at least 5–7 days following cessation of exercise in previously trained subjects, patients with NIDDM have generally not been demonstrated to have improved fasting blood glucose concentrations or improved glucose tolerance with training [33,34]. This has led some to suggest that physical training is ineffective as a means of improving glucose homeostasis in NIDDM. Others, however, have observed that physical training is associated with lower glycosylated hemoglobin levels [3]. Current interpretation is that this may be the cumulative result of decreased blood glucose concentrations associated with repeated bouts of exercise rather than a specific effect of physical training. Since it is known that exercise usually results in a fall of blood glucose concentrations towards normal in hyperglycemic patients with NIDDM and increased insulin-stimulated glucose disposal can be observed for many hours following a single bout of exercise, it is likely that regular exercise 4–7 days a week may result in lower average blood glucose and glycohemoglobin concentrations without a significant effect on fasting blood glucose or glucose responses to meals. Thus, the net effect of exercise repeated on a regular basis would be to improve long-term blood glucose control in patients with NIDDM.

Effects of prior exercise on glucose metabolism

To determine the effects of a single bout of exercise on glucose metabolism and insulin sensitivity and responsiveness during post-exercise recovery, Devlin et al. have conducted a series of studies on basal and insulin-stimulated glucose metabolism during post-exercise recovery in normal subjects and in patients with obesity and insulin resistance or NIDDM [35,36].

The hyperinsulinemic-euglycemic clamp technique, combined with indirect calorimetry and infusion of D-3[^{3}H]glucose, was used to measure basal rates of glucose turnover and oxidation and the response to both submaximal (40 mU/m^2/min) and maximally stimulating (400 mU/m^2/min) concentrations of insulin. Each subject was studied twice, once in the rested state and once 12–14 hours after intermittent, high-intensity cycle exercise performed to muscular exhaustion. The exercise protocol used resulted in a 62% decrease in glycogen content and a 3–4-fold increase in glycogen synthase activity in quadriceps muscle, when measured 12–14 hours after the completion of the exercise with the subjects remaining fasting.

In normal lean volunteers, the basal rate of glucose turnover was decreased following exercise, because of a significant decrease in glucose oxidation and a corresponding increase in lipid oxidation (Fig. 1). Glucose disposal by non-oxidative pathways (NOGD), presumed to represent primarily glycogen synthesis, was increased significantly following exercise, but not enough to compensate fully for the decrease in glucose oxidation. During low-dose insulin infusion, which increased plasma insulin concentrations by approximately 100 mU/l, glucose disposal increased normally to approx. 7 mg/kg fat-free mass/min and was not significantly different in the non-exercised or post-exercise studies. There was, however, a marked difference in the metabolic pathway of glucose disposal. Following exercise, glucose oxidation was lower and NOGD was greater, suggesting that a large portion of the glucose was being utilized for glycogen synthesis. During high-dose insulin infusion, total glucose disposal was increased slightly following exercise. This was associated with a marked increase in NOGD and a moderate decrease in glucose oxidation. Thus, the metabolic response 12–14 hours after high-intensity, glycogen-depleting exercise is a decrease in glucose oxidation, an increase in lipid oxidation and a marked increase in NOGD, which most likely represents increased glycogen synthesis to replete the glycogen stores.

In obese subjects with insulin resistance (Fig. 1) and in patients with NIDDM, qualitatively similar results were obtained. As expected, basal rates of glucose turn-

278

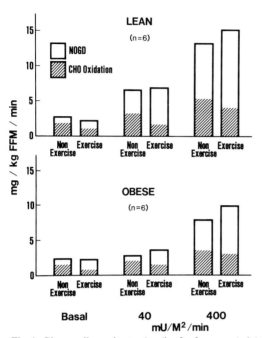

Fig. 1. Glucose disposal rates (mg/kg fat-free mass/min) in lean and obese insulin-resistant subjects with and without prior exercise, in the basal state and during 40 mU/m²/min (low dose) and 400 mU/m²/min (high dose) insulin infusions. Cross-hatched areas represent glucose oxidation and open areas represent non-oxidative glucose disposal (NOGD).

over were normal in the non-diabetic obese subjects and increased in the patients with NIDDM and fasting hyperglycemia. Following exercise, basal glucose turnover did not change but, as in the normal subjects, there was a significant decrease in glucose oxidation and an increase in NOGD. During insulin infusion, total glucose disposal was stimulated to only about 50% of normal, indicating insulin resistance. Following exercise, total insulin-stimulated glucose disposal was increased modestly, associated with a marked increase in NOGD. As in normals, insulin-stimulated glucose oxidation was decreased following exercise (Fig. 2).

When these data are expressed as the metabolic clearance rates of glucose to provide a direct comparison between lean, obese and NIDDM subjects, it is clear that obesity and NIDDM have similar degrees of insulin resistance and that a single bout of exercise results in a modest increase in insulin-stimulated glucose disposal, but does not correct the insulin resistance to normal (Fig. 3). The mechanism for this apparent post-exercise increase in insulin sensitivity and responsiveness appears to be an increase in NOGD associated with increased glycogen synthesis.

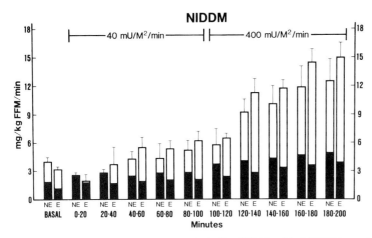

Fig. 2. Rates of total glucose utilization (including SEM bars) in NIDDM men in basal state and during each 20-min interval of low-dose (40 mU/m²/min) and high-dose (400 mU/m²/min) insulin infusions, without (NE) and with (E) prior exercise. Solid areas represent glucose oxidation; open areas represent non-oxidative glucose disposal (from Ref. 36 with permission).

In another set of studies, whole body and regional fuel metabolism was studied in normal volunteers during early post-exercise recovery [37]. These experiments were designed to measure total body glucose turnover, as well as glucose and lipid oxidation rates and NOGD, from approximately 40 minutes to 4 hours following cycle exercise at 70% VO₂max until muscular exhaustion (70–90 min), and to correlate these data with fluxes of metabolic substrates across forearm tissues, in both the ab-

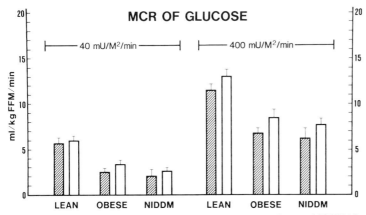

Fig. 3. Metabolic clearance rates (MCR) of glucose in lean, obese and NIDDM men during low-dose (40 mU/m²/min) and high-dose (400 mU/m²/min) insulin infusions, without (hatched bars) and with (open bars) prior exercise. Bars represent SEM (from Ref. 36 with permission).

sence and the presence of insulin infused at 40 mU/m^2/min. After an overnight fast, normal male volunteers either exercised or remained resting in bed prior to the insulin–glucose clamp studies, which were combined with indirect calorimetry to measure rates of glucose, lipid and protein oxidation, and with measurements of the fluxes of glucose, lactate, pyruvate, alanine and branched-chain amino acids (BCAA) across the forearm.

Following exercise, total glucose disposal, in either the absence or the presence of infused insulin, was the same as in the non-exercised state. However, there was a marked shift in the pathways of glucose metabolism, with a decreased rate of glucose oxidation and an increase in NOGD, similar to the pattern seen 12–14 hours post-exercise in the previous studies (Fig. 4). Plasma free fatty acid (FFA) concentrations and lipid oxidation were increased following exercise as was plasma norepinephrine. Before insulin infusion, forearm glucose uptake was the same after exercise as it was in the non-exercised state, but the release of lactate, pyruvate and alanine was increased 2–3-fold, suggesting continued breakdown of glycogen in the forearm muscles (Fig. 5). During insulin infusion without prior exercise, forearm glucose uptake increased approximately 5-fold and there was a slight decrease in the release of 3-carbon compounds and uptake of BCAA. Following exercise, however, insulin infusion failed to increase forearm glucose uptake significantly. This rather striking and somewhat unexpected finding suggests that the forearm muscle, which did not participate in the cycle exercise, becomes insulin-resistant during the early stages of post-exercise recovery and continues to release 3-carbon compounds, presumably coming from

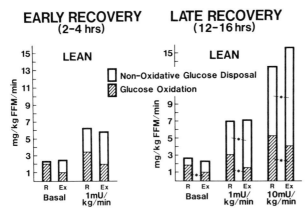

Fig. 4. Glucose disposal rates (mg/kg fat-free mass/min) in lean subjects with (Ex) and without (R) prior exercise in the basal state and during 1 mU/kg/min (low dose) or 10 mU/kg/min (high dose) insulin infusions, either 2–4 hours (early recovery) or 12–16 hours (late recovery) after exercise (or rest). Cross-hatched areas represent glucose oxidation and open areas represent non-oxidative glucose disposal (NOGD).

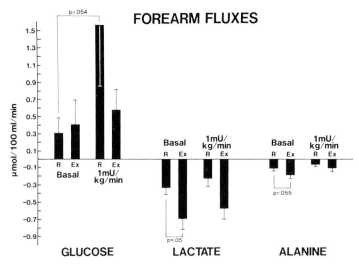

Fig. 5. Fluxes of glucose, lactate and alanine across forearm tissues of lean volunteers 2–4 hours after rest (R) or exercise (Ex) in the basal state and during low-dose insulin infusion (mU/kg/min).

continued glycogenolysis. This, coupled with increased NOGD, suggests that previously exercised and non-exercised muscle groups behave differently during early post-exercise recovery and provide a mechanism whereby metabolic substrates can be shunted from one site to another. Continued glycogenolysis, release of 3-carbon compounds and decreased sensitivity to insulin in non-exercised muscle may provide substrates for hepatic gluconeogenesis via the Cori and glucose-alanine cycles and make more glucose available for uptake in the previously exercised muscles for restoration of glycogen stores. Another interesting finding in these studies was that the rise in plasma BCAA concentrations following exercise was not due to increased release from non-exercised muscle but may have been the result of increased hepatic protein degradation. The increasing BCAA concentrations, combined with uptake of BCAA by forearm muscle, may result in increased rates of BCAA oxidation in muscle following exercise and provide an amino source for the glucose-alanine cycle.

These studies suggest that following exercise a complex and highly integrated pattern of metabolic fuel redistribution and utilization occurs that involves both exercised and non-exercised muscles and probably the liver. It is well known that prior exercise results in increased glucose uptake in skeletal muscle for several hours, particularly in the presence of insulin [38]. It now also appears that non-exercised muscle becomes insulin-resistant following exercise of other muscle groups, a response that serves to limit whole body glucose utilization and provide additional substrates for gluconeogenesis. Whether this response occurs in NIDDM or other insulin-resistant states is not yet known.

282

Conclusions

Based on current knowledge, participation in regular physical exercise can be expected to have many benefits for patients with NIDDM and should be considered an important part of the treatment whenever possible. However, there are also a number of risks of exercise that must be considered before advising a patient with NIDDM to undertake an exercise program. All patients with NIDDM should have a complete medical evaluation to screen for long-term complications of diabetes, with particular attention paid to evaluation of the cardiovascular system and assessment of retinopathy, nephropathy and neuropathy. In some patients, participation in an exercise program may be contraindicated because the risks outweigh the potential benefits. In others, the exercise program must be modified to minimize the risks associated with specific complications of diabetes, whereas in other patients a full exercise program may be undertaken with relative safety. In general, exercise programs should start with a relatively low intensity and duration of exercise and build up gradually as conditioning occurs.

The frequency of exercise should be at least three times weekly, with 4–7 sessions a week being preferred. If this level of exercise is maintained, cardiovascular conditioning will occur and there will be improvement in insulin sensitivity, a lowering of basal and post-prandial insulin concentrations and, in most cases, improved long-term glucose control as measured by a lower glycosylated hemoglobin level. These changes are most probably due to the effects of exercise in lowering blood glucose concentrations acutely and for several hours following exercise and to increased insulin sensitivity following exercise.

During post-exercise recovery, there is a shift in the metabolic pathways of glucose disposal, with a decrease in glucose oxidation and an increase in NOGD, which is thought to represent increased glycogen synthesis in the previously exercised muscles. In NIDDM, this is associated with increased insulin-stimulated glucose disposal rates and may explain the increase in insulin sensitivity that persists for several hours after exercise. In contrast to increased glucose uptake in previously exercised muscles, non-exercised muscle groups exhibit insulin resistance during early post-exercise recovery and continue to release lactate, pyruvate and alanine, which may, in turn, be substrates for hepatic gluconeogenesis. This response during early post-exercise recovery, manifested by decreased insulin-stimulated glucose uptake and continued glycogenolysis and release of 3-carbon compounds in non-exercised muscles and increased glucose uptake and glycogen synthesis in previously exercised muscles, appears to be a homeostatic mechanism whereby unused glycogen stores are mobilized to provide substrates for maintenance of blood glucose and replenishment of glycogen stores in exercised muscle. Whether this mechanism operates normally in patients with NIDDM and how it affects blood glucose regulation following exercise are still to be determined.

References

1. Sushruta SCS. Vaidya Jadavaji Trikamji Acharia. Bombay: Sagar, 1938.
2. Horton ES. Role and management of exercise in diabetes mellitus. Diabetes Care 1988;11:201–211.
3. Schneider SH, Amoroso LF, Khachsdurian AK, Ruderman NB. Studies on the mechanism of improved glucose control during regular exercise in type 2 (non-insulin-dependent) diabetes. Diabetologia 1984;26:355–360.
4. Bjorntorp P, Fahlen M, Grimby G, et al. Carbohydrate and lipid metabolism in middle aged physically well-trained men. Metabolism 1972;21:1037–1042.
5. Bjorntorp P, de Jonge K, Sjostrom L, Sullivan L. The effect of physical training on insulin production in obesity. Metabolism 1970;19:631–637.
6. DeFronzo RA, Ferrannini E, Koivisto V. New concepts in the pathogenesis and treatment of non-insulin dependent diabetes mellitus. Am J Med 1983;74:52–81.
7. DeFronzo RA, Lilly lecture 1987. The Triumvirate: B-cell, muscle, liver – a collusion responsible for NIDDM. Diabetes 1988;37:667–687.
8. Huttunen JK, Lansimies E, Voutilainen E, et al. Effect of moderate physical exercise on serum lipoproteins. Circulation 1979;60:1220–1229.
9. Haskell WL. The influence of exercise training on plasma lipids and lipoproteins in health and disease. Acta Med Scand 1986;Suppl;711:25–37.
10. Kiens B, Lithell H. Lipoprotein metabolism influenced by training induced changes in human skeletal muscle. J Clin Invest 1989;83:558–564.
11. Rotkis TC, Cote R, Coyle E, et al. Relationship between high density lipoprotein cholesterol and weekly running mileage. J Cardiac Rehab 1982;2:109–112.
12. Boyer J, Kasch F. Exercise therapy in hypertensive men. J Am Med Assoc 1970;211:1668–1671.
13. Choquette G, Ferguson R. Blood pressure reduction in borderline hypertensives following physical training. Can Med Assoc J 1973;108:699–703.
14. Krotkiewski M, Mandroukis K, Sjostrom L, et al. Effects of long-term physical training on body fat, metabolism and blood pressure in obesity. Metabolism 1979;28:650–658.
15. Pavlou KN, Steffee WP, Lerman RH, et al. Effects of dieting and exercise on lean body mass, oxygen uptake and strength. Med Sci Sports Exerc 1985;17:466–471.
16. Hill JO, Sparling PB, Shields TW, et al. Effects of exercise and food restriction on body composition and metabolic rate in obese women. Am J Clin Nutr 1987;46:622–630.
17. Bogardus C, Ravussin E, Robbins DC, Wolfe RR, Horton ES, Sims EAH. Effects of physical training and diet therapy on carbohydrate metabolism in patients with glucose intolerance and non-insulin-dependent diabetes mellitus. Diabetes 1984;33:311–318.
18. Warwick PM, Garrow JS. The effect of addition of exercise to a regime of dietary restriction on weight loss, nitrogen balance, resting metabolic rate and spontaneous physical activity in three obese women in a metabolic ward. Int J Obesity 1981;5:25–32.
19. MacDonald MJ. Post-exercise late-onset hypoglycemia in insulin-dependent diabetic patients. Diabetes Care 1987;10:584–588.
20. Mitchell TH, Abraham G, Schiffrin A, et al. Hyperglycemia after intense exercise in IDDM subjects during continuous subcutaneous insulin infusion. Diabetes Care 1988;11:311–317.
21. Mogensen CE, Vittinghus E. Urinary albumin excretion during exercise in juvenile diabetes. Scand J Clin Lab Invest 1975;35:295–300.
22. Viberti GC, Jarrett RJ, McCartney M, Keen H. Increased glomerular permeability to albumin induced by exercise in diabetic subjects. Diabetologia 1978;14:293–300.
23. Storstein L, Jervell J. Response to bicycle exercise testing of long standing juvenile diabetics. Acta Med Scand 1979;205:227–230.

24. Hilsted J, Galbo H, Christensen NJ. Impaired cardiovascular responses to graded exercise in diabetic autonomic neuropathy. Diabetes 1979;28:313–319.
25. Rubler S. Asymptomatic diabetic females: exercise testing. NY State J Med 1981;81:1185–1191.
26. Björntorp P, de Jong K, Sjostrom L, Sullivan L. Physical training in human obesity. II. Effects of plasma insulin in glucose intolerant subjects without marked hyperinsulinemia. Scand J Clin Lab Invest 1973;32:42–45.
27. Sato Y, Iguchi A, Sakamoto N. Biochemical determination of training effects using insulin clamp technique. Horm Metab Res 1984;16:483–486.
28. Yki-Jarvinen H. Koivisto VA. Effects of body composition on insulin sensitivity. Diabetes 1983;32:965–969.
29. Rosenthal M, Haskell WL, Solomon R, Widstrom A, Reaven GM. Demonstration of a relationship between level of physical training and insulin-stimulated glucose utilization in normal humans. Diabetes 1983;32:408–411.
30. Burstein R, Polychronakos C, Toeus CJ, MacDougall JD, Guyda HJ, Posner BI. Acute reversal of the enhanced insulin action in trained athletes. Diabetes 1985;34:756–760.
31. Mikines KJ, Sonne B, Farrell PA, et al. Effect of physical exercise on sensitivity and responsiveness to insulin in humans. Am J Physiol 1988; 254 (Endocrinol Metab 17):E248–E259.
32. Mikines KJ, Sonne B, Tronier B, Galbo H. Effects of acute exercise and detraining on insulin action in trained men. J Appl Physiol 1989;66:704–711.
33. Saltin B, Lindgard F, Houston M, Horlin R, Hygaard E, Gad P. Physical training and glucose tolerance in middle-aged men with chemical diabetes. Diabetes 1978;28(Suppl 1):30–32.
34. Ruderman NB, Ganda OP, Johansen K. The effect of physical training on glucose tolerance and plasma lipids in maturity-onset diabetes. Diabetes 1979;28(Suppl 1):89–92.
35. Devlin JT, Horton ES. Effects of prior high-intensity exercise on glucose metabolism in normal and insulin-resistant men. Diabetes 1985;34:973–979.
36. Devlin JT, Hirshman M, Horton ED, Horton ES. Enhanced peripheral and splanchnic insulin sensitivity in NIDDM men after single bout of exercise. Diabetes 1987;36:434–439.
37. Devlin JT, Barlow J, Horton ES. Whole body and regional fuel metabolism during early post-exercise recovery. Am J Physiol 1989; 256 (Endocrinol Metab 19):E167–E172.
38. Ivy JL, Holloszy JO. Persistent increase in glucose uptake by rat skeletal muscle following exercise. Am J Physiol 1981;241:C200–C203.

© 1989 Elsevier Science Publishers B.V. (Biomedical Division)
Frontiers of diabetes research: current trends in non-insulin-dependent diabetes mellitus
K.G.M.M. Alberti and R. Mazze, editors

CHAPTER 21

Acarbose and related compounds for the treatment of diabetes mellitus

WERNER CREUTZFELDT

Division of Gastroenterology and Endocrinology, Department of Medicine,
Georg August University of Göttingen, F.R.G.

Introduction

Eight years ago I had the privilege to chair and introduce the first International Symposium on Acarbose in Montreux, Switzerland [1]. On that occasion I said that ever since I was confronted with the task of advising patients to eat less and to avoid things they like, I have been thinking about other means of manipulating nutrient entry. As a physician and clinical investigator with interests in endocrinology and gastroenterology I have searched for gastroenterological approaches to this goal. This seemed to become a reality in the 1960s when it became clear that the biguanides had a direct effect on absorption. Since that time my laboratory has been actively involved in these problems, and the leading investigators over the years and still interested in the matter are Wolfgang Caspary and Bernhard Lembcke (both now in Frankfurt) and Reinhold Ebert and Ulrich Fölsch, both still with me.

The biguanides, except metformin, are no longer on the market and their wider use has been limited by systemic side-effects. A less aggressive approach to manipulating food entry than systemic drugs or mutilating operations appeared to be all measures which only delay food assimilation. This approach takes into account gastrointestinal physiology, especially the dependence of the blood glucose response to carbohydrate ingestion on the velocity of digestion and absorption, which is determined by at least six factors, listed in Table 1. While in diabetes mellitus the metabolic and endocrine factors which determine the oral glucose tolerance are at fault, the gastrointestinal factors are undisturbed, except in the case of gut autonomic neuropathy with impaired gastric emptying and intestinal motility, which may eventually lead to severe undernutrition.

286

TABLE 1
Factors determining oral glucose tolerance

1.	**Gastrointestinal functions**
1.1	Number of meals
1.2	Digestibility and composition of food
1.3	Gastric emptying
1.4	Duodenal alpha-amylase activity
1.5	Contact time for digestion and absorption (transit time)
1.6	Intestinal absorption (absorptive surface, hydrolases of the brush border membrane, transport capacity)
2.	**Metabolic and endocrine functions**
2.1	Neural and hormonal B-cell stimulation
2.2	Insulin secretory capacity
2.3	Hepatic glucose uptake
2.4	Hepatic insulin extraction
2.5	Peripheral glucose uptake (insulin action)

The therapeutic principle of delaying absorption [2] is well illustrated in a schematic figure (Fig. 1) from Jenkins [3]. This scheme has been designed to show the consequence of slow digestion and absorption of energy-dilute food in a fibre-rich diet – so-called lente carbohydrates. However, not all will accept such diets. For those unable or unwilling to take the diets new pharmaceutical developments in this field have opened up interesting perspectives.

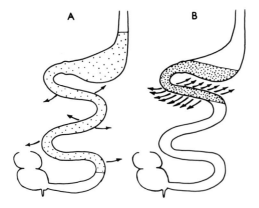

Fig. 1. Schematic representation of stomach and small intestine showing (A) slow digestion and absorption of energy-dilute food in a 'fibre-rich' diet and (B) rapid digestion and absorption of energy-dense food from low-fibre diets (from Ref. 3; with permission).

Development and characteristics of amylase and glucosidase inhibitors

A leading role in the development of substances inhibiting enzymes for carbohydrate digestion (i.e. amylase and glucosidase inhibitors) was played by researchers such as Puls, Schmidt, Keupp and Bischoff from Bayer at Wuppertal [4].

Amylase inhibitors, such as a protein from wheat flour and a disaccharide from microorganisms, did not significantly inhibit the glucose increase after intake of cooked carbohydrate meals. Due to the negative results obtained in clinical studies the further development of these substances was interrupted. However, they have been a necessary step which led to the development of the α-glucosidase inhibitors [5].

More recently, a partially purified amylase inhibitor from beans at a dose of 4–6 g daily has been studied in the Mayo Clinic in volunteers and in diabetics for up to 3 weeks with some effect on postprandial glucose and hormone responses [6]. However, these effects seem to be small if compared with what was demonstrated with inhibitors of α-glucosidases more than 10 years ago in animals, volunteers and diabetic patients [1, 7–9]. Amylopectin and amylose, the main components of starch, are cleaved by pancreatic amylase only to the oligosaccharides α-limit dextrin, maltotriose and maltose (Fig. 2). The final cleavage is done by the α-glucosidases: maltase, glucoamylase (also called gamma-amylase), sucrase, isomaltase (Fig. 3). Lactose is cleaved by the β-galactosidase lactase, which is not inhibited by the known α-glucosidase inhibitors. A prerequisite for the absorption of carbohydrates, i.e. transport into the mucosa cell, is cleavage to monosaccharides, i.e. D-glucose, D-fructose and D-galactose at the surface of the brush border membrane [10]. The advantage of the gluco-

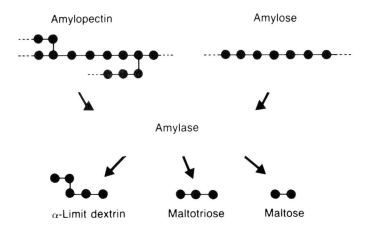

Fig. 2. Enzymatic cleavage of components of starch by pancreatic amylase (from Ref. 10; with permission).

288

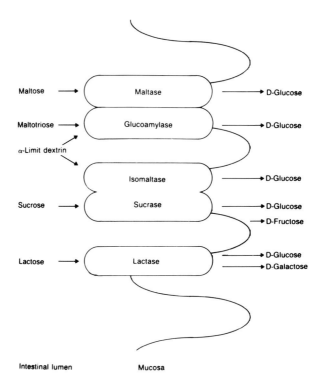

Fig. 3. Digestion and absorption of oligo- and disaccharides at the brush border membrane of the small intestine (from Ref. 10; with permission).

sidase inhibitors over amylase inhibitors is their broader spectrum, which covers starch as well as sucrose, the latter being a major component of daily food.

The most suitable agents for therapeutic use are α-glucosidase inhibitors of a carbohydrate nature. The first thoroughly studied compound was the nitrogen-containing carbohydrate acarbose (BAY g 5421), which has the same molecular size as a tetrasaccharide (Fig. 4). Acarbose is formed by fermentation of certain actinoplantanaceae and is obtained by a complex isolation procedure [11]. The more recently developed nojirimycin derivatives, miglitol (BAY m 1099) and emiglitate (BAY o 1248), are considerably smaller molecules with a remarkable structural similarity to glucose and a nitrogen atom built into the ring (Fig. 5). They are produced by chemical synthesis [11].

The most striking effect of these substances is their binding to the brush border disaccharidases and by this the competitive inhibition of the α-glucosidases glucomaltase, sucrase, maltase and isomaltase in decreasing potency, while trehalase and lactase are not inhibited. This has been demonstrated in human intestinal mucosa [9].

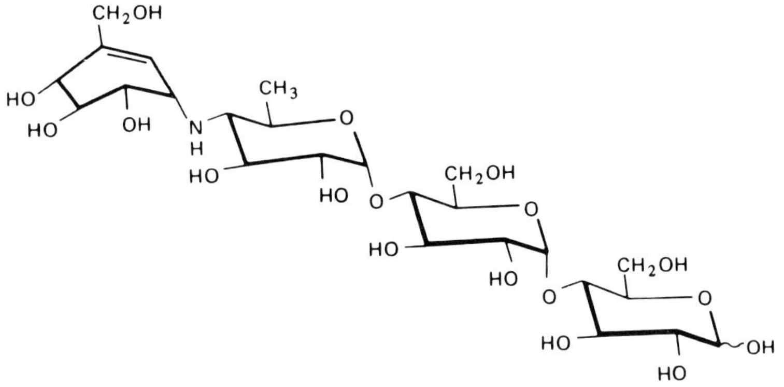

Fig. 4. Chemical structure of acarbose (Bay g 5421).

Miglitol and emiglitate have a 10-times higher affinity for these enzymes and, therefore, are 10-times more effective [12].

The release of the α-glucosidase inhibitors for general therapeutic use has been withheld for several years because of the observation of kidney tumours together with a lower incidence of other tumours after long-term treatment of Sprague-Dawley rats. This event depended on severe malnutrition and could be prevented by glucose feeding. Furthermore, no such effects were observed in Wistar rats or hamsters, and no signs of genotoxicity could be demonstrated [13]. Accordingly, clinical investigations have been resumed and may eventually lead to the introduction of this new therapeutic principle for better control of hyperglycaemia.

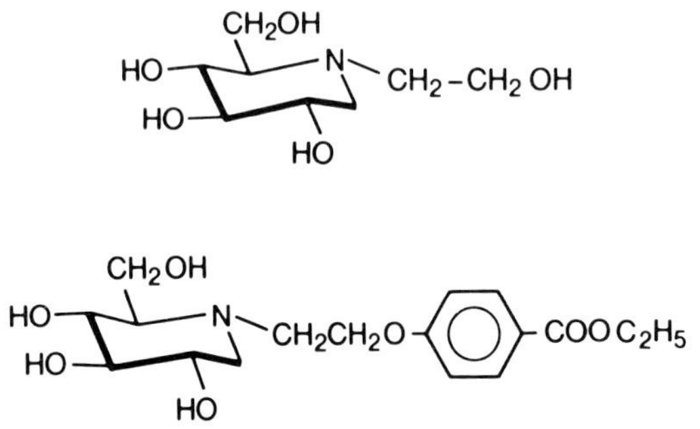

Fig. 5. Chemical structure of the nojirimycin derivatives miglitol (BAY m 1099, upper) and emiglitate (BAY o 1248, lower).

Mechanism of action of α-glucosidase inhibitors in man

Dose-response studies in volunteers have clearly demonstrated that complete, or nearly complete, inhibition of the intestinal α-glucosidases induces maldigestion of complex carbohydrates, which then reach the colon, where they are fermented by

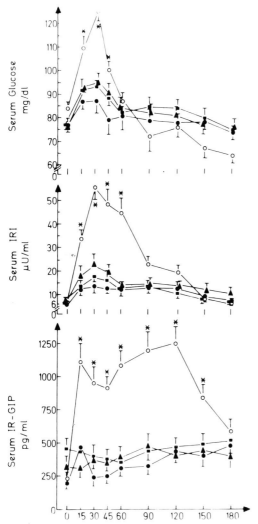

Fig. 6. Responses of serum levels of glucose, insulin, and GIP to ingestion of 100 g sucrose without (○) or with addition of 200 mg acarbose. The effect of the glucosidase inhibitor on the sucrose load was investigated on the first (●), the 28th (■) and the 56th (▲) day of a long-term intake of 3 × 200 mg acarbose by 10 volunteers. *$p < 0.05$ between test and control experiments. IR-GIP, immunoreactive gastric inhibitory polypeptide; IRI, immunoreactive insulin (from Ref. 15; with permission).

bacteria. This results in severe meteorism, abdominal cramps and diarrhea. Such un-acceptable side-effects can be prevented by lowering the acarbose dose. Then, enzyme inhibition is limited to the upper small intestine and absorption can take place in distal intestinal sections; in other words, absorption is only delayed. Milder forms of meteorism usually occur also with small doses of acarbose because of carbohydrate overspill into the colon. However, they are less marked if treatment is started with a low dose for several weeks. In addition, it is the general experience that most volunteers and patients complain less about side-effects after several weeks of treatment.

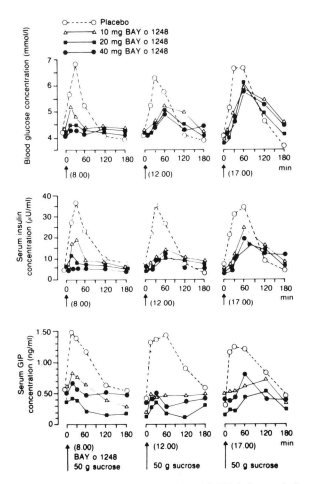

Fig. 7. Serum levels of glucose, insulin and GIP before and after repeated loading with 50 g sucrose at 08.00h, 12.00 h and 17.00 h without or with varying doses (10, 20 and 40 mg) of emiglitate (BAY o 1248) in 8 volunteers. Directly before each loading the subjects received 20 mg metoclopramide to standardize gastric emptying (from Ref. 8; with permission).

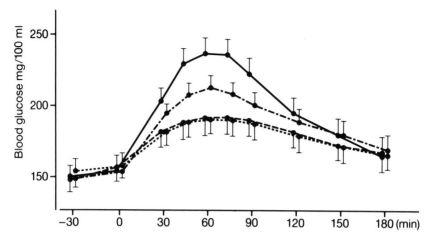

Fig. 8. Fasting and postprandial blood glucose levels in 24 NIDDM patients after a standard breakfast (—), a muesli breakfast (— · — · —), a standard breakfast with 100 mg miglitol (— — —), and a muesli breakfast with 100 mg miglitol (······) (from Ref 16; with permission).

It has been speculated that this is due to an adaptive increase of α-glucosidase concentration in the distal small bowel, as observed in rats [14].

The decreasing abdominal complaints during long-term acarbose intake are not accompanied by a decreasing glucosidase inhibition in the proximal small intestine. We have treated volunteers for 8 weeks with $3 \times$ 200 mg acarbose and investigated the responses to a 100 g sucrose load of the serum levels of glucose, insulin and GIP on the first, the 28th and the 56th day of treatment [15]. All parameters were equally suppressed during the whole acarbose treatment period (Fig. 6). The same observations have been made with miglitol using both sucrose and starch loads.

More recently we have performed dose-response studies with the nojirimycin derivatives miglitol and emiglitate. In these studies the following have been assessed: (1) the dose dependency of the decreased glucose and hormone response to 50 g sucrose (10, 20 and 40 mg miglitol and emiglitate); (2) the prolonged effect of emiglitate in comparison with acarbose and miglitol (glucose and hormone response to sucrose and starch are still lowered at lunch and dinner); (3) the dose-dependent increase of breath hydrogen concentration and the difference in subjective side-effects and H_2 exhalation after sucrose and starch.

Fig. 7 illustrates the effect of emiglitate (BAY o 1248) on glucose and hormone responses to 50 g sucrose after administration of three different doses of the drug before breakfast, and lasting until the sucrose load at 17.00 h.

The H_2 exhalation during the starch or sucrose load does not necessarily mean a

large overspill of undigested carbohydrates into the colon. This test is not quantitative. The absence of diarrhea in our studies suggests the entry into the colon of only
small amounts of undigested carbohydrates.

Treatment of diabetes mellitus with α-glucosidase inhibitors

The therapeutic principle of delaying absorption has been tried in the last 12 years
in diabetic patients under controlled clinical conditions and in out-patients. At first

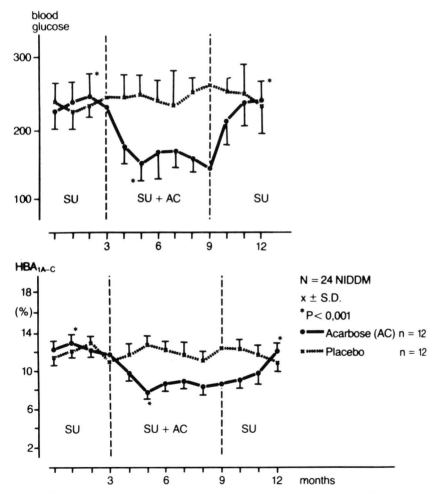

Fig. 9. Effect of acarbose on mean diurnal blood glucose (upper panel) and on HbA$_{1a-c}$ (lower panel) in
NIDDM treated with sulfonylureas (from Ref. 17; with permission).

acarbose was used as an adjuvant in diabetics on diet plus insulin, or on diet plus sulfonylureas. There is general agreement that α-glucosidase inhibitors lower the postprandial blood glucose levels more than a fibre-rich diet with a low glycemic index. This has been best demonstrated by Willms in 24 patients with NIDDM who ingested a standard breakfast or a fibre-rich meal with or without miglitol [16]. Miglitol even lowered the glucose response to a fibre-rich meal (Fig. 8).

The improvement of the 24 h blood glucose profile of diabetic subjects treated with sulfonylureas or insulin has been shown by several authors in double-blind crossover experiments [1, 7]. The compliance in these studies has usually been satisfactory; the side-effects (meteorism and abdominal pains) decreased after several weeks and were not a great problem, especially if compared with fibre-rich diets. Only a small number of patients had to stop acarbose because of diarrhea.

There are only a few long-term studies, partly because of the withholding of these trials as a consequence of the toxicity studies mentioned above. Fig. 9 shows the long-term effects of acarbose vs. placebo in a 6-month trial in patients with poorly controlled NIDDM on sulfonylureas [17]. It also shows an improvement of the HbA$_{1a-c}$ levels in these patients and the deterioration after stopping the acarbose treatment. The effect of acarbose has also been assessed in poorly controlled diabetics in other

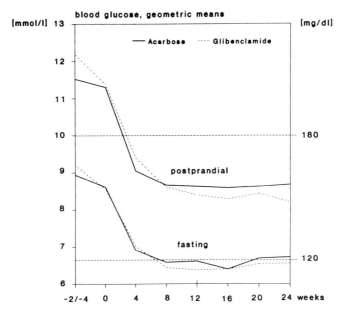

Fig. 10. Fasting and postprandial blood glucose during 6 months treatment with acarbose or glibenclamide (from Ref. 18; with permission).

studies. However, even in patients with sulfonylurea secondary failure a significant improvement of fasting and postprandial blood glucose levels has been achieved with acarbose for up to 12 months [19].

Hypoglycaemic reactions rarely occur and have been reported only in insulin-treated patients before the insulin dose was lowered. Acarbose or other α-glucosidase inhibitors have usually not been used for primary drug treatment of diabetes. Whether this is justified may be questioned. In a recent study the effects of 3×100 mg acarbose were compared with the effects of $1-3 \times 3.5$ mg glibenclamide over a 6-month period. The diagnosis of diabetes mellitus had been made recently in these 55 outpatients and no other treatment except dietary education has been applied. Fig. 10 shows that both therapeutic regimens significantly but equally lowered fasting and postprandial blood glucose levels. The HbA_1 levels also decreased to similar values from 10.8 to 8.5%, and from 11.0 to 8.7% [18].

These new data may start a discussion about whether α-glucosidase inhibitors are for first-line treatment or only indicated if insulin or sulfonylurea treatment does not sufficiently control hyperglycaemia.

Conclusions

1. Delaying absorption of carbohydrates is an attractive principle for treatment of hyperglycaemia.
2. Complete inhibition of digestive enzymes induces malassimilation with unacceptable side-effects; however, smaller doses only delay absorption.
3. α-Glucosidase inhibitors have a broader therapeutic spectrum than amylase inhibitors.
4. The effect of α-glucosidase inhibitors on blood levels of glucose and postprandial hormones does not decrease during long-term treatment, while the intestinal side-effects do.
5. In patients with NIDDM acarbose significantly lowers fasting and postprandial blood glucose levels and HbA_1 concentrations, both during monotherapy and if given in addition to sulfonylureas or insulin.

References

1. Creutzfeldt W. Proceedings First International Symposium on Acarbose. Amsterdam: Excerpta Medica, 1982.
2. Creutzfeldt W, Fölsch UR. Delaying absorption as a therapeutic principle in metabolic diseases. Stuttgart: Thieme, 1983.
3. Jenkins DJA, Taylor RH, Wolever TMS. The diabetic diet, dietary carbohydrate and differences in digestibility. Diabetologia 1982; 23:477–484.

4. Puls W, Bischoff H, Schutt H. Pharmacology of amylase- and glucosidase-inhibitors. In: Creutzfeldt W, Fölsch UR, eds. Delaying absorption as a therapeutic principle in metabolic diseases. Stuttgart: Thieme, 1983;70–76.
5. Fölsch UR. Delaying of carbohydrate absorption by α-amylase inhibitors. In: Creutzfeldt W, Fölsch UR, eds. Delaying absorption as a therapeutic principle in metabolic diseases. Stuttgart: Thieme, 1983;79–85.
6. Boivin M, Flourie B, Rizza RA, Go, VLW, DiMagno EP. Gastrointestinal and metabolic effects of amylase inhibition in diabetics. Gastroenterology 1988;94:387–394.
7. Creutzfeldt W. Acarbose for the treatment of diabetes mellitus. Berlin: Springer, 1988.
8. Fölsch UR, Lembcke B. The clinical use of α-glucosidase inhibitors. In: Caspary WF, ed. Structure and function of the small intestine. Amsterdam: Excerpta Medica, 1987;301–318.
9. Caspary WF. Inhibitors influencing carbohydrate absorption. In: Creutzfeldt W, Lefèbvre, eds. Diabetes mellitus: pathophysiology and therapy. Berlin: Springer, 1989;172–191.
10. Elsenhans B, Caspary WF. Absorption of carbohydrates. In: Caspary WF, ed. Structure and function of the small intestine. Amsterdam: Excerpta Medica, 1987;139–159.
11. Müller L, Puls W. Pharmacology of α-glucosidase inhibitors. In: Caspary WF, ed. Structure and function of the small intestine. Amsterdam: Excerpta Medica, 1987;281–300.
12. Lembcke B, Fölsch UR, Creutzfeldt W. Effect of 1-desoxynojirimycin derivatives on small intestinal disaccharidase activities and on active transport in vitro. Digestion 1985;31:120–127.
13. Schlüter G. Toxicology of acarbose, with special reference to long-term carcinogenicity studies. In: Creutzfeldt W, ed. Acarbose for the treatment of diabetes mellitus. Berlin: Springer, 1988;5–14.
14. Creutzfeldt W, Fölsch UR, Elsenhans B, Ballmann M, Conlon JM. Adaptation of the small intestine to induced maldigestion in rats. Scand J Gastroenterol 1985;20 (Suppl 112):45–53.
15. Fölsch UR, Ebert R, Creutzfeldt W. Response of serum levels of gastric inhibitory polypeptide (GIP) and insulin to sucrose ingestion during long-term application of acarbose. Scand J Gastroenterol 1981;16:629–632.
16. Willms B. Acarbose in non-insulin-dependent diabetes mellitus: short-term studies in combination with oral agents. In: Creutzfeldt W, ed. Acarbose for the treatment of diabetes mellitus. Berlin: Springer, 1988;79–91.
17. Sachse G. Acarbose in non-insulin-dependent diabetes – long-term studies in combination with oral agents. In: Creutzfeldt W, ed. Acarbose for the treatment of diabetes mellitus. Berlin: Springer, 1988;92–101.
18. Spengler M, Hänsel G, Boehme K. Efficacy of 6 months monotherapy with glucosidase inhibitor acarbose versus sulphonylurea glibenclamide on metabolic control of dietary treated type II diabetics. (a) Eur J Clin Invest 1989;19:A71. (b) Horm Metab Res (Suppl.) 1989; in press.
19. Rosak C. Acarbose treatment and sulfonylurea secondary failure. In: Creutzfeldt W, ed. Acarbose in the treatment of diabetes mellitus. Berlin: Springer, 1988;156–161.

Frontiers of diabetes research: current trends in non-insulin-dependent diabetes mellitus
K.G.M.M. Alberti and R. Mazze, editors

The role of inhibitors of lipolysis and lipid oxidation in the treatment of non-insulin-dependent diabetes

G.R. FULCHER and K.G.M.M. ALBERTI

Department of Medicine, University of Newcastle upon Tyne, The Medical School, Framlington Place,
Newcastle Upon Tyne, NE 1 4LP, U.K.

Introduction

Although abnormalities in carbohydrate metabolism are the hallmark of patients with non-insulin-dependent diabetes (NIDDM), it is clear that lipid regulation is also abnormal. Circulating non-esterified fatty acid levels (NEFA) are raised, and hyperlipidaemia is common [1]. Not only is this important as a risk factor for macrovascular disease [2], but there is both in vitro and in vivo evidence that abnormal levels of blood and tissue lipids may be an important contributing factor to insulin resistance, and therefore glycaemic control (vide infra). Treatment which lowers plasma lipids, in particular NEFA, could theoretically, therefore, provide additional therapeutic benefit in the diabetic. Thus glycaemic control may be improved, and morbidity and mortality from macrovascular disease may be lowered. In this paper the evidence for the glucose–fatty acid association in NIDDM will first be reviewed, followed by consideration of the role of nicotinic acid, an inhibitor of lipolysis, in the management of diabetes. Preliminary data on one of the newer antilipolytic agents, acipimox, will then be reviewed, and finally the potential use of the inhibitors of fatty acid metabolism will be briefly discussed.

Background

In vitro studies – the glucose–fatty acid cycle

In the early 1960s Randle et al. [3] proposed that substrate competition between fatty acids and glucose could produce insulin resistance in muscle. They demonstrated, in

298

vitro, that the addition of fatty acids to the perfusion medium of isolated rat muscle produced defects in glucose transport and phosphorylation, glycolysis and pyruvate oxidation. They found that these were similar to changes which were seen in the muscle of diabetic animals [4]. In further studies [5, 6] they demonstrated that an intracellular accumulation of by-products of fatty acid oxidation, namely citrate and acetyl-CoA, inhibited key enzymes of glycolysis and pyruvate oxidation. They concluded that 'accelerated fatty acid oxidation is a primary event in the development of these defects in glucose metabolism in the diabetic muscle' [7]. The regulatory effect of fatty acids on glucose metabolism is termed the glucose–fatty acid cycle [3], and its increased activity in NIDDM has been shown to contribute to (although probably not primarily cause) insulin resistance. It is probably worth adding that ketone bodies can have the same effect, and Newsholme has referred to it as the glucose–ketone body–fatty acid cycle [8].

In vivo studies – evidence in man

Abnormal levels of plasma non-esterified fatty acids (NEFA) are found in both obese and non-obese diabetic subjects. In studies from Reaven's group [9], both fasting and post-prandial changes in plasma glucose, NEFA and insulin were measured over an 8-hour period and compared with normal controls (Fig. 1). Both non-obese and obese subjects had a significant elevation of both plasma glucose and NEFA values, while insulin levels were similar. In addition a significant correlation was shown between fasting plasma NEFA levels, fasting plasma glucose, and endogenous hepatic glucose production. These findings have been extended recently by Groop et al. [10], who showed a positive correlation of NEFA oxidation and lipid oxidation with hepatic glucose production in the basal and hyperinsulinaemic state. These data indicate that defects in the regulation of both carbohydrate and fat metabolism coexist in patients with NIDDM, and that a causal relationship could exist between the two. The nature of this interaction has been further explored in vivo in both the basal and insulin-stimulated state.

The basal state
The relationship between fasting plasma NEFA levels, lipid oxidation, endogenous hepatic glucose production and fasting plasma glucose levels was examined in a controlled study of non-insulin-dependent diabetic subjects. Bogardus et al. [11] showed that a strong correlation exists between fasting plasma NEFA and lipid oxidation, and both fasting plasma glucose values and endogenous hepatic glucose production. They proposed that increased basal fatty acid oxidation stimulated gluconeogenesis, and therefore (in the presence of an increased supply of gluconeogenic precursors to the liver) basal hepatic glucose production.

The insulin-stimulated state

Ferrannini et al. [12] have studied normal subjects under hyperglycaemic and eugly-caemic, hyper-insulinaemic clamp conditions. They showed that an Intralipid infusion during the clamp caused an increase in plasma NEFA levels and decreased insulin-mediated glucose disposal. From these data, they extrapolated that in NIDDM, where circulating NEFA levels are chronically raised, substrate competition could explain insulin resistance in the insulin-stimulated state. They thus provided in vivo evidence, albeit indirect, for the operation of the glucose–fatty acid cycle in diabetic man.

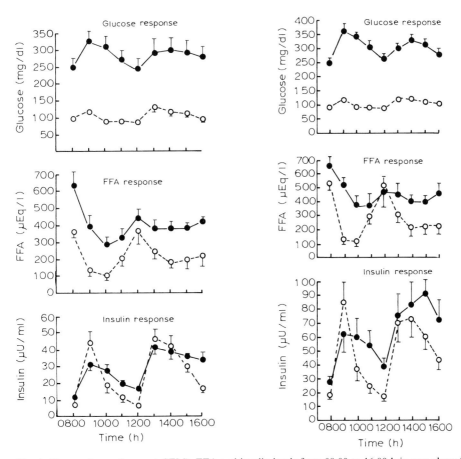

Fig. 1. Plasma glucose (mean ± SEM), FFA and insulin levels from 08.00 to 16.00 h in non-obese (left-hand panels) and obese (right-hand panels) individuals with either normal glucose tolerance (open circles) or NIDDM (closed circles). Breakfast was eaten at 08.00 and lunch at noon. Reproduced from Golay A, Swislocki ALM, Chen Y-DI, Reaven GM [9] with permission.

It is therefore clear that NEFA may worsen blood glucose control by two independent mechanisms. Firstly, in the basal state, reducing equivalents derived from fatty acid oxidation can drive gluconeogenesis and increase hepatic glucose production. Secondly, in the insulin-stimulated state, through mechanisms elucidated by Randle, peripheral glucose uptake into muscle is reduced, and insulin resistance is increased. Although it has been disputed that increased glucose–fatty acid cycle activity is the prime cause of insulin resistance in some or all non-insulin-dependent diabetics, e.g. normal-weight diabetics [13,14], it nevertheless appears to be a significant factor in many.

The role of inhibitors of lipolysis and lipid oxidation

It follows that drugs which can inhibit lipolysis and/or fatty acid oxidation may prove useful in lowering blood glucose, both by increasing peripheral glucose disposal and by decreasing the rate of gluconeogenesis (Table 1). For this to happen a number of conditions would have to be met. Firstly, adequate suppression of fatty acid oxidation, either directly or indirectly (via inhibition of lipolysis), must be achieved, and sustained. This is particularly relevant overnight, when insulin levels are lower and hepatic glucose production is highest. To obtain a significant improvement in fasting blood glucose (strongly correlated with hepatic glucose production) [11], control of either plasma NEFA production or fatty acid oxidation in the early hours of the morning may be vital. Secondly, in the insulin-stimulated state, when the supply of NEFA to muscle is decreased and glycolysis is stimulated, blood glucose should serve as the preferential alternative fuel. Thirdly, the fall in blood glucose should not be compensated by a counter-regulatory increase in glycogenolysis.

Inhibitors of lipolysis

To date, although many studies *have* been able to demonstrate an acute fall in blood

TABLE 1
Effects of inhibitors of lipid metabolism

Inhibition of hepatic gluconeogenesis
1. Inhibitors of carnitine acyltransferase (CAT)
2. Inhibitors of beta oxidation
3. Inhibitors of lipolysis (indirect)

Stimulation of peripheral glucose uptake
1. Inhibitors of lipolysis
2. ? Inhibitors of CAT and beta oxidation.

---

glucose concentration following antilipolytic therapy, results have been inconsistent, and the routine use of such treatment for the purpose of improving diabetic control has not become established medical practice. This may relate more to the characteristics of the drug most widely investigated, nicotinic acid, than to basic flaws in the theory.

Nicotinic acid

Of the many hypolipidaemic agents which have been shown to have a hypoglycaemic effect (Table 2), nicotinic acid is the most widely investigated [15]. It has been used for the treatment of hyperlipidaemia since the mid-1950s, and produces a rapid, although variable, suppression of plasma NEFA. Unfortunately it is limited by a short duration of action (1–2 h), a marked rebound in the drug washout period, and significant side-effects [16]. It is clear from this pharmacokinetic profile that either suppressed, normal or elevated plasma NEFA levels can accompany its use [17].

Acute effects on blood glucose   The acute effect of nicotinic acid on blood glucose has been variable, with decreased [18,19] and increased [20,21] levels reported following its use. The reason for this variability is not always clear. Plasma NEFA and ketone body levels were not always measured [20,21], and it is possible that a considerable inter-study variation in plasma NEFA and fatty acid oxidation occurred. Although this would explain the variable levels of blood glucose in terms of the glucose–fatty acid cycle, this can only be conjecture. Conclusions cannot readily be drawn from much of this early work regarding the effects of NEFA lowering on blood glucose levels. Recently, however, Reaven et al. [22] have shown a significant acute hypoglycaemic effect of nicotinic acid in streptozotocin-induced diabetic rats.

TABLE 2

Hypolipidaemic compounds with hypoglycaemic effects

---

1. Fibric acid derivatives
  Clofibrate
  Bezafibrate

2. Nicotinic acid related compounds
  Nicotinic acid (pyridine-3-carboxylic acid)
  Acipimox (5-methylpyrazine carboxylic acid 4-oxide)
  3,5-Dimethylpyrazole
  B-pyridylcarbinol

3. Others
  Phenylisopropyladenosine
  Glycodiazine

They were able to demonstrate both a decrease in hepatic glucose production, and an increase in peripheral glucose uptake, related to the antilipolytic effect of the drug. Although these results are encouraging they have not been accompanied by demonstrated benefit on long-term diabetes control in humans.

Long-term effects on blood glucose   In the long term nicotinic acid has most consistently been shown to aggravate glycaemic control, an effect that was universal in one group of patients reported by Molnar et al. [23]. Indeed, it has recently been suggested that nicotinic acid therapy should not be used in NIDDM patients because of worsened glycaemia and the development of hyperuricaemia [24]. This can be clearly explained when one examines the results of 24-hour metabolic profiles measured on patients taking this drug [25]. Plasma NEFA levels are clearly not decreased overall, either during the day, when acute rebound of NEFA cancels the suppressive effect of each dose, or overnight, when clearly elevated levels are seen, again in the drug washout period. The rise in plasma NEFA at this time is accompanied by a tendency to hyperglycaemia, even in normal subjects. This is consistent with the data of Molnar et al. [23], where elevation of both circulating fatty acids and ketone bodies accompanied the worsening of diabetes control. These findings provide supportive evidence (albeit indirect) for the operation of the glucose–fatty acid cycle in man, and indicate that incomplete suppression of fatty acids overnight is not sufficient if blood glucose is to be lowered. At the same time they explain and reinforce the unsuitability of nicotinic acid as a hypoglycaemic, hypolipidaemic agent in NIDDM.

Acipimox
Acipimox (Fig. 2) is a recently introduced, well-tolerated analogue of nicotinic acid. It is rapidly absorbed, achieving peak drug levels within 2 hours, and produces a sustained suppression of NEFA for up to 8 hours. Rebound of plasma NEFA levels is significantly less than with nicotinic acid [26].

The effect of lowering plasma NEFA values in non-insulin-dependent diabetic subjects has been studied with acipimox under a variety of experimental conditions, including both the insulin-stimulated and basal states.

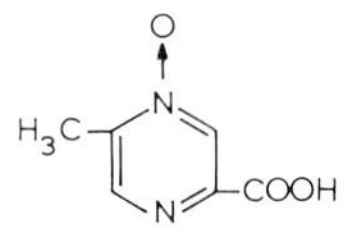

Acipimox
5-methylpyrazinecarboxylic acid 4-oxide

Fig. 2. Structural formula of acipimox.

Effects of acipimox on blood glucose in the insulin-stimulated state   Studies performed in the insulin-stimulated state include an assessment of the effect of NEFA lowering on the oral glucose tolerance test (OGTT), the glucose-insulin-infusion test (GIIT) and the glycaemic response to a mixed meal. A consistent and significant improvement in glucose tolerance, insulin sensitivity (Piatti and Monti, unpublished observations) and the glycaemic response to a mixed meal (Fulcher et al., unpublished observation) has been found. In these studies complete suppression of NEFA was obtained, which persisted throughout the tests. These findings are consistent with the theory that a decrease in NEFA availability results in increased glucose utilization and improves glycaemic control. In a further study, overnight metabolic profiles were measured in non-obese diabetic subjects, following acipimox and a mixed meal. Mean overnight plasma NEFA levels were lower, although complete suppression was not achieved. Significantly, however, no rebound occurred. In addition the mean 12-hour blood glucose concentration was also significantly lower, although fasting blood glucose was unchanged.

Effects of acipimox on blood glucose in the basal state   Although some studies in diabetic rats have demonstrated that nicotinic acid can profoundly lower fasting blood glucose levels [22], this has not been a universal finding, and has not been clearly established in man. On the contrary, Balasse et al. [27] demonstrated that when plasma NEFA levels were lowered with nicotinic acid, although peripheral uptake of glucose was increased, a compensatory increase in hepatic glucose production occurred and blood glucose was unchanged. They proposed that hormonal changes associated with antilipolysis could have mediated this response, and the finding that a rise in both glucagon [27] and cortisol [16] has been shown to accompany antilipolysis is consistent with this proposal. An increase in hepatic glycogenolysis has been demonstrated to occur with nicotinic acid by a number of authors [18,19,28], although this was not necessarily accompanied by a rise in blood glucose [19]. This indicates that peripheral

TABLE 3
Fatty acid oxidation inhibitors

1. Carnitine acyltransferase inhibitors
2-Tetradecylglycidate
Methylpalmoxirate
Etomoxir
POCA

2. Beta-oxidation inhibitors
Hypoglycin
Pent-4-enoate
Valproate

uptake can occur to a greater extent than the compensatory rise in glucose production. To explore this relationship further seven obese diabetic subjects were studied overnight. Acipimox (250 mg) was administered at 7 p.m., 1 a.m. and 6 a.m., and fasting (6 a.m.) plasma NEFA and blood glucose levels were measured. A significant decrease in both fasting NEFA and blood glucose values was found. One can extrapolate from these data that it is essential for antilipolytic agents to be completely active overnight, and sustained-release preparations may be necessary if a significant long-term improvement in blood glucose is to be achieved.

Inhibitors of fatty acid oxidation

Drugs which inhibit fatty acid oxidation can be broadly separated into two groups (Table 3): first, those that inhibit the transport of fatty acid across the mitochondrial membrane (carnitine acyltransferase 1 (CAT1) inhibitors), and second, those that inhibit beta oxidation at various intermediate steps.

Inhibitors of beta oxidation

Drugs in this latter category include hypoglycin, pent-4-enoate and valproate. None of these is a clinically useful hypoglycaemic agent. Hypoglycin and pent-4-enoate are poisons, while valproate has only minimal efficacy at therapeutic doses [30].

Inhibitors of carnitine acyltransferase

The hypoglycaemic effect of drugs which inhibit carnitine acyltransferase 1 (CAT1) has been investigated for a number of years. Such agents include 2-tetradecylglycidate [31], methylpalmoxirate [32], 2-[5-(4-chlorophenyl)pentyl]-oxirane-2-carboxylate (POCA) [33–35] and etomoxir [36]. These drugs act by decreasing the transfer of fatty acids into the mitochondria, thereby reducing fatty acid oxidation, the generation of reducing equivalents and hence, in the liver, gluconeogenesis. Methylpalmoxirate has been shown to decrease plasma glucose, lessen ketosis, and cause a depletion of liver glycogen in diabetic animals [37], and a similar effect has been shown for POCA [34]. Studies in streptozotocin-diabetic rats have shown that the acute use of etomoxir is accompanied by a striking decrease in plasma glucose, which is further lowered by the addition of nicotinic acid [38]. Both plasma NEFA and triglyceride levels rose when etomoxir was used alone, but in combination with nicotinic acid this did not occur. Etomoxir alone in normal man produced similar changes, but a fall in blood glucose did not occur [37]. The rise in plasma NEFA and triglyceride values is a worrying side-effect of such agents and obviously limits their usefulness as sole agents in the treatment of NIDDM. The idea of combining an inhibitor of lipolysis with an inhibitor of lipid oxidation is an interesting therapeutic approach, and worthy of further investigation.

Conclusion

Increased NEFA oxidation may significantly interfere with glucose metabolism and worsen diabetic control. Agents which lower NEFA have been shown to lower blood glucose values in the insulin-stimulated state under a variety of experimental conditions. Complete overnight suppression of NEFA can lower fasting blood glucose, in spite of the fact that an acute counter-regulatory hormonal response to antilipolysis has been demonstrated with nicotinic acid. Drugs which inhibit lipid oxidation significantly lower blood glucose in rodents, but further research is needed in man. It has yet to be firmly established that long-term treatment with NEFA-lowering agents significantly improves diabetic control. The value of such an approach may have been confounded by the early use of nicotinic acid, whose unfavourable metabolic profile has made it an unsuitable agent to use in this context. Although the role of antilipolytic and antilipid oxidation therapy for blood glucose control is yet to be clearly defined, nevertheless it is likely that correction of the lipid abnormalities that characterize NIDDM will have a favourable effect on carbohydrate metabolism.

References

1. Reaven GM, Greenfield MS. Diabetic hypertriglyceridemia. Evidence for three clinical syndromes. Diabetes 1981;30, Suppl 12:66–75.
2. Brown WV. Diabetes mellitus and arteriosclerosis: risk factors, mechanisms, and management. In: Peterson CM, ed. Diabetes management in the '80s. New York: Praeger 1982;Ch. 5:40–55.
3. Randle PJ, Garland PB, Hales CN, Newsholme EA. The glucose-fatty acid cycle. Its role in insulin sensitivity and the metabolic disturbances of diabetes mellitus. Lancet 1963;i:785–789.
4. Randle PJ, Newsholme EA, Garland PB. Regulation of glucose uptake by muscle. 8. Effects of fatty acids, ketone bodies and pyruvate, and alloxan diabetes and starvation, on the uptake and metabolic fate of glucose in rat heart and diaphragm muscles. Biochem J 1964;93:652–665.
5. Garland PB, Newsholme EA, Randle PJ. Regulation of glucose uptake by muscle. Effects of fatty acids and ketone bodies, and of alloxan diabetes and starvation, on pyruvate metabolism and on lactate/pyruvate and L-glycerol-3-phosphate/dihydroxyacetone phosphate concentration ratios in rat heart and rat diaphragm muscles. Biochem J 1964;93:665–678.
6. Garland PB, Randle PJ. Regulation of glucose uptake by muscle. 10. Effects of alloxan diabetes, starvation, hypophysectomy and adrenalectomy, and of fatty acids, ketone bodies and pyruvate, on the glycerol output and concentrations of free fatty acids, long chain fatty acyl-coenzyme A, glycerol phosphate and citrate-cycle intermediates in rat heart and diaphragm muscles. Biochem J 1964;93:678–687.

306

7. Randle PJ, Garland PB, Hales CN, Newsholme EA, Denton RM, Pogson CI. Interactions of metabolism and the physiological role of insulin. Rec Prog Horm Res 1966;22:1–44.

8. Newsholme EA, Leech AR. Integration of carbohydrate and lipid metabolism. Biochemistry for the medical sciences. London: Wiley, 1988;Ch. 8:336–356.

9. Golay A, Swislocki ALM, Chen Y-DI, Reaven GM. Relationships between plasma free fatty acid concentration, endogenous glucose production, and fasting hyperglycaemia in normal and non-insulin-dependent diabetic individuals. Metabolism 1987;36:692–696.

10 Groop LC, Bonadonna RC, Delprato S, et al. Glucose and free fatty acid metabolism in non-insulin dependent diabetes mellitus. Evidence for multiple sites of insulin resistance. J Clin Invest 1989;84:205–213.

11. Bogardus C, Lillioja S, Howard BV, Reaven G, Mott D. Relationships between insulin secretion, insulin action, and fasting plasma glucose concentration in nondiabetic and non-insulin dependent diabetic subjects. J Clin Invest 1984;74:1238–1245.

12. Ferrannini E, Barrett EJ, Bevilacqua S, DeFronzo RA. Effect of fatty acids on glucose production and utilisation in man. J Clin Invest 1983;72:1737–1747.

13. DeFronzo RA. The triumvirate: B-cell, muscle, liver. A collusion responsible for NIDDM. Diabetes 1988;37:667–687.

14. Golay A, DeFronzo RA, Ferrannini E, et al. Oxidative and non-oxidative glucose metabolism in non-obese Type 2 (non-insulin dependent) diabetic patients. Diabetologia 1988;31:585–591.

15. Gey KF, Carlson LA, eds. The metabolic effects of nicotinic acid and its derivatives. Bern: Huber, 1970.

16. Pereira JN. The plasma free fatty acid rebound induced by nicotinic acid. J Lip Res 1967;8:239–244.

17. Carlson LA. Nicotinic acid: its metabolism and its effects on plasma free fatty acids. In: Gey KF, Carlson LA, eds. The metabolic effects of nicotinic acid and its derivatives. Bern: Huber, 1970; 157–165.

18. Root MA, Ashmore J. The hypoglycaemic activity of nicotinic acid in rats. Naunyn Schmeidebergs Arch Pharmacol Exp Pathol 1964;248:117–123.

19. Ammon HPT, Estler CJ, Heim F. Alteration of carbohydrate metabolism in liver, skeletal muscle and brain by nicotinic acid in mice. In: Gey KF, Carlson LA, eds. Metabolic effects of nicotinic acid and its derivatives. Bern: Huber, 1970;799–809.

20. Dzedin T, Svedmyr N, Lundholm L. Influence of nicotinic acid on the carbohydrate metabolism: relationship with adrenergic receptors. In: Gey KF, Carlson LA, eds. Metabolic effects of nicotinic acid and its derivatives. Bern: Huber, 1970;747–751.

21. Gaut ZN, Solomon HM, Miller ON. The influece of antilipemic doses of nicotinic acid on carbohydrate tolerance and plasma insulin levels in man. In: Gey KF, Carlson LA, eds. Metabolic effects of nicotinic acid and its derivatives. Bern: Huber, 1970;923–927.

22. Reaven GM, Chang H, Ho H, Jeng C-Y, Hoffman BB. Lowering of plasma glucose in diabetic rats by antilipolytic agents. Am J Physiol 1988;254:E23–E30.

23. Molnar GD, Berge KG, Rosevear JW, McGuckin WF, Achor WP. The effect of nicotinic acid in diabetes mellitus. Metabolism 1964;13:181–190.

24. Garg A. Nicotinic acid therapy for treatment of dyslipidaemia in non-insulin dependent diabetes mellitus. Advantages and drawbacks. Atherosclerosis 1988;8:581a.

25. Froberg SO, Boberg J, Carlson LA, Eriksson M. Effect of nicotinic acid on the diurnal variation of plasma levels of glucose levels of glucose, free fatty acids, triglycerides and cholesterol and of urinary excretion of catecholamines. In: Gey KF, Carlson LA, eds. Metabolic effects of nicotinic acid and its derivatives. Bern: Huber, 1970;167–181.

26. Fuccella LM, Goldaniga G, Lovisolo P, et al. Inhibition of lipolysis by nicotinic acid and by acipimox. Clin Pharmacol Ther 1980;28:790–795.

27. Balasse EO, Neef MA. Influence of nicotinic acid on the rates of turnover and oxidation of plasma glucose in man. Metabolism 1973;22:1193–1204.

28. Luyckx AS, Lefebvre PJ. Arguments for a regulation of pancreatic glucagon secretion by circulating plasma free fatty acids. Proc Soc Exp Biol Med 1970;133:524–528.

29. Nikkila EA, Pykalisto O. Induction of adipose tissue lipoprotein lipase by nicotinic acid. Biochim Biophys Acta 1968;152:421–423.

30. Sherratt HSA, Bartlett K, Turnbull DM. Four hypoglycaemic compounds that inhibit beta oxidation: 2-[5-(4-chlorophenyl)pentyl]oxirane-2-carboxylate (POCA), hypoglycin, pent-4-enoate and valproate: a comparison of their mechanisms of action. In: Kabara JJ, ed. The pharmacological effects of lipids. Champaign, IL: American Oil Chem. Soc. 1985;Vol. 2:247–262.

31. Tutwiler GF, Kirsch T, Mohrbacher R, Ho W. Pharmacological profile of methyl 2-tetradecylglycidate (McN 3716) – an orally effective hypoglycaemic agent. Metabolism 1978;27:1539–1556.

32. Tutwiler GF, Dellevigne P. Action of the oral hypoglycaemic agent 2-tetraglycidic acid on hepatic fatty acid oxidation and gluconeogenesis. J Biol Chem 1979; 254:2935–2941.

33. Wolf HPO, Engel DW. Decrease of fatty acid oxidation, ketogenesis and gluconeogenesis in isolated perfused rat liver by phenylalkyl oxirane carboxylate (B 807-27) due to inhibition of CPT 1 (EC 2.3.1.21). Eur J Biochem 1985;146:359–363.

34. Wolf HPO, Eistetter K, Ludwig G. Phenylalkyl oxirane carboxylic acids, a new class of hypoglycaemic substances: hypoglycaemic and hypoletonaemic effects of sodium 2-[5-(4-chlorophenyl)-pentyl]oxirane-2-carboxylate (B 807-27) in fasted animals. Diabetologia 1982;22:456–463.

35. Turnbull DM, Bartlett K, Younan IM, Sherratt HSA. The effects of 2-[5-(4-chlorophenyl)pentyl]oxirane-2-carbonyl-CoA on mitochondrial oxidations. Biochem Pharmacol 1984;33:475–481.

36. Wolf HPO, Eistetter K, Ludwig O. Phenyloxirane carboxylic acids, a new class of hypoglycaemic substances. Diabetologia 1981;21:344.

37. Young JC, Treadway JL, Fades EI, Caslin RF. Effects of oral hypoglycaemic agent methylpalmoxirate on exercise capacity of streptozotocin diabetic rats. Diabetes 1986;35:744–748.

38. Reaven GM, Chang H, Hoffman BB. Additive hypoglycaemic effects of drugs that modify free-fatty acid metabolism by different mechanisms in rats with streptozotocin-induced diabetes. Diabetes 1988;37:28–32.

39. Selby PL, Bartlett K, Sherratt HSA, Alberti KGMM. Prolonged inhibition of ketogenesis in man by etomoxir. Diabetologia 1987;30:581A.

© 1989 Elsevier Science Publishers B.V. (Biomedical Division)
Frontiers of diabetes research: current trends in non-insulin-dependent diabetes mellitus
K.G.M.M.Alberti and R. Mazze, editors

The clinical significance of insulin resistance in NIDDM: studies with continuous subcutaneous insulin infusion

EROL CERASI[1], BENJAMIN GLASER[1], GRAZIANO DEL RIO[3],
SHLOMO SASSON[2] and LUCIANO DELLA CASA[3]

Departments of [1]Endocrinology and Metabolism and
[2]Pharmacology, Hebrew University Hadassah Medical Center, Jerusalem, Israel and
[3]Department of Metabolic Diseases, University of Modena Medical School, Modena, Italy

Introduction

For the last decade-and-a-half, diabetologists have been exposed to massive amounts of data which suggest that severe insulin resistance is the main trait of type 2, non-insulin-dependent diabetes (NIDDM). In addition to implications regarding the pathogenesis of the disease, this has led to the adoption of negative attitudes regarding insulin treatment in NIDDM. Indeed, if the data from hyperinsulinemic clamp studies can be extrapolated to the clinical situation of NIDDM, only formidable doses of insulin should be able to reduce the blood glucose in these patients.

We and others [1–3] have consistently presented data indicating that insulin output is severely reduced in NIDDM, and suggested that the alleged hyperinsulinemia of this disease is a reflection of the hyperglycemia, rather than the indication of hyper-function of beta-cells [4]. The recent demonstration by Hales and co-workers [5] that much of the circulating insulin-like material in NIDDM consists of proinsulin and its cleavage intermediates certainly reinforces our view that NIDDM is a hypoinsu-linemic state.

The above considerations do not negate the presence of insulin resistance in NIDDM. In this paper evidence will be presented which points to the possibility that such insulin resistance results from the response of a physiological regulatory mecha-nism to hyperglycemia. It will be shown that this phenomenon is rapidly reversible, allowing optimal control of blood glucose with moderate doses of insulin in lean as well as obese NIDDM patients.

Correspondence: Prof. E. Cerasi, Department of Endocrinology and Metabolism, Hadassah University Hospital, 91120 Jerusalem, Israel.

310

Material and methods

Patients

The main characteristics of the patients studied are shown in Table 1. Group I consisted of 10 Italian patients with newly diagnosed NIDDM. Despite several weeks of diet treatment, they were hyperglycemic on acceptance to the study. Seven were obese (BMI 27–33), while three had normal body weight (BMI 20–24). None had ever received insulin or oral antidiabetic agents. Group II comprised 11 Israeli NIDDM patients with secondary failure with oral agents. Seven were obese (BMI 26–32), four lean (BMI 20–23). NIDDM was diagnosed 1–25 years before the study. None could be adequately controlled with maximal dose oral treatment (20 mg glibenclamide and 1700 mg metformin daily). Six patients were on conventional insulin treatment, but were still grossly hyperglycemic. Two patients had previously received insulin; the treatment was abandoned because of persistent hyperglycemia. At admission, all patients were poorly controlled as judged by the high fasting blood glucose (240–470 mg/dl; 13.3–26.1 mmol/l) and HbA_{1c} levels (10.7–20.5%). All medication was discontinued several days before the study.

Clinical studies

All patients were hospitalized and given a weight-maintaining diet (ca. 30 kcal/kg). Blood glucose control was determined by measuring glucose before and 2 h after each meal and at 23.00 h for 2 days (7 determinations per day). Following this 2-day control period, insulin treatment by continuous subcutaneous infusion (CSII) was initiated in Group I. Group II patients were further investigated before CSII by i.v. glucose infusion test, and i.v. glucagon test, performed on two consecutive days. In the glucose infusion test, an i.v. bolus of glucose (0.3 g/kg) was injected rapidly; immedi-

TABLE 1
Characteristics of NIDDM patients

		n	Age (years)	BMI (kg/m²)	FBG (mg/dl)	HbA_{1c} (%)
New-onset	Obese	7	52 ± 3	29 ± 0.7	218 ± 16	10.7 ± 1.0
(Group I)	Lean	3	52 ± 3	22 ± 1.2	211 ± 26	12.0 ± 0.9
Secondary failure	Obese	7	53 ± 4	29 ± 0.9	306 ± 25	14.0 ± 1.3
(Group II)	Lean	4	59 ± 3	21 ± 0.8	321 ± 10	12.4 ± 1.6

ately thereafter, a 10 mg/min infusion of glucose was started and continued for 60 min. Multiple plasma samples were obtained for glucose and insulin determinations over 150 min. C-peptide response to glucagon was determined after an overnight fast. Plasma glucose concentrations were normalized before the test using i.v. insulin or CSII. Insulin was withdrawn at least 45 min before glucagon administration. After obtaining two basal blood samples, 1 mg of glucagon was rapidly injected i.v. Glucose and C-peptide were measured 2, 5, 10, 15, 20 and 30 min after the injection. These tests were repeated after discontinuation of CSII.

In both groups, near normoglycemia was achieved by CSII following 2–4 days of adaptation. CSII was continued for a further 14 days; thus all patients were near-normoglycemic for at least 2 weeks. Near normoglycemia is defined as fasting blood glucose (measured from capillary blood with a glucometer) < 110 mg/dl (6.1 mmol/l), and mean of 7 daily measurements < 140 mg/dl (7.8 mmol/l).

In vitro studies

Young male albino rats (40–70 g) of the Sabra strain (Hebrew University, Jerusalem) were maintained at constant temperature (23°C) with a 12-h light-dark cycle. They received standard laboratory chow and water ad libitum. Their serum glucose concentrations at death ranged between 150 and 180 mg/dl (8.3–10.0 mmol/l). The rate of glucose utilization through the glycolytic pathway in isolated rat soleus muscles was assessed with [5-^{3}H]glucose according to the method described by Zawalich and Matschinsky [6]. The rats were killed by cervical dislocation, and the soleus muscles were quickly removed and incubated in 10 ml DMEM supplemented with glucose at the desired concentration. The incubation media were continuously gassed with O_2/CO_2 (95:5 vol/vol) in a metabolic shaker (40 cycles/min) at 37°C. At the end of the first incubation period (2.5–3.0 h), each muscle was washed for 5 min at 37°C in glucose-free Krebs-Ringer bicarbonate buffer (KRB, pH 7.4) supplemented with 10 mmol/l HEPES. It was then transferred to 0.5 ml KRB with 5 μCi [5-^{3}H]glucose and unlabeled glucose (5.0 mmol/l). The [5-^{3}H]glucose was dried before the assay to remove ^3H_2O. At the end of a 5-min incubation the muscle was quickly removed, blotted lightly, frozen in liquid N_2, and stored at -80°C until assayed. The content of ^3H_2O in the incubation medium was determined as previously described [6].

The effect of glucose on muscle hexose transport was studied in detail using the rat skeletal myocyte line L8, originally established by D. Yaffe, Weizmann Institute of Science (Rehovot, Israel) and obtained through his courtesy. The cells were grown as previously described [7]. In brief, mononucleated myogenic cells were plated in 35-mm gelatin-coated tissue culture plates (10^5 cells/plate) in Waymouth medium supplemented with 15% (v/v) fetal calf serum. In order to investigate the effect of varying glucose concentrations, the medium was changed 18–20 h before the experiment to glucose-free DMEM containing serum supplemented with glucose at the desired concentration. The myocytes in culture were then rinsed 8 times with 2 ml KRB. After rinsing, 1 ml KRB containing 1.0 μCi 2-[^{3}H]deoxyglucose (dGlc) and unlabeled dGlc (0.5 mmol/l) was added to the plates (in triplicates). After 5 min at room temperature the incubation was terminated by aspirating the medium and rinsing the cells 5 times with 2 ml ice-cold KRB. After digestion of the cells with 1 ml 1 N NaOH (60 min at 37°C) and neutralization with concentrated HCl, aliquots of 800 μl were taken for liquid scintillation counting. Extracellular space was determined in parallel incubations with 1.0 μCi [^{14}C]sucrose. The data were calculated on the basis of cell number with correction for extracellular space. Cytochalasin B (5–10 μM) effectively inhibited the uptake of dGlc when added before the hexose. Usually the noninhibitable uptake of dGlc was similar to the dGlc content of the extracellular space as determined by [^{14}C]sucrose.

Analytical methods

Plasma glucose was determined with a Beckman glucose analyser (Fullerton, CA). Insulin levels were determined by double-antibody RIA. Labelled insulin (> 300 μCi/ μg) was purchased from CIS (St-Quentin-Yvelines, France), human standard insulin from Novo Research Laboratories (Bagsvaerd, Denmark) and antibodies from Linco Research Inc. (Eureca, MO). The minimal detectable concentration was 1.2 μU/ml; intra- and inter-assay CV were 5.2% and 7.3%, respectively. Plasma C-peptide concentrations were measured by radioimmunoassay using the antibody M 1221 and other reagents purchased from Novo. Intra- and inter-assay CV were 5% and 7.3%, respectively. Insulin antibodies which were present in some patients did not interfere with the C-peptide assay, but did render the insulin determinations unreliable.

Statistical methods

Data are expressed as means $\pm$ SEM. Paired samples were compared using the Wilcoxon Rank test or the paired t-test, whereas unpaired samples were compared using the Mann-Whitney U-test.

Results and discussion

Increasing clinical evidence suggests that the insulin resistance and reduced peripheral glucose utilization of the diabetic may be related to hyperglycemia itself. However, in vivo data are difficult to interpret since any modification of the patients' blood glucose is always accompanied by profound changes in the hormonal and metabolic

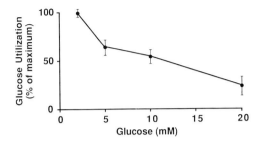

Fig. 1. Influence of preincubation glucose concentration on glucose utilization of skeletal muscle. Rat so-leus muscles were incubated in the presence of the glucose concentrations shown for 3 h at 37°C. The muscles were then washed for 5 min in glucose-free KRB, and the glucose utilization rate assessed with [5-³H]glucose in the presence of 5 mmol/l glucose as described previously (6, 9). Results are presented as per cent of glycolysis in muscles preincubated with 2 mmol/l glucose, which was 85.5 ± 4.3 nmol/g·min⁻¹. Mean ± SEM of 3–5 experiments.

milieu of the peripheral tissues. For this reason, we decided to investigate the effect of modifications of the glucose concentration alone on the in vitro glucose metabo-lism of the main peripheral tissue, skeletal muscle.

Our studies showed that glucose itself indeed has a major regulatory role on muscle glucose metabolism, as shown in Figs. 1 and 2 (for full details, the reader should see Refs. 8 and 9). Using the isolated rat soleus muscle, it could be demonstrated that the glucose concentration of the incubation medium had a profound effect on the rate of glucose utilization (Fig. 1): for each mmol/l increase in the glucose concentra-tion, glycolysis diminished by ca. 3%. Translated into the clinical situation (and as-suming that human muscle behaves like rat muscle), these findings suggest that by

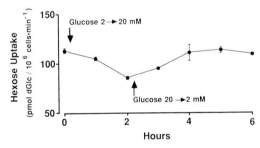

Fig. 2. Time-scale of the glucose effect on muscle glucose uptake. L8 myocytes, grown to confluency, were incubated overnight in DMEM containing 2 mmol/l glucose. At 0 time the medium was changed to DMEM with 20 mmol/l glucose. After a further 2-h incubation, the glucose was again changed to 2 mmol/l. At the end of each incubation period, batches of culture dishes were rinsed 8 times, and the [³H]deoxyglu-cose uptake rate was determined as described [8]. Means ± SEM of three experiments (where not shown, the SE was smaller than the size of the symbol).

the sheer virtue of hyperglycemia a NIDDM patient with blood glucose levels in the 300–400 mg/dl (16.7–22.2 mmol/l) range may reduce his peripheral glucose utilization by ca. 40%. We have demonstrated in extensive studies that the reduction of glucose utilization under these conditions is entirely accountable by the reduction of glucose transport into the muscle cells, rather than by modification of the phosphorylation and further metabolism of the hexose [8]. Furthermore, only the maximal velocity of transport was modulated by glucose, the affinity of transporters for glucose remaining constant [8]. From such studies we concluded that glucose regulates the number of glucose transporters on muscle cell membranes with a finely tuned negative feed-back system. This effect of glucose is specific for glucose transport, since amino acid transport into muscle was not influenced by the hyperglycemic incubation milieu [8,9].

The mechanism by which hyperglycemia down-regulates the glucose uptake and metabolism of muscle is not clear, and is currently under intensive investigation by our group. Of importance for NIDDM, however, is the fact that this glucose effect is fully reversible. Fig. 2 presents results of in vitro experiments which emphasize the dynamics of the glucose autoregulation. The glucose uptake of muscle cells was up-regulated by exposing the cultures to hypoglycemic levels of glucose (2 mmol/l), then changing the media to hyperglycemic levels (20 mmol/l). As shown in Fig. 2, within 2 h a significant reduction of the glucose transport was apparent (other experiments show that the maximal effect of hyperglycemia expresses itself following 4–5 h of exposure). At this time the glucose level was reduced back to 2 mmol/l; it is seen clearly that the transport-reducing effect of hyperglycemia was totally reversed within 2 h.

It may be questioned to what extent results from in vitro studies on rodent tissues or cell lines represent the complex events that occur in vivo in man under physiological and pathological conditions. Despite this concern, it is tempting to suggest that the in vitro studies described above predict the insulin resistance and reduced peripheral glucose utilization of NIDDM to be readily reversed (by up-regulating the muscle glucose uptake) once hyperglycemia is controlled. Since our studies in NIDDM show these patients to be low insulin responders [1,2] we also hypothesized that, if given in a physiological mode, modest doses of insulin should be sufficient to control the blood glucose. These ideas were tested by attempting to induce near-normoglycemia in NIDDM patients with the help of CSII.

Group I patients, who were newly diagnosed NIDDM subjects, responded remarkably well to CSII despite the presence of obesity. A dramatic improvement in blood glucose levels was observed within 1–4 days of initiating CSII, almost normal values being obtained with continued treatment (e.g., on day 17 fasting blood glucose was 83 ± 4 mg/dl (4.6 ± 0.2 mmol/l), while the mean of the highest postprandial level recorded in each subject was 157 ± 8 mg/dl (8.7 ± 0.4 mmol/l)). This is reflected in the mean blood glucose values (mean of 7 determinations daily) presented in Fig.

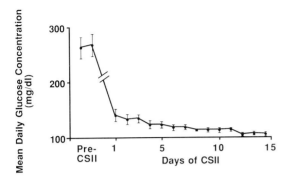

Fig. 3. Effect of CSII therapy on blood glucose control in new-onset NIDDM. Group I patients were monitored by 7 daily blood glucose measurements, the mean of which is shown. After two days without treatment, CSII was initiated (broken curve). Day 1 is the first day where mean blood glucose level was below 140 mg/dl (7.8 mmol/l) (usually 2–4 days after initiation of CSII). Values are means ± SEM of daily mean blood glucose levels in 10 patients.

3: most values were below 125 mg/dl (6.9 mmol/l). Table 2 gives the mean daily insulin dose needed to achieve the degree of blood glucose control. It appears quite clearly that modest amounts of insulin (in the vicinity of 0.5 U/kg/24 h, divided equally between a constant basal dose and three pre-meal bolus doses) were sufficient. We wish to draw attention to the fact that normal subjects secrete 0.6–1.2 U/kg/24 h insulin, and that most lean IDDM subjects require 0.6–0.7 U/kg/24 h by CSII, and significantly more by conventional injections [10–12].

Group II, which consisted of NIDDM patients with secondary failure with oral antidiabetics, and where a substantial proportion of subjects had previously received

TABLE 2

CSII insulin dose at beginning and end of normoglycemic period in NIDDM

| | | | Daily insulin dose | | | |
| | | | Initial | | Final | |
		n	U	U/kg	U	U/kg
New-onset	Obese	7	42 ± 6	0.52 ± 0.09	38 ± 6	0.49 ± 0.09
(Group I)	Lean	3	37 ± 9	0.55 ± 0.09	29 ± 6	0.43 ± 0.04
Secondary failure	Obese	7	69 ± 12	0.88 ± 0.12	69 ± 13	0.87 ± 0.13
(Group II)	Lean	4	42 ± 15	0.65 ± 0.07	38 ± 13	0.60 ± 0.03

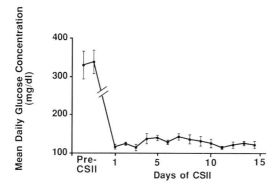

Fig. 4. Effect of CSII therapy on blood glucose control in NIDDM patients with secondary failure. Group II patients were treated as group I patients (see text of Fig. 3). Means ± SEM of daily mean blood glucose levels in 11 patients.

conventional insulin treatment, also responded to CSII with excellent blood glucose control, as shown in Fig. 4. The insulin dose needed to obtain near-normoglycemia was somewhat higher in this group (about 0.6–0.9 U/kg/24 h; Table 2), but still comparable to the normal insulin production rate, and not very different from doses used in insulin-dependent diabetics. We assume that the difference in insulin requirements between Groups I and II is due to the presence of insulin antibodies in many Group II patients, and to the fact that the latter were some severely diabetic (for full details, see Ref. 13).

In both groups of patients, CSII treatment was given without caloric restriction. In spite of this, body weight remained constant in Group I over the nearly 3 weeks of insulin administration (body weight change: + 0.2 ± 0.17 kg). Group II patients had more severe diabetes; in these, CSII led to a modest weight gain (+ 1.9 ± 0.8 kg). This is similar to findings in Type 1 diabetics given intensified insulin treatment, and probably reflects the reversal of catabolic metabolism [14].

The above results in two populations of mildly obese NIDDM patients, with different ethnic backgrounds, dietary habits and degrees of severity of diabetes, clearly demonstrate that whatever insulin resistance prevails in NIDDM, it is not of the magnitude to prevent induction of normoglycemia by insulin, at least when given in a near-physiological mode of treatment (CSII, possibly also multiple injection regimens). If one takes into consideration that most of our patients were obese, where in addition to the post-receptor defect of NIDDM decreased sensitivity to insulin due to obesity per se is expected to be present, it is striking that as low doses of insulin as the ones used here could regulate the blood glucose level. This is in contradiction with the findings from many euglycemic hyperinsulinemic clamp studies in NIDDM

[15–17]. This contradiction is presumably due to two facts. (1) The post-receptor defect is a secondary event generated by hyperglycemia; following insulin administration and reduction of the hyperglycemia, the resistance is rapidly reversed, allowing for the full effect of insulin therapy. (2) NIDDM patients are hypoinsulinemic [1–5] and therefore, even when obese, relatively insulin-sensitive; hence the excellent response of blood glucose to modest insulin doses. This latter statement is obviously in discord with the present dogma of insulin resistance in NIDDM; we do believe, however, that future clinical studies may clarify to what extent insulin efficiency is modified in diabetes, and what its implications are for the treatment of NIDDM.

Over recent years much interest has been focused on the so-called toxic effect of glucose on the pancreatic beta-cell [17–19]. This issue was investigated in our Group II patients. These severe NIDDM patients had markedly impaired beta-cell function as evidenced by low mean C-peptide levels in the face of very high mean blood glucose levels over the day (Fig. 5), low C-peptide response to glucagon (Table 3) and minimal first-phase insulin response to i.v. glucose administration (Table 3). These parameters of beta-cell function were re-evaluated following two weeks of normoglycemia, after cessation of CSII. As shown in Fig. 5, in the absence of any treatment, the mean blood glucose of the daily profiles was now significantly lower, C-peptide was higher, and the C-peptide-to-glucose ratio, which gives a measure of beta-cell sensitivity to glucose, was twice as high. In a similar fashion, C-peptide response to glucagon was significantly higher (Table 3). Finally, following the period of normoglycemia, a small but significant first-phase insulin response to glucose reappeared (Table 3). We wish to stress that while the demonstrated improvement of beta-cell function was significant, the CSII-induced normoglycemic period did not normalize the insulin secretory capacity in these patients (for further data on the effect of CSII on beta-cell function, see Ref. 13). However, the improvement in insulin output was

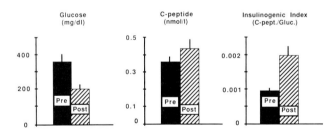

Fig. 5. Effect of normoglycemia on daily profiles of glucose and C-peptide in NIDDM patients with secondary failure. Following CSII treatment (see Fig. 4) insulin was discontinued, and the patients were monitored for 2 further days without treatment. Each bar gives the mean (+ SEM) of 7 daily determinations (pre- and postprandial) of plasma glucose and C-peptide for 2 days before (Pre) and after (Post) CSII in 11 patients. Insulinogenic index refers to the ratios of C-peptide over plasma glucose levels for each sampling time.

TABLE 3

Effect of normoglycemia on beta-cell function in NIDDM

		Incremental insulin response (mU/l)	Incremental C-peptide response (nmol/l)
Glucose	Before CSII	11 ± 3.8	0.11 ± 0.03
		(n = 4)	(n = 5)
	After CSII	31 ± 19	0.28 ± 0.06
Glucagon	Before CSII		0.13 ± 0.05
			(n = 8)
	After CSII		0.21 ± 0.03

important enough to enable 6 out of 11 patients with demonstrated secondary failure with oral agents to be controlled without insulin for 1–20 months after termination of the study.

Conclusions

It seems ironical that studies spanning a quarter of a century [1–5, 20] should be necessary to convince diabetologists that in all stages of NIDDM beta-cell function is deficient, and that hyperinsulinemia proper probably seldom occurs [5] in this disorder. We feel our claims that NIDDM starts on the basis of reduced insulin output are fully justified [21,22]. Insulin resistance, which has been the center of so much attention over the past 15 years, seems to us to be of secondary and perhaps minor importance against the background of the above data and discussion. We are far from denying the beneficial effects of measures that increase insulin sensitivity (weight reduction, exercise) in NIDDM; however, we feel those measures are effective as long as insulin output remains low. When insulin is replaced, their role seems to be minimal. This is clearly shown by the fact that blood glucose could be normalized in obese, new onset NIDDM patients with as little as 0.5 U/kg/24 h insulin without caloric restriction or increased physical activity. It would not be logical to advocate the general use of insulin in all NIDDM patients. Too many patients are, however, left poorly controlled because of the belief that they are hyperinsulinemic and that addition of exogenous insulin cannot but be deleterious. The question of whether hyperinsulinemia per se is atherogenic has been much debated but remains unanswered (for a recent review, see Ref. 23). A recent study shows that insulin therapy induces antiatherogenic changes in serum lipoproteins in NIDDM patients [24]. Furthermore, doses of insulin such as those used in this study hardly cause hyperinsulinemia [11,12]. Therefore, we do feel that selected NIDDM patients should more readily be transferred to insulin treatment. An additional issue raised by our study (partly also from the study of Gormley et al. [25]) is the continued beneficial effect of insulin treatment after termination of CSII. Our results are too limited to allow more general conclusions. However, it is possible that short courses of CSII or other measures which induce normoglycemia could be of therapeutic value, allowing significant periods of good metabolic control with oral agents or diet alone.

To summarize, NIDDM seems to be initiated by insulin deficiency, followed by hyperglycemia-induced reduction in peripheral glucose utilization, and 'glucose toxicity', which further reduces insulin output. This vicious cycle which aggravates and perpetuates the hyperglycemia can be broken by insulin treatment. In our hands, genuine insulin resistance is a rare phenomenon in NIDDM; therefore insulin treatment also seems to be a realistic alternative in non-insulin-dependent diabetes.

Acknowledgements

Some of the studies summarized in this report were supported by grants from the Wolfson Family Charitable Fund, the George Grandis Endowment for Medical Research, and Servier Research Institute. We are grateful to the staff of the Endocrine Laboratories in Jerusalem and Modena for the various determinations, and to our nursing staff for superb clinical care. Our thanks to Ms. Liza Granot for secretarial help.

References

1. Cerasi E, Efendic S, Luft R. Dose-response relation between plasma insulin and blood glucose levels during oral glucose loads in pre-diabetic and diabetic subjects. Lancet 1973;i:794–797.
2. Nesher R, Della Casa L, Litvin Y, Sinai J, Del Rio G, Pevsner B, Wax Y, Cerasi E. Insulin deficiency and insulin resistance in Type 2 (non-insulin-dependent) diabetes: quantitative contributions of pancreatic and peripheral responses to glucose homeostasis. Eur J Clin Invest 1987;17:266–274.
3. Ward KW, Bolgiano DC, McKnight B, Halter JB, Porte D. Diminished B cell secretory capacity in patients with noninsulin-dependent diabetes mellitus. J Clin Invest 1984;74:1318–1328.
4. Cerasi E, Nesher R. Assessment of insulin secretion dynamics. In: Clarke WL, Larner J, Pohl SL, eds. Methods in diabetes research, Vol II: Clinical methods. New York: John Wiley & Sons, 1986;77–90.
5. Temple RC, Carrington CA, Luzio SD, Owens DR, Schneider AE, Sobey WJ, Hales CN. Insulin deficiency in non-insulin-dependent diabetes. Lancet 1989;i:293–295.
6. Zawalich WJ, Matschinsky FM. Sequential analysis of the releasing and fuel function of glucose in isolated perifused pancreatic islets. Endocrinology 1977;100:1–8.
7. Yaffe D. Cellular aspects of muscle differentiation in vitro. Curr Top Dev Biol 1969;4:37–77.

8. Sasson S, Cerasi E. Substrate regulation of the glucose transport system in rat skeletal muscle: characterization and kinetic analysis in isolated soleus muscle and skeletal muscle cells in culture. J Biol Chem 1986;261:16827–16833.

9. Sasson S, Edelson D, Cerasi E. In vitro autoregulation of glucose utilization in rat soleus muscle. Diabetes 1987;36:1041–1046.

10. Kruszynska TY, Home PD, Hanning I, Alberti KGMM. Basal and 24-h C-peptide and insulin secretion rate in normal man. Diabetologia 1987;30:16–21.

11. Olsson PO, Arnqvist HJ, Von Schenk HV. Free insulin profiles during intensive treatment with biosynthetic human insulin. Diabet Metab (Paris) 1988;14:253–258.

12. Marshall SM, Taylor R, Home PD, Alberti KGMM, Intermediary metabolism, insulin sensitivity and insulin receptor status under comparable long-term therapy with insulin injections and continuous subcutaneous insulin infusion. Acta Endocrinol (Copenh) 1988;177:417–427.

13. Glaser B, Leibovich G, Nesher R, Hartling S, Binder C, Cerasi E. Improved beta-cell function after intensive insulin treatment in severe non-insulin-dependent diabetes. Acta Endocrinol (Copenh) 1988; 118:365–373.

14. The DCCT Research Group. Weight gain associated with intensive therapy in the diabetes control and complications trial. Diabetes Care 1988;11:567–573.

15. De Fronzo RA, Deibert D, Hendler R, Felig P, Soman V. Insulin sensitivity and insulin binding to monocytes in maturity-onset diabetes. J Clin Invest 1979;63:939–946.

16. Olefsky JM, Kolterman OG. Mechanism of insulin resistance in obesity and non-insulin-dependent (Type II) diabetes. Am J Med 1981;70:151–168.

17. Garvey WT, Olefsky JM, Griffin J, Hamman RF, Kolterman OG. The effect of insulin treatment on insulin secretion and insulin action in type II diabetes mellitus. Diabetes 1985;34:222–234.

18. Leahy JL, Cooper HE, Deal DA, Weir GC. Chronic hyperglycemia is associated with impaired glucose influence on insulin secretion. A study in normal rats using chronic in-vivo glucose infusions. J Clin Invest 1986;77:908–915.

19. Hoenig M, Macgregor LC, Matschinsky FM. In-vitro exhaustion of pancreatic beta cells. Am J Physiol 1986;250:E502–511.

20. Cerasi E, Luft R. Plasma insulin response to sustained hyperglycaemia induced by glucose infusion in human subjects. Lancet 1963;ii:13599–13561.

21. Cerasi E, Luft R, Efendic S. Decreased sensitivity of the pancreatic beta cells to glucose in prediabetic and diabetic subjects. A glucose dose-response study. Diabetes 1972;21:224–234.

22. Cerasi E. Insulin secretion in diabetes mellitus. In: Lefèbvre PJ, Pipeleers DG, eds. The pathology of the endocrine pancreas in diabetes. Berlin: Springer-Verlag, 1988;191–218.

23. Jarrett RJ. Is insulin atherogenic? Diabetologia 1988;31:71–75.

24. Taskinen MR, Kuusi T, Helve E, Nikkilä EA, Yki-Jarvinen H. Insulin therapy induces antiatherogenic changes of serum lipoproteins in noninsulin-dependent diabetes. Arteriosclerosis 1988;8:168–177.

25. Gormley MJJ, Hadden DR, Weeds R, Sheridan B, Andrews WJ. One month's insulin treatment of type II diabetes: the early and medium-term effects following insulin withdrawal. Metabolism 1986;35:1029–1036.

Conclusions

© 1989 Elsevier Science Publishers B.V. (Biomedical Division)
Frontiers of diabetes research: current trends in non-insulin-dependent diabetes mellitus
K.G.M.M. Alberti and R. Mazze, editors

Four decades of clinical research and care: reflections of a clinical diabetologist

HAROLD RIFKIN

35 E. 75th Street, New York, NY 10021, U.S.A.

Prologue

The original assignment given to me by the editors and members of the coordinating committee was to prepare a paper which would serve as a summation of this two-day conference which stressed 'the total care of the patient with NIDDM.' To give myself some leeway, I asked if the title could be changed to: 'Four decades of clinical research and care: reflections of a clinical diabetologist.'

I began medical school in 1936 and relatively soon afterwards became interested and involved with the study of diabetes and metabolism as a career. The major factors which led to my interest in diabetes were fourfold: (1) an introductory course in physiology and biochemistry under the direction of a Professor who was intimately and enthusiastically involved with the investigations of Doctors Banting and Best and the biochemists and physiologists at the University of Toronto; (2) the development or at least the diagnosis of diabetes in three intimate members of my family, father, brother and paternal grandmother; (3) two monumental publications in 1936 – which have since influenced and stimulated basic scientists, clinical researchers and clinical diabetologists – the first by Professor Himsworth in the Lancet, entitled 'Diabetes mellitus: a differentiation into insulin-sensitive and insulin-resistant types' and the second by Drs. Kimmelstiel and Wilson, entitled 'Intercapillary lesions in glomeruli of the kidney'; and (4) subsequent to medical school graduation, the work of Professor Louis Leiter, a colleague and good friend of Rachmiel Levine, a renal physiologist, clinician and professor of medicine at the University of Chicago, who had expertise in metabolism as well as nephrology. He subsequently became Director of Medicine at the Montefiore Medical Center in New York City, where I became his chief resident and fellow, learning at first hand the then existing fundamentals of acid–base balance, metabolic diseases and nephrology.

Overview

Reflecting on the changes in the medical practice of diabetes over the ensuing years, one is struck by the following: the introduction of reflectance meters for the instant measurement of blood glucose, the development of newer techniques in insulin delivery, the use of glycosylated hemoglobin for assessing long-term glycemic control, and newer pharmacological agents; additionally, the development of the diabetic team including physicians with expertise in various medical and surgical disciplines, nurse educators, nutritionists, pharmacists, social workers and psychologists, as well as the introduction of computer programs to interpret patient-collected clinical data, which has led to either subtle or overt changes in management of the diabetic patient; finally, the appreciation of the importance of treating hypertension, obesity and hyperlipidemia early and adequately, in addition to attempting adequate glycemic control.

Space will not permit a complete exposition of current knowledge of the diagnosis and treatment of type II diabetes. This chapter is therefore meant to highlight a few salient features covered more fully in the text of this symposium.

Genetic factors play a distinct role in the causation of NIDDM. It is apparent, however, that the significant diabetogenic genes, including the insulin gene, the insulin receptor gene and the glucose receptor gene, have not yet been identified. This may be the result of late age-of-onset and incomplete penetration, as well as the clinical and probable genetic heterogeneity of NIDDM. A brief statement regarding the magnitude and ramifications of NIDDM and its complications is in order. In the last 10–15 years, sufficient data have been accumulated regarding the distribution and determinants of the two main forms of diabetes, namely IDDM and NIDDM. This is largely due to the original observations of the late Kelly West, and subsequent studies by students and colleagues, including Harry Keen, John Jarret, Paul Zimmet, Peter Bennett and so many others. Noteworthy observations include:

1. NIDDM is more common in many other parts of the world than in Western countries. The prevalence of NIDDM affecting adults in most western countries is in the neighborhood of 3–7%, in contrast to the increased prevalence among populations in various Pacific islands, Native American Indians, Australian Aborigines, and various Asian Indian populations.

2. Variations in the prevalence of NIDDM are observed in different populations liv-

ing in the same country – note the prevalence of NIDDM (20–25%) in the Pima Indians. This prevalence increases with age, and is higher in Black and Hispanic, particularly Mexican, Americans.

3. Both microvascular and macrovascular complications have come to be of great concern to third-world countries, and are no longer restricted to highly industrialized nations. The etiology of mortality in NIDDM varies in different areas of the world, with cardiovascular disease as the major causative factor in Western countries. In areas such as Afro-Caribbean communities, Hong Kong and Japan, renal disease appears to occupy a more significant role.

4. Additionally, hypertension, proteinuria and microalbuminuria, after adjustment for age, sex and duration of diabetes, now emerge as predictive factors for increased mortality for lethal coronary artery disease as well as nephropathy. Noteworthy is the fact that impaired glucose tolerance is associated with a doubling of mortality from coronary artery disease in some populations but with a relatively small risk from microvascular disease.

Emerging newer concepts underlying the genesis of NIDDM involve decreased secretion as well as diminished action of insulin in both peripheral and hepatic tissues. In patients with mild hyperglycemia, the principal peripheral tissue defect of diminished sensitivity or responsiveness to glucose is observed in peripheral tissues, primarily muscle, whereas augmented gluconeogenesis with increased hepatic production and output is noted with progressive elevations in plasma glucose. Although the early insulin response is lost when plasma glucose exceeds 115–120 mg/dl, basal insulin concentrations may be normal or elevated, reflecting an increased basal rate of insulin secretion which in turn is responding to an elevated fasting plasma glucose concentration. With intermediate fasting plasma glucose levels, of the order of 120–180 mg/dl, the total plasma insulin response may be normal, increased or decreased, again inversely correlated with the level of fasting hyperglycemia. With plasma glucose levels of the order of 180–300 mg/dl, both the early and late phases of insulin secretion become markedly impaired.

It has become increasingly apparent that therapeutic intervention, including weight reduction, with calorie restriction, exercise and behavior modification, sulfonylurea therapy and intensive exogenous insulin therapy, even for relatively short periods of time, is capable of normalizing these various defects responsible for the metabolic abnormalities. Additionally, these therapies may completely normalize increased hepatic glucose production and output, but will not totally normalize the insulin secretory defect or the peripheral tissue insulin resistance. A report in this symposium challenges the view that insulin resistance is a major etiological defect in NIDDM, demonstrating that insulin responsiveness to glucose is reduced to less than 20% of normal, and that, when administered by CSII, insulin is effective even in obese patients with NIDDM. It appears that once hyperglycemia develops and persists, it may ultimately lead to further impairment and accentuation of both insulin secretion and resistance. The term 'glucotoxicity' is now becoming part of the diabetic vocabulary. Previous studies by Drs. Olefsky and Kolterman and associates have demonstrated that glycemic control with intermittent periods of insulin administration for 10–14 days will lead to significant improvement in endogenous insulin secretion, decreased hepatic glucose output and decreased resistance at the periphery. A study from the Hadassah University Medical Center also indicates that two weeks of near normoglycemia were sufficient to induce a significant increase in endogenous insulin secretion in some patients, enabling them to return to their original therapy with oral hypoglycemic agents.

Another paper in the symposium thoroughly reviews the regulation of glucose transport. In insulin-resistant states, maximally stimulated glucose transport activity is decreased. This insulin-resistant glucose transport is associated with an apparent depletion of glucose transporters in the basal state in the intracellular pool of muscle and adipose tissue, with a corresponding decrease in translocation of glucose transporters from this pool to the plasma membrane, where they are ordinarily activated in response to insulin.

Patients with NIDDM are also resistant to insulin suppression of plasma FFA concentrations. Such elevated FFA levels can provide the source of intracellular energy for activation of gluconeogenesis via fatty acid oxidation, resulting in increased hepatic glucose production and output with resultant increased concentrations of fasting plasma glucose levels. Increased plasma FFA concentrations can be prevented if increased amounts of insulin can be secreted. However, hyperinsulinemia, if present, may play a significant role in the pathogenesis of hypertension, because of either increased sympathetic activity and/or increased renal tubular reabsorption of sodium and volume. Hence, insulin resistance, hyperglycemia, hyperinsulinemia and perhaps hyperproinsulinemia, in a setting of increased VLDL triglycerides and decreased HDL cholesterol concentrations, may be important factors in the pathogenesis of coronary artery disease (Syndrome X of Reaven).

It has now become more obvious that physicians will be obliged to pay increasingly closer attention to therapeutic manoeuvres in the treatment of elevated plasma glucose levels not only in NIDDM, but in patients with impaired glucose tolerance. This should be instigated early and continued as persistently as possible. Interventional therapy directed towards the management of systolic and diastolic hypertension and hyperlipidemia is important.

Regarding diet, the results of studies from Stanford and Dallas are intriguing, challenging somewhat the recommendations of the American, British, Canadian and European Diabetes Associations, pertaining particularly to the distribution of food energy between fat and carbohydrate. The investigations from Dallas and Stanford indicate that a regimen of high-carbohydrate, low-fat intake may lower levels of LDL cholesterol, but may increase VLDL triglycerides and decrease plasma high-density lipoprotein cholesterol levels for periods of at least 4–6 weeks. However, studies from Oxford indicate that a low-fat, high-carbohydrate diet will decrease both LDL cholesterol and plasma glucose, without necessarily increasing the plasma triglyceride concentrations. The Dallas group employed diets substituting monosaturated fatty acids for saturated fats and containing decreased amounts of carbohydrates, of the order of 35%. Preliminary results from this group further indicate that partial replacement of complex carbohydrates with monosaturated fatty acids (olive oil), equivalent to 37% of the total energy intake, does not increase the level of LDL, may actually improve glycemic control, and does not increase levels of plasma VLDL triglycerides. Prolonged multicenter clinical trials become necessary and perhaps mandatory, in spite of the formidable expense, and it is premature to make specific changes or formal recommendations at the moment.

Examining exercise, the consensus report of the European NIDDM policy group, representing diabetologists from 14 European countries, is in close agreement with other groups reporting on the overall benefits of exercise, including decreasing hyperinsulinemia, enhancing insulin sensitivity, reducing weight and hypertension and improving lipoprotein profiles. Consideration must be given to the state of diabetic control, the effects of aging and the existence of diabetic complications. Absolute or relative insufficiency, leading to a decrease in peripheral glucose disposal, an increase in hepatic glucose production and increased lipolysis, may be disastrous in terms of increasing hyperglycemia and ketosis. Also, hepatic glucose production may not increase sufficiently, relative to the exercise-induced increased glucose disposal, leading to possible hypoglycemia. Specific precautions and directions to patient and family regarding the type and duration of exercise, timing of exercise in relationship to meals, appropriate adjustments of insulin, intermediate or long-acting oral hypoglycemic agents, and sites of insulin injection relative to the type and timing of exercise should be considered in both the insulin-dependent patient and the insulin-using patient with NIDDM. The possible deleterious effects of exercise in the presence of proliferative retinopathy, peripheral and/or autonomic neuropathy and coronary artery disease, i.e. acute myocardial infarction, arrhythmias, sudden death, become vital therapeutic considerations for the clinician and patient.

Newer modalities of therapy based on a variety of physiological mechanisms are reviewed and their consequences detailed in this volume. Among them are modifiers of carbohydrate digestion and absorption such as soluble and insoluble alpha-glucosidase inhibitors (miglitol, emiglitate and acarbose), and the effects of inhibitors of lipolysis and fatty acid oxidation on gluconeogenesis, with decreased hepatic glucose production and output. Other avenues being explored around the world are the use of inhibitors of counter-regulatory hormones (somatostatin and glucagon analogues), and the possible re-introduction of the biguanidines, particularly metformin, in the U.S.A., since this agent has a short life span, is not metabolized by the liver, is not bound to serum proteins and rarely leads to lactic acidosis.

Data are accumulating which indicate that hypertension, whether in IDDM or NIDDM, may not be the end result of established diabetic nephropathy, but in point of fact may be etiologically related, albeit genetically predetermined, to the actual development of diabetic renal disease. Reduction in blood pressure will lead to diminished glomerular hyperperfusion, hyper-filtration and microalbuminuria. Measuring genetic markers for hypertension, such as red blood cell sodium-lithium countertransport velocity and the degree of microalbuminuria, may become actualities of future practice with diabetic patients. However, pertinent questions do remain: What constitutes microalbuminuria – 15 μg/min or 30 μg/min or 50 μg/min? What collection periods should one employ? What assays are available and have they stood the test of time? At what level of blood pressure does one begin to treat: 160/95, 140/90 or 135/85? Considerations of the quality of life and the side-effects of anti-hypertensive agents, as well as the expense involved in terms of cost-benefit, become of primary importance. Other considerations should include modification of diet in terms of restriction of protein and phosphorus.

The microvascular and macrovascular complications of NIDDM, the interrelationships of genetic factors, degree of glycemic control, duration of diabetes, hypertension, hyperlipidemia, apoprotein abnormalities, obesity, cigarette smoking, hyperinsulinemia, hyperproinsulinemia, disturbed proteoglycan metabolism and increased platelet adhesiveness and aggregation have been stressed as important factors, particularly in the genesis of macrovascular disease. Randomized controlled trials of antiplatelet therapy following stroke or myocardial infarction have indicated a reduction in vascular mortality of 15% but also a reduction in subsequent stroke or myocardial infarction of 30%.

In addition to anti-hypertensive therapy and other therapeutic modalities, a recent multicenter randomized controlled clinical trial conducted in two French and United Kingdom centers indicates that aspirin (330 mg three times daily) with or without dipyridamole significantly slows the development of microaneurysm in early diabetic retinopathy. Antiplatelet agents, at present, perhaps should be considered as ancillary therapy, and not detract from other preventive measures directed at the aforementioned major vascular risk factors.

Finally, we are beginning to see a more systematic approach to the treatment of type II diabetes. Reported in this symposium is a novel approach to organizing and delivering health care services to the person with NIDDM. Recognizing that the majority of diabetes is treated at the primary care level, this study demonstrates that a systematic approach using computer-assisted clinical decision-making can provide the primary care physician with the means of managing 'routine' diabetes, and establish the standards by which co-management with an endocrinologist is appropriate. Such a system, relying on verified self-monitored blood glucose data from patients using memory-based reflectance meters and linking these devices via telephone modem to the primary care physician, will ensure immediate and accurate communications, enhancing the therapeutic alliance between patient and health care provider.

Author index

Alberti, K.G.M.M., 297

Barrett-Connor, E., 177
Bennett, P.H., 89
Bergenstal, R., 223
Björntorp, P., 61

Cerasi, E., 309
Colwell, J.A., 193
Costagliola, D., 71
Creutzfeldt, W., 285
Cushman, S.W., 155

Del Rio, G., 309
Della Casa, L., 309
Devlin, J.T., 271
Dowse, G.K., 37

England, J.D., 141
Eschwège, E., 71
Etzwiler, D., 223

Fontbonne, A., 71
Fulcher, G.R., 297

Glaser, B., 309
Goldstein, D.E., 141

Harris, M.I., 119
Hollander, P., 223
Home, P.D., 215
Horton, E.S., 271

Kahn, B.B., 155

Keen, H., 3
Knowler, W.C., 89

Lacroux, A., 71
Little, R.R., 141

Mazze, R., 223
McKenzie, E., 141

Nathan, D.M., 133
Nelson, R.G., 89

Papoz, L., 71
Pettitt, D.J., 89

Reaven, G.M., 167
Rifkin, H., 323

Sasson, S., 309
Serjeantson, S.W., 21
Spencer, M., 223
Strock, E., 223

Tattersall, R., 263
Tuomilehto, J., 101

Vinik, A.I., 233

Watkins, P.J., 207
Wiedmeyer, H.-M., 141

Zimmet, P.Z., 21, 37